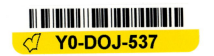

1994
YEAR BOOK OF
DENTISTRY®

Statement of Purpose

The YEAR BOOK Service

The YEAR BOOK series was devised in 1901 by practicing health professionals who observed that the literature of medicine and related disciplines had become so voluminous that no one individual could read and place in perspective every potential advance in a major specialty. In the final decade of the 20th century, this recognition is more acutely true than it was in 1901.

More than merely a series of books, YEAR BOOK volumes are the tangible results of a unique service designed to accomplish the following:

- to *survey* a wide range of journals of proven value
- to *select* from those journals papers representing significant advances and statements of important clinical principles
- to provide *abstracts* of those articles that are readable, convenient summaries of their key points
- to provide *commentary* about those articles to place them in perspective.

These publications grow out of a unique process that calls on the talents of outstanding authorities in clinical and fundamental disciplines, trained literature specialists, and professional writers, all supported by the resources of Mosby, the world's preeminent publisher for the health professions.

The Literature Base

Mosby subscribes to nearly 1,000 journals published worldwide, covering the full range of the health professions. On an annual basis, the publisher examines usage patterns and polls its expert authorities to add new journals to the literature base and to delete journals that are no longer useful as potential YEAR BOOK sources.

The Literature Survey

The publisher's team of literature specialists, all of whom are trained and experienced health professionals, examines every original, peer-reviewed article in each journal issue. More than 250,000 articles per year are scanned systematically, including title, text, illustrations, tables, and references. Each scan is compared, article by article, to the search strategies that the publisher has developed in consultation with the 270 outside experts who form the pool of YEAR BOOK editors. A given article may be reviewed by any number of editors, from one to a dozen or more, regardless of the discipline for which the paper was originally published. In turn, each editor who receives the article reviews it to determine whether or not the article should be included in the YEAR BOOK. This decision is based on the article's inherent quality, its probable usefulness to readers of that YEAR BOOK, and the editor's goal to represent a balanced picture of a given field in each volume of the YEAR BOOK. In addition, the editor indicates when to include figures and tables from the article to help the YEAR BOOK reader better understand the information.

Of the quarter million articles scanned each year, only 5% are selected for detailed analysis within the YEAR BOOK series, thereby assuring readers of the high value of every selection.

The Abstract

The publisher's abstracting staff is headed by a physician-writer and includes individuals with training in the life sciences, medicine, and other areas, plus extensive experience in writing for the health professions and related industries. Each selected article is assigned to a specific writer on this abstracting staff. The abstracter, guided in many cases by notations supplied by the expert editor, writes a structured, condensed summary designed so that the reader can rapidly acquire the essential information contained in the article.

The Commentary

The YEAR BOOK editorial boards, sometimes assisted by guest commentators, write comments that place each article in perspective for the reader. This provides the reader with the equivalent of a personal consultation with a leading international authority—an opportunity to better understand the value of the article and to benefit from the authority's thought processes in assessing the article.

Additional Editorial Features

The editorial boards of each YEAR BOOK organize the abstracts and comments to provide a logical and satisfying sequence of information. To enhance the organization, editors also provide introductions to sections or individual chapters, comments linking a number of abstracts, citations to additional literature, and other features.

The published YEAR BOOK contains enhanced bibliographic citations for each selected article, including extended listings of multiple authors and identification of author affiliations. Each YEAR BOOK contains a Table of Contents specific to that year's volume. From year to year, the Table of Contents for a given YEAR BOOK will vary depending on developments within the field.

Every YEAR BOOK contains a list of the journals from which papers have been selected. This list represents a subset of the nearly 1,000 journals surveyed by the publisher and occasionally reflects a particularly pertinent article from a journal that is not surveyed on a routine basis.

Finally, each volume contains a comprehensive subject index and an index to authors of each selected paper.

The 1994 Year Book Series

Year Book of Allergy and Clinical Immunology: Drs. Rosenwasser, Borish, Gelfand, Leung, Nelson, and Szefler

Year Book of Anesthesia and Pain Management: Drs. Tinker, Abram, Kirby, Ostheimer, Roizen, and Stoelting

Year Book of Cardiology®: Drs. Schlant, Collins, Engle, Gersh, Kaplan, and Waldo

Year Book of Chiropractic: Dr. Lawrence

Year Book of Critical Care Medicine®: Drs. Rogers and Parrillo

Year Book of Dentistry®: Drs. Meskin, Currier, Kennedy, Leinfelder, Berry, and Roser

Year Book of Dermatologic Surgery: Drs. Swanson, Glogau, and Salasche

Year Book of Dermatology®: Drs. Sober and Fitzpatrick

Year Book of Diagnostic Radiology®: Drs. Federle, Clark, Gross, Madewell, Maynard, Sackett, and Young

Year Book of Digestive Diseases®: Drs. Greenberger and Moody

Year Book of Drug Therapy®: Drs. Lasagna and Weintraub

Year Book of Emergency Medicine®: Drs. Wagner, Burdick, Davidson, McNamara, and Roberts

Year Book of Endocrinology®: Drs. Bagdade, Braverman, Poehlman, Kannan, Landsberg, Molitch, Morley, Odell, Rogol, Ryan, and Nathan

Year Book of Family Practice®: Drs. Berg, Bowman, Davidson, Dietrich, and Scherger

Year Book of Geriatrics and Gerontology®: Drs. Beck, Reuben, Burton, Small, Whitehouse, and Goldstein

Year Book of Hand Surgery®: Drs. Amadio and Hentz

Year Book of Hematology®: Drs. Spivak, Bell, Ness, Quesenberry, and Wiernik

Year Book of Infectious Diseases®: Drs. Keusch, Wolff, Barza, Bennish, Gelfand, Klempner, and Snydman

Year Book of Infertility®: Drs. Mishell, Lobo, and Sokol

Year Book of Medicine®: Drs. Bone, Cline, Epstein, Greenberger, Malawista, Mandell, O'Rourke, Utiger

Year Book of Neonatal and Perinatal Medicine®: Drs. Klaus and Fanaroff

Year Book of Nephrology®: Drs. Coe, Favus, Henderson, Kashgarian, Luke, Myers, and Curtis

Year Book of Neurology and Neurosurgery®: Drs. Bradley and Crowell

Year Book of Neuroradiology: Drs. Osborn, Eskridge, Grossman, and Harnsberger

Year Book of Nuclear Medicine®: Drs. Hoffer, Gore, Gottschalk, Rattner, Zaret, and Zubal

Year Book of Obstetrics and Gynecology®: Drs. Mishell, Kirschbaum, and Morrow

Year Book of Occupational and Environmental Medicine: Drs. Emmett, Frank, Gochfeld, and Hessl

Year Book of Oncology®: Drs. Simone, Longo, Ozols, Steele, Glatstein, and Bosl

Year Book of Ophthalmology®: Drs. Laibson, Adams, Augsburger, Benson, Cohen, Eagle, Flanagan, Nelson, Rapuano, Reinecke, Sergott, and Wilson

Year Book of Orthopedics®: Drs. Sledge, Poss, Cofield, Frymoyer, Griffin, Hansen, Johnson, Simmons, and Springfield

Year Book of Otolaryngology–Head and Neck Surgery®: Drs. Paparella and Holt

Year Book of Pain: Drs. Gebhart, Haddox, Jacox, Payne, Rudy, and Shapiro

Year Book of Pathology and Clinical Pathology®: Drs. Gardner, Bennett, Cousar, Garvin, and Worsham

Year Book of Pediatrics®: Dr. Stockman

Year Book of Plastic, Reconstructive, and Aesthetic Surgery: Drs. Miller, Cohen, McKinney, Robson, Ruberg, and Whitaker

Year Book of Podiatric Medicine and Surgery®: Dr. Kominsky

Year Book of Psychiatry and Applied Mental Health®: Drs. Talbott, Frances, Breier, Meltzer, Perry, Schowalter, and Yudofsky

Year Book of Pulmonary Disease®: Drs. Bone and Petty

Year Book of Rheumatology: Drs. Sergent, LeRoy, Meenan, Panush, and Reichlin

Year Book of Sports Medicine®: Drs. Shephard, Drinkwater, Eichner, Sutton, Torg, Col. Anderson, and Mr. George

Year Book of Surgery®: Drs. Copeland, Deitch, Eberlein, Howard, Luce, Ritchie, Seeger, Souba, and Sugarbaker

Year Book of Thoracic and Cardiovascular Surgery: Drs. Ginsberg, Lofland, and Wechsler

Year Book of Transplantation: Drs. Ascher, Hansen, and Strom

Year Book of Ultrasound: Drs. Merritt, Babcock, Carroll, Goldstein, and Mittelstaedt

Year Book of Urology®: Drs. Gillenwater and Howards

Year Book of Vascular Surgery®: Dr. Porter

1994

The Year Book of
DENTISTRY®

Editor-in-Chief
Lawrence H. Meskin, D.D.S., Ph.D.

Editors
Thomas G. Berry, D.D.S., M.A.
G. Fräns Currier, D.D.S., M.S.D., M.Ed.
James E. Kennedy, D.D.S., M.S.
Karl F. Leinfelder, D.D.S., M.S.
Steven M. Roser, M.D., D.M.D.
Kenneth L. Zakariasen, D.D.S., M.S., Ph.D.

Guest Editors
Denise K. Kassebaum, D.D.S., M.S.
Andrea Schreiber, D.M.D.

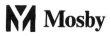

St. Louis Baltimore Boston Chicago London Madrid Philadelphia Sydney Toronto

Vice President and Publisher, Continuity Publishing: Kenneth H. Killion
Director, Editorial Development: Gretchen C. Murphy
Developmental Editor: Amy L. Reynaldo
Illustrations and Permissions Coordinator: Maureen A. Livengood
Senior Project Manager: Max F. Perez
Project Supervisor: Tamara L. Smith
Senior Production Editor: Wendi Schnaufer
Production Editor: Sandra Rogers
Editorial Coordinator: Rebecca Nordbrock
Manager, Literature Services: Edith M. Podrazik, R.N.
Senior Information Specialist: Terri Santo, R.N.
Information Specialist: Nancy R. Dunne, R.N.
Senior Medical Writer: David A. Cramer, M.D.
Proofreading Supervisor: Barbara M. Kelly
Vice President, Professional Sales and Marketing: George M. Parker
Marketing and Circulation Manager: Barry J. Bowlus
Marketing Coordinator: Lynn Stevenson

1994 EDITION
Copyright © July 1994 by Mosby–Year Book, Inc.

Printed in the United States of America
Composition by International Computaprint Corporation
Printing/binding by Maple-Vail

Mosby–Year Book, Inc.
11830 Westline Industrial Drive
St. Louis, MO 63146

Editorial Office:
Mosby–Year Book, Inc.
200 North LaSalle St.
Chicago, IL 60601

International Standard Serial Number: 0084-3717
International Standard Book Number: 0-8151-5877-7

Table of Contents

Mosby Document Express

Copies of the full text of the original source documents of articles abstracted or referenced in this publication are available by calling Mosby Document Express, toll-free, at **1 (800) 55-MOSBY**.

With Mosby Document Express, you have convenient, 24-hour-a-day access to literally every article on which this publication is based. In fact, through Mosby Document Express, virtually any medical or scientific article can be located and delivered by FAX, overnight delivery service, international airmail, electronic transmission of bitmapped images (via Internet), or regular mail. The average cost of a complete, delivered copy of an article, including up to $4 in copyright clearance charges and first-class mail delivery, is $12.

For inquiries and pricing information, please call the toll-free number shown above. To expedite your order for material appearing in this publication, please be prepared with the code shown next to the bibliographic citation for each abstract.

Journals Represented

Mosby subscribes to and surveys nearly 1,000 U.S. and foreign medical and allied health journals. From these journals, the Editors select the articles to be abstracted. Journals represented in this YEAR BOOK are listed below.

Acta Cytologica
Acta Odontologica Scandinavica
American Journal of Dentistry
American Journal of Neuroradiology
American Journal of Orthodontics and Dentofacial Orthopedics
Australian Dental Journal
British Dental Journal
Caries Research
Cleft Palate-Craniofacial Journal
Clinical Infectious Diseases
Community Dentistry and Oral Epidemiology
Compendium of Continuing Education in Dentistry
Dental Economics
Deutsche Medizinische Wochenschrift
Endodontics and Dental Traumatology
General Dentistry
Illinois Dental Journal
International Journal of Adult Orthodontic and Orthognathic Surgery
International Journal of Oral and Maxillofacial Implants
International Journal of Oral and Maxillofacial Surgery
International Journal of Prosthodontics
Journal of Clinical Periodontology
Journal of Craniofacial Genetics and Developmental Biology
Journal of Dental Education
Journal of Dental Research
Journal of Dentistry
Journal of Dentistry for Children
Journal of Endodontics
Journal of Long-Term Effects of Medical Implants
Journal of Oral Pathology and Medicine
Journal of Oral and Maxillofacial Surgery
Journal of Orofacial Pain
Journal of Periodontal Research
Journal of Periodontology
Journal of Prosthetic Dentistry
Journal of the American Dental Association
Journal of the American Medical Association
Journal of the California Dental Association
Journal of the Canadian Dental Association
Journal of the Dental Association of South Africa
Journal of the Maryland State Dental Association
Journal of the National Cancer Institute
New England Journal of Medicine
New York State Dental Journal
Oral Surgery, Oral Medicine, Oral Pathology
Pediatric Dentistry
Quintessence International
Scandinavian Journal of Dental Research

Standard Abbreviations

The following terms are abbreviated in this edition: acquired immunodeficiency syndrome (AIDS), the central nervous system (CNS), cerebrospinal fluid (CSF), computed tomography (CT), electrocardiography (ECG), human immunodeficiency virus (HIV), magnetic resonance (MR) imaging (MRI), and temporomandibular joint (TMJ).

Introduction

Major changes in America's health-care system are anticipated, although the extent of dentistry's involvement remains unanswered. Nevertheless, regardless of the eventual construct of health-care reform, dentistry will be impacted. Current political emphasis on cost control and quality guarantees future challenges to every aspect of dental practice. This 1994 YEAR BOOK OF DENTISTRY is specifically designed to assist its readers in effectively participating in health-care restructuring. For example, transfer of technology, especially in the area of new dental material, has been given additional attention. This year's section on "hands-on" restorative dentistry complements an enlarged selection of information on dental materials. With 40% of the 1994 YEAR BOOK OF DENTISTRY devoted to discussions of restorative dentistry, our readers should be well positioned to incorporate this information into their dental practices. Additionally, new chapters dedicated to providing information on the use of lasers and radiologic devices have been included in anticipation that the area of emerging mechanical technologies needs to be an integral part of the YEAR BOOK'S offerings.

However, not all of what is new in dentistry is limited to the restorative field. Indeed, major changes in practice philosophy, based on clinical evidence demonstrating the advantages of nonsurgical treatment of carious and periodontally involved teeth, may be forthcoming. Interest in providing a risk-free environment for patients and health-care workers continues to be a primary concern of practice management. Meanwhile, new advances in implantology and the treatment of temporomandibular disorders accentuate an explosive increase in interest in these emerging subjects.

It is obvious that dental practice continues to change at a spectacular rate. The importance of selecting pertinent literature to address these changes cannot be overemphasized. To achieve this goal, the primary rationale in selecting an article for inclusion in the 1994 YEAR BOOK OF DENTISTRY has been based on the article's clinical relevancy to the dental practitioner. The editors of the YEAR BOOK OF DENTISTRY intend to pursue this policy vigorously.

Lawrence H. Meskin, D.D.S., Ph.D.

1 Practice Management

Introduction

"We are in," said the outgoing president of the American Dental Association, Jack Harris, when referring to the National Health Care Reform Bill submitted by the Clinton administration. To what degree dentistry will be "in" will not be known until the final health-care reform votes are counted. The potential impact on dental practice of each proposed dental component of health reform will dominate practice management discussions in the forthcoming year. As a prelude to these discussions, publications that assessed quality in dental delivery have been selected for inclusion in this YEAR BOOK OF DENTISTRY. The importance of continued vigilance in control of infection has also been given prominence in the YEAR BOOK OF DENTISTRY, as new information suggests possible cross-contamination from saliva ejectors, dental carts, dental unit water lines, and ultrasonic cleaning solutions, as well as impressions and prostheses received by the dental laboratory. Because of an improving economy, attention has also been directed to publications that provide financial information pertinent to the practitioner. Included in this discussion is the high prevalence of upper extremity neuropathy, which appears to be a major source of disability and lost income among dental practitioners.

Lawrence H. Meskin, D.D.S., Ph.D.

Quality of Practice

What Is BS5750?

Davies L (Davies Assoc Practice Support Services)
Br Dent J 174:298–299, 1993   105-94-1–1

Background.—BS5750 is a British Standard given to organizations that can demonstrate that they have quality management systems. The 20 requirements include all main components of a management system, from contracting with patients to handling patient complaints. Quality may be defined as "fitness for purpose, reliability, and value for money."

Achieving BS5750.—Achieving the standard involves 3 main elements: a quality systems manual that includes a quality policy statement and quality aims and objectives; a procedures manual outlining the practice's working procedures; and, if needed, a more detailed manual of work instructions. Proof is obtained by internal audit or review and by external evaluation.

Benefits of BS5750.—The benefits of achieving the standard are enormous. It is the ultimate marketing tool. It can also lead to better patient understanding and satisfaction, team involvement and commitment, and improved uses of time and resources. Changes can be made as often as desired as long as they are made according to the documented system.

▶ BS5750, by itself only a combination of meaningless letters and numbers, represents an important construct that has the potential to vastly improve all components of a dental practice. Total quality management (TQM) has been used by major industries in the United States to enhance their entire business operation. Some characterize it as the ultimate marketing tool, because it is concerned with changing the organization by involving all members of the work force in a concerted effort to do things right the first time—being proactive rather than reactive. This article challenges the dental practitioner to consider implementing such a system in his or her dental office. The TQM system calls for a program that documents what you do. It then assesses whether you have accomplished that goal and then requires proof. Everything is documented, everything is evaluated, and everyone participates. The dental practice becomes an entity that strives to avoid errors. By doing so, it provides a better service to the patient and brings greater economies to the practice. With health-care reform on the horizon, implementing a program such as TQM may become the critical factor that determines how successful a practitioner of the future will be.—L.H. Meskin, D.D.S., Ph.D.

A Unique Manual for Self-Assessment by Dental Practitioners
James DW (Cardiff, Wales)
Quintessence Int 23:701–704, 1992   105-94-1-2

Background.—The *Self-Assessment Manual and Standards (SAMS)*, produced by the Faculty of General Dental Practitioners of the Royal College of Surgeons of England and the Department of Health, provides a method for clinicians to assess themselves against generally accepted norms. The manual is designed to raise standards of patient care.

Content.—The *SAMS* is a prototype, not a complete reference. Its aim is to provoke discussion, challenge, and reassessment, by which it can be revised and updated. The manual is divided into 3 sections: an introduction, clinical sections, and case studies. The clinical sections contains tables of clinical standards. The case studies describe typical situations in general practice. Each case leads to a grid of treatment choices. The manual states that self-assessment requires discipline to initiate the process and to be honest with oneself. A practice sheet template appears on the last page.

Conclusion.—The *SAMS* can be used in several ways: as a textbook, for group work, or for peer review. Clinicians may start with a case study and progress through the relevant sections, and clinicians may use the practice sheet to assess their performance.

▶ One of the sought-after rewards of becoming a dentist is "being one's own boss." Dentists have enjoyed that status essentially by remaining in a solo practitioner–dominated profession that has only recently expanded its domain by adding dental associates and the occasional dental partner. This arrangement creates a situation in which assessment of dental quality rests almost totally on self-assessment. To assist dentists in this process, this article describes the efforts of organized dentistry in Britain to develop standards of care by which practitioners can assess themselves. This type of process allows for a nonthreatening evaluation of the practitioner's treatment programs. Outcomes, not procedures, are assessed. Unfortunately, this innovative effort does not appear to have been adopted by other countries. Efforts to develop standards relating to outcomes of dental care are at a virtual standstill in the United States. Fear that development of such standards might limit a practitioner's right to provide treatment of their choosing appears to be the basis for the resistance.—L.H. Meskin, D.D.S., Ph.D.

Assessing Quality in Dentistry: Dental Boards, Peer Review Vary on Disciplinary Actions
Damiano PC, Shugars DA, Freed JR (Univ of Iowa, Iowa City; Univ of North Carolina, Chapel Hill; Univ of California, Los Angeles)
J Am Dent Assoc 124(5):113–131, 1993   105-94-1–3

Introduction.—State licensure is the primary method used to certify the quality of care provided by dental practitioners. Across jurisdictions, however, entry-level quality assurance appears to be inconsistent. The disciplinary activities of state boards of dental examiners and state peer review committees were examined.

Dental Boards and Peer Review.—State boards or similar disciplinary bodies administer entrance examinations and police the performance of licensed practitioners. Peer review committees review or mediate complaints concerning dental care. Reports of inconsistencies to entry-level examinations and variations in available disciplinary mechanisms suggest that the processes of boards and peer review need to be improved. Questionnaires mailed to state boards yielded data on the variation in disciplinary rates within and among states and the results of peer review analyses.

Survey Results.—Twenty-one of 40 responding states provided at least 5 years of data for 1979–87. In 10 states, the year-to-year disciplinary rates were significantly different. The 11 states in which disciplinary rates did not differ significantly over time generally disciplined few providers. Rates varied widely among states, from more than 10 per 1,000 practi-

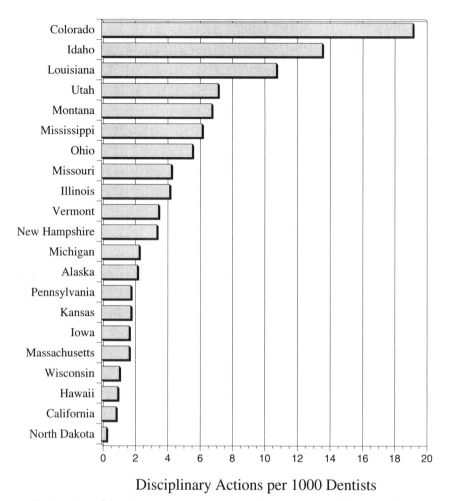

Disciplinary Actions per 1000 Dentists

Fig 1-1.—Rate of disciplinary actions by state boards of dental examiners. (Courtesy of Damiano PC, Shugars DA, Freed JR: *J Am Dent Assoc* 124(5):113-131, 1993.)

tioners yearly to less than 1 per 1,000 (Fig 1-1). The rate of response from peer review committees was 88%. In 1988, 3,991 new peer review cases were initiated in 44 states (Fig 1-2). States varied considerably in their level of peer review activity, from zero cases in Virginia to 109 cases per 1,000 dentists in Arizona. Most cases were initiated by patients (86%) and were related to quality of care (80%). Overall, 43% of decisions favored the patients and 31% favored the dentists. Of those peer review cases that were decided against the treating dentist, 3.8% were subsequently referred to the state board for further review (table).

Conclusion.—These findings raise questions about the ability of state dental boards and peer review committees to provide a consistent national system of quality assurance. Some states may have more resources than others, and many states rely on patient complaints rather than on

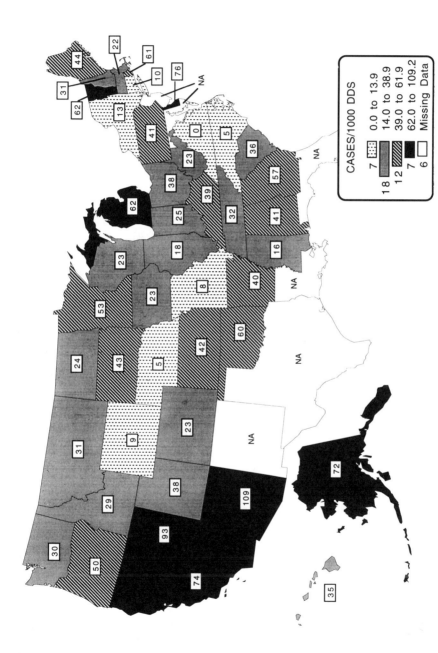

Fig 1–2.—The number of peer review cases brought in 1988 per 1,000 dentists. (Courtesy of Damiano PC, Shugars DA, Freed JR: *J Am Dent Assoc:* 124(5):113–131, 1993.)

Results of the Peer Review Analysis

Total number of cases brought in 1988	3,881
Total number of cases completed in 1988	2,497
Reason for claims	
Quality	63%
Appropriateness	17%
Fees	11%
Other	9%
Source of claims	
Patient	86%
Dentist (other than treating dentist)	7%
Dentist (other than treating dentist) excluding California and Pennsylvania (which account for 75% of such cases)	2%
Other	7%
Outcomes of cases	
Settled in mediation	28%
Settled by full committee	38%
Not resolved	20%
Voluntarily dropped	14%
Referrals to a State Board of Dental Examiners	
Percentage of decisions against the dentist that were referred (n=62)	3.8%
Percentage of decisions against the dentist that were referred excluding Georgia and Missouri (which account for 34 of the 62 cases)	2.1%

(Courtesy of Damiano PC, Shugars DA, Freed JR: *J Am Dent Assoc* 124(25):113–131, 1993.)

formal mechanisms for quality assessment. A system combining education with sanctions, when appropriate, is recommended.

▶ Perhaps no subject generates as much heated discussion among dentists as does the subject of dental licensure. For years, dentists have been critical of inconsistencies in entry-level examinations that are used to test new graduates and already licensed dentists desiring to relocate. If entry-level examinations are not consistent, then policing the performance of already licensed practitioners takes on added importance. This study demonstrates that the effectiveness of state board disciplinary procedures and state peer review systems is open to question. The inconsistencies that occur between states and within states during different time intervals point out the need for a different assessment mechanism to measure quality. A nonpunitive method to assess and improve competency, if necessary, needs immediate development. The concept of self-assessment described in previous abstracts may provide the answer if dentists would accept the concept of continuous improvement as a mandatory requirement for continued dental practice.—L.H. Meskin, D.D.S., Ph.D.

Whistle Blowing: The Ethics of Revealing Professional Incompetence Within Dentistry

Doyal L, Cannell H (London Hosp and St Bartholomew's Med Colleges, London)
Br Dent J 174:95–101, 1993   105-94-1-4

Background.—The professional literature stresses the importance of not undermining trust in other colleagues and, consequently, in the profession itself. But when does this duty begin to conflict with other moral responsibilities? What should students or dentists do when a colleague is placing patients at immediate risk and is unwilling to change negligent practice or the personal circumstances causing it?

The Moral Basis of Professional Rights and Duties.—An analysis of the rights and responsibilities of practitioners should begin with a discussion of the rights of the patients. Patients are entitled to good quality care and to act as the moral guardians of their own bodies. Clinicians have a duty to protect the life and health of their patients and to respect their patients' autonomy. A dentist's obligation not to criticize publicly the work of other dentists stems from the moral duty to help all others, including patients, avoid serious harm. This obligation does not derive from any inherent right of colleagues to be protected from their mistakes. The accusation of incompetence may seriously harm the professional and personal lives of the accused and may constitute libel or slander. Although there are circumstances in which the fault of colleagues should be exposed, there is considerable moral indeterminacy in deciding when this should be.

Conclusion.—When there is a high risk of serious harm, colleagues should discuss the grounds of disagreement with other professionals who have no vested interest in the outcome. Fear of becoming involved in litigation tends to constrain discussions of errors from which much could be learned. When dentists and patients perceive their relationship as a moral partnership rather than as a financial contract, patients will be more likely to accept honest mistakes without seeking legal redress.

▶ Self-regulation is one of the more important activities of a highly developed profession. Self-regulation takes on even greater responsibility in a health profession in which the professional ethic dictates that practitioners striving to do good (beneficence) will first—and above all—do no harm (nonmaleficence). The American Dental Association's Principle of Ethics and Code of Conduct is clear in its requirement that "dentists shall be obliged to report to the appropriate reviewing agency . . . instances of gross or continual faulty treatment by other dentists." Whistle-blowing is the ugly term used to publicly describe the action of a professional citing the questionable practices of another professional. Fear of recrimination, legal action, or unfavorable professional criticism may cause health professionals to abrogate their ethical responsibilities. Society becomes the victim of such inaction. Considering that society has granted a group of health professionals a virtual monopoly to deliver a specific health service, society, in turn, must depend on the profession to ensure that the service is of the highest quality. Whistle-blowing, as difficult as the process may be, is the ethical responsibility of the health professional to maintain quality. For if not the professional, then who?—L.H. Meskin, D.D.S., Ph.D.

Requests for Treatment: Ethical Limits on Cosmetic Dentistry
Chiodo GT, Tolle SW (Oregon Health Sciences Univ, Portland)
Gen Dent 41:16–20, 1993   105-94-1–5

Introduction.—The legal and ethical limits of a patient's right to refuse treatment are clearly defined, but a patient's right to request specific treatment has been less thoroughly explored. Because of our increasingly consumer-oriented society, the latter issue is receiving more attention, as demonstrated by a patient who requested cosmetic dental treatment that could not be justified on a physiologic or biological basis.

Case Report.—Man, 32, a mechanical engineer with dental insurance, had emigrated from the Soviet Union to the United States 7 years earlier and required the restoration of only 3 small carious lesions after never having received routine dental care. Because of his admiration for a financially successful uncle in the Soviet Union who had a gold crown on an anterior tooth, he asked the dentist to make him a similar gold crown for his front tooth. The dentist explained that the tooth was healthy and did not need a crown, and he asked the patient to reconsider. When the patient returned 2 weeks later to have the 3 amalgam restorations placed, he remained firm in his request for an anterior gold crown strictly for cosmetic purposes.

Discussion.—Requests by patients for aesthetic dental treatment for conditions such as tetracyline- or fluoride-stained teeth are usually honored without question. It is recognized that the cosmetic treatment in these cases will have no physiologic value but may have psychological benefit. The dentist in this case may believe strongly that placing a gold crown on a sound front tooth for cosmetic purposes is wrong, but he may grant the patient's wishes ethically. The dentist may also ethically refuse to grant the patient's wishes, in which case he or she is obligated to refer the patient elsewhere.

▶ As this article indicates, the patient's right to refuse treatment has been adequately documented. What about the patient's right to request treatment that a dentist believes is unwarranted or could result in an adverse health condition? The doctrine of "do no harm" competes with the right of individuals to determine what should be done to their bodies. It is the obligation of the dentist to direct the patient away from treatments that may be harmful. It is clear that patient requests for futile or unproved treatment can be ethically refused. For example, when patients wish to have their amalgam restorations removed because they consider them a source of toxic substances to the body, the dentist must explain the absence of scientific evidence for such a procedure. The dentist must further explain that the removal of the restorations may cause damage to the teeth as well as release high levels of mercury. What if the patient persists in the request? Because only a dentist can legally perform dental procedures, can the dentist be forced to remove the amalgam restorations? Ethicists would probably state that the dentist could still refuse treatment, citing that there are standards of care regarding this issue. Compromising those standards would undermine the integrity of the profession.—L.H. Meskin, D.D.S., Ph.D.

Economics

Is Now a Good Time to Boost Practice Size?

Nash KD (ADA's Bureau of Economic and Behavioral Research)
J Am Dent Assoc 124(3):99–101, 1993   105-94-1–6

Introduction.—The economy now appears to be recovering, and dental patient visits are increasing (Fig 1–3). Many dentists may be considering expanding their practices through capital investment and hiring.

Is This A Good Time to Grow?—A survey by the American Dental Association shows that median gross billings reached $250,000 for general practitioners in the past year (table). The data in the table can be used as a yardstick by which dentists can measure their utilization of operatories with the utilization rates of their colleagues. In addition to operatory utilization, dentists must consider inflation in dental fees when contemplating practice expansion. Dentists should examine current size relative to patient visits and gross billings and have a solid projection of what to expect in the future.

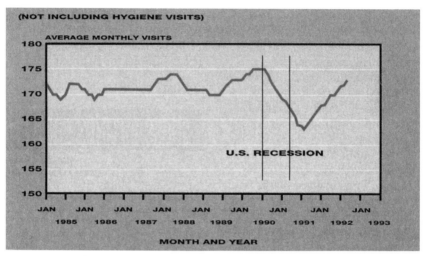

Fig 1–3.—Monthy visits to the dentist, excluding hygiene visits. Source: American Dental Association, Quarterly Survey of Dental Practice. (Courtesy of Nash KD: *J Am Dent Assoc* 124(3):99–101, 1993.)

Conclusion.—Striking a balance between patient load and practice size can be difficult, but it is possible. The decision to expand one's practice should always be based on hard facts.

▶ Suffering from reduced patient loads and fee levels that have barely kept up with inflation, dentists have turned to practice efficiencies to increase income. For example, after adjusting for inflation, the average gross billing for a square foot of dental office space increased from $188 in 1987 to $221 in 1990. With patient visits now increasing, dentists may wonder whether adding an additional operatory would facilitate future practice growth. The table can give dentists a "broad" guideline as to how they stand in relationship to other practitioners. The table demonstrates that if a dentist has 2 operatories and gross billings of $106,000, 75% of dentists with 2 operatories are billing more than his or her office. This dentist should be able to handle many more patients without increasing the number of operatories. Caution must be exercised in using this table because it was assembled from national data. Wide geographic variations in fees often result in higher or lower gross income reports. Still, without a more exacting data set, the full text of this publication can assist the practitioner who is considering a capital expenditure increase in his or her practice.—L.H. Meskin, D.D.S., Ph.D.

Patient Billings and Practice Size
General Practitioners
(Thousands of 1991 Dollars)

Size	1st Quartile	2nd Quartile	Median	3rd Quartile	4th Quartile
One	< 65	65-85	85	85-121	> 121
Two	< 106	106-140	140	140-196	> 196
Three	< 188	188-240	240	240-304	> 304
Four	< 270	270-350	350	350-437	> 437
Five	< 327	327-412	412	412-525	> 525
Six +	< 441	441-500	500	500-626	> 626

(Courtesy of Nash KD: J Am Dent Assoc 124(3):99–101, 1993.)

Financing Oral Health Care: Can Dentistry Diversify the Portfolio?
Niessen LC (Baylor College of Dentistry, Dallas)
N Y State Dent J 58:35–40, 1992   105-94-1–7

Background.—Demand for dental services has long been correlated with income and education. The greater one's income and education level, the more dental services one consumes. Currently, 98% of all dental expenditures are reimbursed through the private sector, including out-of-pocket expenses and private dental insurance. However, circumstances (e.g., income reductions or increased health-care costs) can effectively limit the amount of discretionary income available to purchase dental services, thus impacting on when and how much dental care will be consumed. In its present state, oral health-care services are primarily based on the ability to pay. It was suggested that it is time to integrate oral health and medical care.

Discussion.—At least 3 of the currently proposed national health-care plans include dentistry, with the extent of dental coverage varying by bill. Disaggregating oral health-care services into acute, primary care, and rehabilitative services is 1 suggested method for structuring policy options. If separated into these categories, each component would effectively be correlated with other comparable health services. One positive consequence of this proposed method is that dentistry will become allied with other health-care constituencies and consumer groups. In addition, health care in general will improve as it becomes more comprehensive.

The connection between oral and systemic care is clear. For example, oral health services should be considered a primary component of care for patients with diabetes, patients with head and neck tumors who are about to undergo radiotherapy, patients with HIV infection, and patients with any other systemic diseases with demonstrated oral manifestations. In addition, patients at high risk for having oral complications caused by medical treatment (e.g., steroid therapy) would benefit from an integrated approach to oral and medical care.

Conclusion.—Even if dentistry was not included in any health-care reform proposal, organized dentistry should actively support health-care reform legislation. If the population can be protected from major health-care expenditures, consumers will be better able to access necessary oral health-care services.

▶ As the 1994 YEAR BOOK OF DENTISTRY goes to press, the debate on health-care reform continues. Dentistry, viewed as a luxury commodity by many, may be included, but perhaps only in a peripheral manner. Some in our profession would rejoice if dentistry was not included in the final health-care reform package. Niessen argues otherwise, maintaining that oral health care must be integrated with medical care. The dental profession has failed to convince the public that oral health care is an essential health service, not a luxury. Health-care policymakers must understand that dentistry must be given equal priority with other essential health services, even in the face of competing needs. The dental profession has done an excellent job promoting sound health principles; it must now challenge its undeserved reputation as an "expendable" health service.—L.H. Meskin, D.D.S., Ph.D.

Compensating Associates

Manji I (Experdent)
J Can Dent Assoc 59:344–346, 1993   105-94-1–8

TABLE 1.—Potential Costs Involved in Taking on an Associate

	Year One ($)	Year Two ($)	Year Three ($)
Associate Collection Net of Lab	150,000	200,000	250,000
Office Dental Supplies at 8%	12,000	16,000	20,000
Reserve Funds	12,000	12,000	12,000
Professional Fees	4,800	Discretionary	Discretionary
Facility Improvements/Enhancements (amortized over 5 years)	12,000	12,000	12,000
Additional staff	Full-time assistant Part-time recept. 42,000	Full-time assistant Full-time recept. 54,000	Full-time assist. & recept. with 6% increase 57,240
Risk factor	24,000	10,000	---
Marketing costs	3,000	Discretionary	Discretionary
Total expenses	109,800	104,000	101,240

(Courtesy of Manji I: *J Can Dent Assoc* 59:344–346, 1993.)

TABLE 2.—Calculation of Net Profit or Loss

	Associate Collection Net of Lab	Expenses	Associate Compensation	Net Profit/Loss
Year One	150,000	109,800	25% = 37,500	2,700
	150,000	109,800	30% = 45,000	-4,800
	150,000	109,800	35% = 52,500	-12,300
	150,000	109,800	40% = 60,000	-19,800
Year Two	200,000	104,000	25% = 50,000	46,000
	200,000	104,000	30% = 60,000	36,000
	200,000	104,000	35% = 70,000	26,000
	200,000	104,000	40% = 80,000	16,000
Year Three	250,000	101,240	25% = 62,500	86,260
	250,000	101,240	30% = 75,000	73,760
	250,000	101,240	35% = 87,500	61,260
	250,000	101,240	40% = 100,000	48,760

(Courtesy of Manji I: J Can Dent Assoc 59:344-346, 1993.)

Introduction.—Senior dentists are frequently unsure of how to compensate their associates. By sharing information on how a particular compensation package has been determined, subsequent misunderstandings can be avoided. The factors to be considered in paying an associate were discussed.

Motivation.—Dentists may decide to hire associates for financial or psychological reasons. Economic motives include increased revenue and reduced overhead. Dentists whose primary motivation is to reduce their workload may be satisfied with only a small increase in their net earnings. The financial package offered a potential associate will be influenced by the senior dentist's motivation.

Financial Considerations.—The bottom line is to find out what your practice can afford to offer an associate. Practice financials consist of operating costs, or overhead, and true profit. Overhead for the last 2 or 3 years can help to forecast future overhead costs. Potential costs involved in taking on an associate include supplies, reserve funds, professional fees, facility improvements, additional staff, and start up and marketing costs (Table 1). Net profit or loss will depend on the associate's earnings, expenses from the collection, and the percentage paid to the associate (Table 2). An associate can be paid on a percentage basis only, or he or she can be offered a guaranteed minimum base salary or a fixed percentage, whichever is higher.

Conclusion.—The goal is to reach a break-even point within 1 or 2 years. Although the initial period may not be profitable, the senior dentist may get relief from the reduced workload, and practice goodwill may build. Because the figures will vary from practice to practice, the examples offered should be considered guidelines for compensating associates.

▶ With dental students graduating with education debt that can exceed $100,000, the desire to be one's own boss and open a dental practice shortly after graduation is often an impossible dream. Each year, the number of graduates seeking an associate position increases. Reduction of financial debt may be a primary rationale for becoming an associate, but what these new professionals seek most is the ability to work in an environment in which they can continue to increase their dental knowledge. This article sets out some pertinent financial considerations that both the dentist and prospective associate must consider before any contract is signed. Although this article stresses the importance of new fixed costs, it gives little attention to the "social costs" borne by the dentist who must take on the role of director of an individualized general practice residency after hiring the new associate. Many excellent dentists may not have the patience necessary to teach procedures that "every dental graduate should know." "We didn't learn it that way in dental school" may eventually cause both parties to wonder why they ever agreed to their association. Interpersonal relationships between dentist and future associate should have equal, perhaps even greater, consideration as the financial numbers before the final contract is signed.—L.H. Meskin, D.D.S., Ph.D.

Prevalence of Upper Extremity Neuropathy in a Clinical Dentist Population

Stockstill JW, Harn SD, Strickland D, Hruska R (Univ of Nebraska, Lincoln; St Elizabeth's Hosp, Lincoln, Neb)
J Am Dent Assoc 124(8):67–72, 1993   105-94-1–9

Background.—Acute and chronic cervical and back pain is a significant problem in the population at large, a problem usually linked to the

Site of Neuropathy	
Location	(%)
Cervical	45.7
Arm (unspecified side)	24.3
Left arm	11.4
Right arm	13.3
Forearm (unspecified side)	26.4
Left forearm	12.7
Right forearm	19.4
Elbow (unspecified side)	11.4
Left elbow	4.9
Right elbow	7.6
Hand (unspecified)	55.8
Left hand	32.0
Right hand	44.2
Thumb	30.2
Index finger	25.6
Middle finger	22.8
Ring finger	22.3
Smallest finger (fifth digit)	19.8

(Courtesy of Stockstill JW, Harn SD, Strickland D, et al: *J Am Dent Assoc* 124(8):67–72, 1993.)

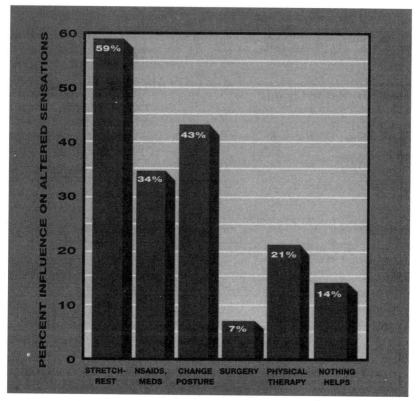

Fig 1–4.—Resolutions of altered sensations by respondents. (Courtesy of Stockstill JW, Harn SD, Strickland, et al: *J Am Dent Assoc* 124(8):67–72, 1993.)

biomechanics of work-related movement. Thoracic outlet syndrome is a common disorder associated with back and neck pain. It refers to the compression of nerves between the base of the neck and the uppermost part of the thorax and axilla. Another common disorder is carpal tunnel syndrome, often associated with repetitive movement of the hands and wrists. Members of professions that are most dependent on upper body movement, such as dentistry, are highly susceptible to such problems. The incidence of upper extremity neuropathy in dentists and how this condition is influenced by work-related conditions were investigated.

Method.—Dentists were asked whether they experienced peripheral neuropathy, which is characterized by altered sensation in the hands, forearm, arms, and neck. They were asked to describe the sensation—pain, numbness, tingling, or loss of muscle control—and to locate the specific site. The severity of the disorder was measured by calculating the frequency and duration of symptoms and the number of workdays missed.

Results.—Of the 1,016 dentists interviewed, 29% experienced peripheral neuropathy. The locations of the symptoms are outlined in the table. Frequency of this disorder did not appear to be significantly related to age, years in practice, or patient position. However, more frequent symptoms were commonly associated with certain procedures, notably crowns and bridges. When asked how they relieved symptoms of peripheral neuropathy, dentists provided a number of responses (Fig 1–4).

Discussion.—The only condition that seemed to affect symptomatic status was dominant hand factor: right-handed dentists were more likely to have peripheral neuropathy than were left-handed dentists. A clinical study investigating the relationship between subjective symptom reporting and nerve conduction studies in affected dentists is now under way.

▶ With almost one third of dentists reporting some form of upper extremity neuropathy, attention to the prevention and relief of these symptoms is critical. A continuing education course from the University of Minnesota may be the answer. Using the combined skills of an orthopedic surgeon, a physical therapist, a specialist in hand rehabilitation, and a member of the operative dentistry department, course attendees learned how to (1) minimize occupational risk, (2) manage pain and discomfort, (3) heed warning signs and take precautions to prevent disability, and (4) modify the work and home environment to prevent further occupational pain. Using the example of risk management, perhaps the disability insurance companies might underwrite the tuition of these courses or even sponsor the courses directly.—L.H. Meskin, D.D.S., Ph.D.

Infection Control

Infection Control in the Dental Laboratory: Concerns for the Dentist
Merchant VA (Univ of Detroit, Mercy)
Compend Contin Educ Dent 14:382–390, 1993   105-94-1–10

Background.—Current Occupational Safety and Health Administration (OSHA) regulations stipulate that all dental office and laboratory personnel must be protected against blood-borne pathogens. Dental impressions and other related prosthodontic items that are routinely transported between the office and laboratory have the potential to transmit infectious microorganisms when contaminated with blood or saliva. Proper procedures for the control of infection and adequate communication with the dental laboratory regarding handling of such items are important concerns for the dental clinician.

Discussion.—Although OSHA does allow shipping of contaminated items when properly packaged and labeled, the American Dental Association (ADA) and the Centers for Disease Control recommend that dental impressions and prostheses undergo disinfection before handling, adjusting, or shipping. In fact, if the proper disinfection methods and

Sterilization-Disinfection of Prosthodontic Materials, Instruments, and Polishing Agents

Prosthodontic Materials, Instruments, Polishing Agents	Sterilization/Disinfection Method*
Articulators/Facebows	Spray-wipe-spray†
Bowls/water baths	
Stainless steel	Dry heat, chemical vapor, autoclave
Rubber	Spray-wipe-spray
Burs	
Carbon steel	Dry heat, chemical vapor, ethylene oxide
Steel	Dry heat, chemical vapor, ethylene oxide, autoclave
Tungsten-carbide	Dry heat, ethylene oxide, autoclave, chemical vapor
Facebow forks	Autoclave, chemical vapor, ethylene oxide
Impression Trays	
Aluminum	Autoclave, chemical vapor, ethylene oxide, dry heat
Chrome-plated	Autoclave, dry heat, chemical vapor, ethylene oxide, chemical sterilization/disinfection

(continued)

materials are used, there should be little concern about adverse effects to these items.

In its 1991 update, the ADA recommended that all impressions undergo disinfection with an appropriate, approved tuberculocidal (TB) disinfectant. Impressions should be rinsed thoroughly to remove any

Table (continued)

Custom acrylic resin	Discard‡, ethylene oxide
Plastic	Discard, ethylene oxide, chemical sterilization/disinfection
Polishing points, wheels, disks, and brushes	
Garnet and cuttlefish	Discard, ethylene oxide
Rubber	Discard, ethylene oxide, autoclave
Rag	Autoclave, ethylene oxide, chemical vapor
Brushes	Autoclave, ethylene oxide, chemical vapor
Shade guides	Chemical sterilization/disinfection, spray-wipe-spray, ethylene oxide
Spatulas/Knives	Spray-wipe-spray
Stones	
Diamond	Dry heat, chemical vapor, ethylene oxide, autoclave
Abrasive (polishing)	Autoclave, chemical vapor, ethylene oxide, dry heat
Wax rims/Wax bites	Spray-wipe-spray

* Preferred method listed first.
† Spray-wipe-spray with surface disinfectant.
‡ For disposable items.
(Courtesy of Merchant VA: *Compend Contin Educ Dent* 14:382–390, 1993.)

blood or saliva before immersion, should not remain in a solution for longer than the time required for TB disinfection, and should be rinsed again after disinfection. For removable prostheses, the ADA advises sterilization by exposure to ethylene oxide or disinfection by immersion in iodophor or chlorine compound. Prostheses should not be stored in a disinfectant before insertion. After disinfection and rinsing, acrylic items may be kept in diluted mouthwash until insertion. In addition, denture cleansers, including ultrasonic solutions, should not be used as substitutes for disinfectant solutions. The ADA recommends an iodophor spray-wipe-spray method for wax rims and wax bites, although rinse-spray-rinse-spray techniques may be more appropriate for wax bites. These items should remain wet for the recommended TB disinfection time. Stone casts can be disinfected by spraying until wet or by immersing in a 1:10 sodium hypochlorite dilution or an iodophor. Custom acrylic resin impression trays can be disinfected by spraying with a surface disinfectant or by immersion in 1:213 iodophor or 1:10 sodium hypochlorite. The table summarizes recommendations for sterilizing and disinfecting selected prosthodontic materials, instruments, and polishing agents.

Conclusion.—The dental office and laboratory should possess a clear understanding of each other's infection control procedures. Effective communication between these facilities can aid in eliminating possible duplication of infection control measures and may reduce potential adverse effects to the dental items involved.

▶ With an increasing number of HIV-positive individuals seeking dental care, dentists are disturbed that many of the infected are unwilling to disclose their status, fearing the dentist will not treat them. Considering these circumstances, each patient must be treated as if he or she were HIV positive, and the dental laboratory must consider that each impression and prosthesis they receive is from an HIV-positive individual. Even though the ADA has recommended disinfection of impression materials since 1985, 2 relatively recent studies indicate a 50% noncompliance rate. In 1990, 41 California dental laboratories reported receiving bloody material from 50% of their dental clients. A survey of dentists published in 1992 indicated than less than half are disinfecting dental impressions (1). Dentists must protect their dental laboratories: disinfection works!—L.H. Meskin, D.D.S., Ph.D.

References

1. Reis-Schmidt T: *Dental Products Report*, pp 85–102, April 1992.

Possibility of Cross-Contamination Between Dental Patients by Means of the Saliva Ejector
Watson CM, Whitehouse RLS (Academy Dental Group, Edmonton, Alta, Canada; Univ of Alberta, Edmonton, Canada)
J Am Dent Assoc 124(4):77–80, 1993   105-94-1-11

Background.—Much attention has recently been devoted to the safety of various dental procedures. However, interpatient contamination through the saliva ejector has not been studied.

Methods and Findings.—Twenty dental units in 10 locations were tested to assess the saliva ejector as a possible vehicle for cross-contamination among patients. Backflow was possible, and oral bacteria were able to survive in the vacuum hose. In a survey of 117 dental offices, 91% reported that patients were asked to close their lips around the saliva ejector tip, which creates the seal that causes fluid backflow. Only 23% of the offices surveyed rinsed or disinfected suction lines between patients. Forty-one percent rinsed or disinfected the lines daily; 9% rinsed or disinfected the lines twice a week; and 27% rinsed or disinfected the lines once a week.

Conclusion.—The risk of cross-contamination among patients through the saliva ejector needs to be reduced. As an immediate, temporary measure, patients can be told not to close their lips around the ejector tip. However, patients may accidentally close their mouths, forming a seal around the tip. Vacuum tubes must therefore be rinsed and disinfected after being used for each patient.

▶ "Suck-back," which is not a pretty term, has been characterized by the authors of this paper as a possible source of cross-contamination among dental patients. Their red dye studies and bacterial culturing of fluid in vacuum lines connected to the saliva ejector present convincing evidence that bacteria and perhaps viruses could be transferred from patient to patient; however, there are no clinical cases of disease that have been traced to this form of contamination. Without clear-cut evidence that contaminated saliva ejectors present a threat of disease, should dental researchers and policymakers give priority to this subject? Considering the large numbers of bacteria that appear to be available for patient-to-patient transfer, it is difficult to believe that at least some infectivity has not occurred, especially in the medically compromised patient. In our profession's present desire to achieve zero risk for dental patients, it should be our responsibility to demonstrate that current procedures are safe, not the opposite. As a starting point, the authors' suggestion that patients be told not to close their lips around the saliva ejector appears to have merit.—L.H. Meskin, D.D.S., Ph.D.

Modes of Potential Cross-Contamination With the Dental Cart
Ioset SM, Rossmann JA (Fort Ritchie Dental Clinic, Md; Univ of Texas Health Sciences Ctr, Houston)
Gen Dent 41:150–155, 1993   105-94-1-12

Background.—The increased attention focused on infection control has produced a number of studies on the proper use of barrier techniques and disinfection of environmental surfaces and handpieces. However, few studies have examined how aseptic techniques can be adapted to the dental office. In an effort to identify and quantify contacts and actions that potentiate cross-contamination among patients, the dental

Contacts That Violated Aseptic Technique, by Category

Category	No. of CVATs observed	% of CVATs
Return of contaminated item to place of storage	40	23.5
Contaminated gloved hands in drawers/place of storage	38	22.3
Failure to disinfect work field and its contents	36	21.2
Ungloved contamination of instruments	22	12.9
Use of contaminated forceps to retrieve items from place of storage/bulk storage	18	10.6
Gloved handling of nondisinfected objects or surfaces	14	8.4
Cart drawer(s) open during production of air-water aerosol	2	1.1
Total	170 out of 564 contacts	

(Courtesy of Ioset SM, Rossmann JA: *Gen Dent* 41:150–155, 1993.)

cart and dental assistant's contact with it were examined from the perspective of infection control.

Methods.—Eleven dental assistants trained in infection control according to American Dental Association, Occupational Safety and Health Administration, and standard operating procedure guidelines were included in this study. A video camera was used to record 19 contacts between the dental cart and the various dental assistants during the performance of routine operative procedures. To determine the adequacy of disinfection between patients, recordings were begun with seating of the patient and concluded with the assistant's actions after the completion of the procedure and before seating the next patient. Contacts that violated aseptic technique (CVAT) and provided a possible cross-contamination route were noted.

Results.—For all dental assistants, the average number of contacts was 34, with a range of 17 to 68. The average number of CVATs was 11, with a range of 2.5 to 27. The mean percentage of CVATs among total contacts was 33%, with a range of 8.3% to 57.5%. The number of contacts per observation ranged from 11 to 68, and the range for number of CVATs was 1 to 27. From a total of 564 observed contacts, 170 were found to be CVATs. The most frequently seen violation was the return of contaminated items to their place of storage, followed by placement of contaminated gloves into drawers or places of storage and failure to disinfect the work field and its contents (table).

Conclusion.—The observed violations have simple solutions that are applicable to all cart systems, such as disinfection of all contaminated items before being returned to storage, dispensing unit-dose items onto the work field before seating the patient, methodical disinfection of the work field, changing gloves before disinfection and again before setup, and closing cart drawers to protect against aerosol. Training and increased awareness of aseptic procedures among dental employees will aid in reducing potential cross-contamination among patients.

▶ This is an excellent, well-designed study with immediate implications for the training and retraining of dental office personnel. The study results indicated that 33% of all dental cart contacts by highly trained dental assistants violated aseptic principles. This information, coupled with the knowledge that many pathogens can live on inanimate objects for extended periods of time, should provide the stimulus for the entire dental team to periodically reexamine their sterile techniques. In-service training, using a video camera, appears to be an effective and inexpensive method to achieve this goal.—L.H. Meskin, D.D.S., Ph.D.

Tuberculosis in the 1990s: Current Implications for Dentistry
Molinari JA, Cottone JA, Chandrasekar PH (Univ of Detroit, Mercy; Univ of Texas Health Science Ctr, San Antonio; Wayne State Univ, Detroit)
Compend Contin Educ Dent 14:276–292, 1993   105-94-1–13

Background.—Tuberculosis (TB) has reemerged in the United States and is rapidly reaching epidemic proportions within certain populations. Traditional medical and dental approaches to treatment are being reassessed because of increased concern about the airborne route of mycobacterial transmission through microdroplet nuclei. The implications of the current TB outbreak for dentistry were discussed.

TABLE 1.—Patient History: Suspicion of Active TB

* Productive cough (> 3 weeks)--for pulmonary TB

* Other symptoms (fever, chills, night sweats, fatigue, etc.)

* 15% of cases--extrapulmonary TB

* Patients with TB and HIV--40% to 75% have extrapulmonary TB and pulmonary TB

* History of TB exposure and/or previous TB infection (active disease)

(Courtesy of Molinari JA, Cottone JA, Chandrasekar PH: *Compend Contin Educ Dent* 14:276-292, 1993.)

TABLE 2.—Persons at Increased Risk for TB

* **Persons with HIV infection**

* **Close contacts with infectious patients**

* **Persons with medical conditions that increase risk of TB**

* **Persons from TB-prevalent countries**

* **Low-income populations**

* **Alcoholics; parenteral drug abusers; high-risk minorities**

* **Prisoners; long-term care patients**

* **Local risk: health-care workers in certain areas**

(Courtesy of Molinari JA, Cottone JA, Chandrasekar PH: *Compend Contin Educ Dent* 14:276-292, 1993.)

Etiology and Pathogenesis.—Contrary to popular belief, TB is not highly contagious. *Mycobacterium tuberculosis* infection usually requires extended close contact of a susceptible host with an infectious source. In most human transmissions, affected persons have inhaled mycobacteria-laden respiratory microdroplets, with nuclei 1–5 μm in diameter. Repeated exposure to air contaminated by droplets from a TB-infected individual can predispose others to TB infection. Most individuals with M. *tuberculosis* infection do not progress to clinical disease.

Risk Factors.—Infection with HIV is a common risk factor for TB infection. The increase in the number of people emigrating to the United States from countries with high prevalence rates of TB infection has had an impact. A variety of compromising medical conditions can predispose a person to clinical TB after M. *tuberculosis* infection, including prolonged immunosuppression, diabetes mellitus, silicosis, and chronic malabsorption syndrome (Tables 1 and 2).

Implications for Dentistry.—Dental professionals are currently considered to be at minimal risk of TB transmission from patients. There have been no confirmed cases of occupational transmission of TB from patients to dental workers. One cluster of dentist-to-patient transmission of TB has been reported.

Recommendations.—Recommendations for dental professionals include TB education and training, patient assessment, surveillance, and minimizing splash and spatter in work practices (Table 3). Universal precautions for bloodborne pathogens should also provide protection against TB transmission.

TABLE 3.—1993 TB Recommendations for Dentristry

1. Understand TB transmission, pathogenesis, signs and symptoms, risk groups.

2. Refer high-risk patients exhibiting TB signs and symptoms for medical evaluation.

3. Annual PPD skin testing of all dental-care providers.

4. Minimize droplet nuclei formation:

    a. minimize splash and spatter

    b. use rubber dam

    c. use high-volume evacuation

    d. careful use of sonic, ultrasonic devices

5. Infection-control procedures for TB:

    a. use universal precautions

    b. change masks and gloves for each patient

    c. appropriate use of other personal protective equipment

    d. instrument sterilization

    e. tuberculocidal surface disinfection

(Courtesy of Molinari JA, Cottone JA, Chandrasekar PH: *Compend Contin Educ Dent* 14:276–292, 1993.)

Conclusion.—Dental professionals should become knowledgeable about M. *tuberculosis,* raise their index of suspicion for patients who may need treatment for undiagnosed TB, and receive annual skin testing. Work practices that decrease the potential for generation of microdroplet nuclei should be incorporated as well as infection-control recommendations for preventing TB transmissions in health-care facilities.

▶ More infection control regulations are forthcoming! In 1990, the Centers for Disease Control (CDC) adopted guidelines to reduce the transmission of tuberculosis in health-care facilities. Last year, the National Institute for Occupational Safety and Health published its recommendations, which called for at-risk health-care workers to wear personal respiratory devices. These devices are bulky and costly, and they can interfere with the interpersonal relationship between provider and patient. Few complied with their suggestions. The CDC is in the process of issuing new guidelines that call for risk assessment and early identification and isolation of patients with infectious TB. The guidelines include effective engineering controls, an appropriate respiratory protection program, and education of health-care workers regarding TB. For those in dental offices, the CDC recommends that if TB is suspected, treatment should be delayed until an infectious determination is made.—L.H. Meskin, D.D.S., Ph.D.

Viral Infections in the Dental Setting: Potential Effects on Pregnant HCWs
Glick M, Goldman HS (Temple Univ, Philadelphia; Morristown Mem Hosp, NJ)
J Am Dent Assoc 124(6):79–86, 1993   105-94-1-14

Introduction.—Universal precautions against disease transmission will minimize the risk of transmission, but they will not eliminate disease-causing agents. The viral agents that may be transmitted to pregnant dental professionals are discussed.

Risk of Infection.—Because pregnant women are immunologically suppressed, they and their fetuses are more suspectible to intracellular bacterial and viral infections. Most infections affecting offspring occur during gestation. Viruses that can affect pregnant dental professionals include herpes, hepatitis, HIV, respiratory viruses, human parvovirus B19, rubella, mumps, and measles.

Herpes viruses.—About half of women of childbearing age are seropositive for cytomegalovirus, fetal infection may occur when primary maternal infection occurs in gestation. Approximately 4% to 5% of pregnant women are susceptible to varicella-zoster infection. Congenital varicella syndrome occurs in about 4% of the fetuses of infected mothers. Approximately 5% of pregnant women are susceptible to primary infection with Epstein-Barr virus, which is associated with congenital malformations. The effect of herpes simplex virus type 1 on pregnancy outcomes and fetuses is not clear.

Hepatitis Virus.—Infection with hepatitis A during pregnancy apparently does not pose a risk for mother or fetus. The risk of hepatitis B infection among dental workers is 3–5 times that of the general population. Women with acute viral hepatitis have an increased risk of spontaneous abortion during the first trimester. About 60% of women acquiring hepatitis B infection close to their delivery date transmit the virus to the neonate, and 85% of infected children become chronic carriers, which increases the chance of childhood liver disease, liver cirrhosis, and cancer. The prevalence of hepatitis C in health-care workers is higher than that in the general population, and it is highest in workers with direct patient contact. Oral surgeons have the highest prevalence of hepatitis C exposure (9.3%) among dental professionals. Although there are not enough data to assess the risk of hepatitis C in pregnancy, any risk is significant, because hepatitis C virus results in chronic hepatitis in

Common Viruses

Virus	Essential modes of transmission		Possible complication
	Saliva	Blood	
Cytomegalovirus	X	X	Birth defects
Varicella zoster	X		Birth defects
Epstein-Barr virus	X		Birth defects
Herpes simplex virus	X		Maternal infection
Hepatitis A		X	Maternal infection
Hepatitis B	X	X	Spontaneous abortions, chronic carrier state of the child
Hepatitis C	X	X	Maternal infection
Hepatitis D		X	Maternal infection
Hepatitis E		X	Maternal fatality
Human immunodeficiency virus		X	Chronic carrier state of the child
Influenza	X		Stillbirth, maternal risk, adult onset schizophrenia
Human parvovirus B19	X	X	Spontaneous abortion, intrauterine death
Rubella	X		Congenital rubella syndrome
Mumps	X		Spontaneous abortion
Measles	X		Prematurity

(Courtesy of Glick M, Goldman HS: *J Am Dent Assoc* 124(6):79-86, 1993.)

50% of infected persons, 10% of whom will die of associated complications.

Human Immunodeficiency Virus.—The risk of HIV transmission appears low in dental settings. Maternal transmission of HIV is common, and about 4,000 children have had AIDS develop by maternal transmission.

Upper Respiratory Tract Infection.—Human parvovirus B19 causes erythema infectiosum. Human parvovirus B19 infection has not been associated with congenital defects in liveborn infants. Persons in close contact with children of preschool and school age are at high risk for infection.

Childhood Diseases.—Congenital defects have been associated with maternal rubella. Most rubella infections are subclinical and are easily misdiagnosed as mild measles or human parvovirus B19. The severity of rubella's effects on the fetus depends on the stage of gestation when the infection is acquired. Deafness is the most common manifestation of congenital rubella infection. When infection occurs during the first 10 weeks of pregnancy, there is also a high incidence of mental retardation, cardiac malformations, and ocular defects. Although gestational mumps have not been associated directly with fetal abnormalities, there is an increased risk of spontaneous abortion. Gestational measles may be associated with premature labor, but teratogenic effects are not commonly related to maternal measles.

Conclusion.—Some of the viral diseases to which dental professionals are exposed can affect pregnancy outcomes (table). Pregnant workers need to be aware of the risks and take necessary precautions.

▶ Although well written, this review of viral pathology only examines the sequelae of viral agents that may be transmitted to the pregnant dental healthcare worker (DHCW) in the dental office setting. The reader must ask about the incidence of viral infections in pregnant DHCWs. If the frequency of infection in DHCWs is found to be higher than that in the normal population, what actions must be instituted to lower the risk of infectivity? If there are no available data to answer this question, research should be instituted to clarify this issue.—L.H. Meskin, D.D.S., Ph.D.

Changing Dental Requirements for Glove Selection and Hand Protection
Fay MF, Sullivan RW, Markovic ER (Regent Hosp Products, Greenville, SC)
Gen Dent 40:489–494, 1992   105-94-1-15

Background.—Glove usage among dental professionals has increased significantly in the past 5 years, mainly to protect against transmission of infectious agents.

Clinical Considerations.—The type of glove selected depends on the length of time the glove is to be worn, the type of procedure being done, the stresses to which the glove will be subjected, and wearer and patient sensitivity to the glove material (Fig 1–5). Sterile gloves meet the greatest tensile strength requirements, because they are subjected to greater in-use stress over time. Many clinicians believe that a thinner glove does not provide the level of protection needed over time for general dental use.

Allergies and Injury.—Because dentistry is a high-risk profession for skin irritation and contact allergy, allergies may affect dentists and other dental personnel. Latex may be an important factor in occupational skin disease (Figs 1-6 to 1-8). Latex sensitivity has a delayed onset and is chronic. Persons with latex sensitivity should use hypoallergenic gloves.

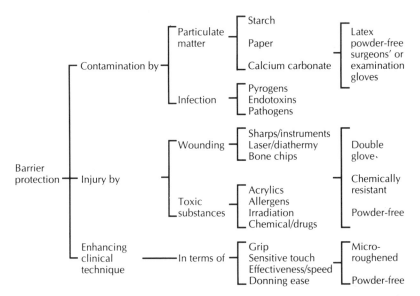

Fig 1–5.—Clinical criteria for dental glove selection. (Courtesy of Fay MF, Sullivan RW, Markovic ER: *Gen Dent* 40:489–494, 1992.)

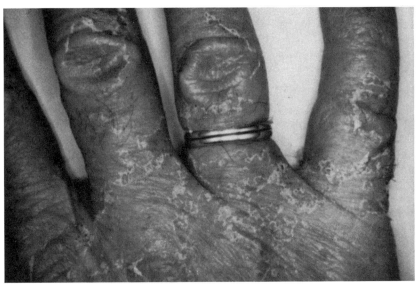

Fig 1–6.—Severe latex thiuram-starch allergy. The reaction was controlled in 10 days with cortisone therapy and use of Biogel D hypoallergenic, powder-free gloves. (Courtesy of Fay MF, Sullivan RW, Markovic ER: *Gen Dent* 40:489–494, 1992.)

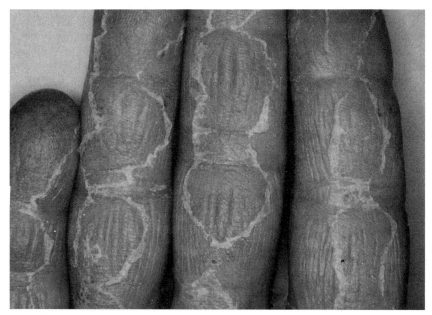

Fig 1–7.—Chapped, dry skin can lead to skin eruptions. (Courtesy of Fay MF, Sullivan RW, Markovic ER: *Gen Dent* 40:489–494, 1992.)

Powder-free hypoallergenic latex gloves are appropriate for chemically sensitized persons. Latex-free gloves can be used in extreme cases.

Subjective Criteria.—Finger-tip grip and feel are critical to endodontists handling broaches, files, and reamers. Fit, thickness, and pliability are critical features for general dentists. Periodontists tend to prefer gloves that do not impair dexterity and that minimize hand fatigue. Because latex gloves may tear when excessive pressure is applied during wear, a longer, stronger cuff with a beaded edge may be preferable. Glove texture and type of lubricant should be considered when assessing a glove's sensory characteristics. Gloves may become slippery when moistened by perspiration, so most dentists prefer gloves with roughened surface.

Conclusion.—Because gloves are a part of infection control, dentists should be knowledgeable about the characteristics of different gloves and should establish objective, clinical, and subjective criteria for glove selection.

▶ During a 4-year period, the Food and Drug Administration noted 1,118 reported cases of latex reactions. Nineteen involved rubber dams, and more than 400 were attributed to examination gloves. Reactions to latex may be as minimal as a local contact allergic reaction or as severe as anaphylaxis. Addressing that subject, a recent international conference dedicated to latex sensitivity in medical devices supplied useful information for dental provid-

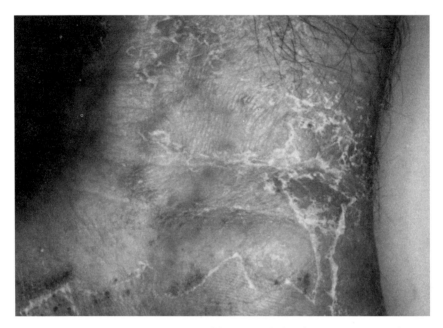

Fig 1–8.—Glove or starch dermatitis should be suspected when skin eruptions stop at the wrist. (Courtesy of Fay MF, Sullivan RW, Markovic ER: *Gen Dent* 40:489–494, 1992.)

ers. All medical questionnaires for dental patients should include questions about latex sensitivity. The appearance of a rash or wheezing after inflating a balloon may be a good question to include. It was also suggested that if latex sensitivity is suspected but not documented, the provider should substitute gloves made of alternate materials and consider advising patients with established sensitivity to wear a bracelet or medallion with that information.—L.H. Meskin, D.D.S., Ph.D.

Presence of Microorganisms in Used Ultrasonic Cleaning Solutions
Miller CH, Riggen SD, Sheldrake MA, Neeb JM (Indiana Univ, Indianapolis)
Am J Dent 6:27–31, 1993   105-94-1-16

Background.—Saliva, blood, or dental materials not removed from contaminated instruments may shield underlying microorganisms against sterilizing agents or disinfecting materials. To ensure adequate microbial killing, precleaning of contaminated dental instruments before sterilization or disinfection is essential. Hand scrubbing and ultrasonic cleaning are both commonly used for instrument cleaning. Hand scrubbing can cause problems, though, because it involves handling of sharp, contaminated instruments. Ultrasonic cleaning allows instruments to be placed in a basket or in specially designed instrument cassettes, eliminating the need for direct handling. However, because numerous batches of instru-

Microbiological Characteristics of Used Ultrasonic Cleaning Solutions

Dental office	Cleaning solution*	Pre-treatment	No. instrument batches processed	Bacteria in the used solution ($\log_{10}$ CFU/ml)	Antibacterial activity of used solution ($\log10$ reduction in CFU/ml)	
					S. aureus	*P. aeruginosa*
1	A	None	17	3.54	0.75	0
2	A	Water scrub	18	1.00	4.82[+]	3.62[+]
3	A	None	7	4.00	0.17	0.28
4	A	Glutaraldehyde	5	2.54	4.82[+]	1.78
5	A	None	27	1.60	4.82[+]	1.36
6	A	None	12	4.00	#	#
7	B	None	8	2.83	1.58	0.06
8	B	Iodophor	5	2.86	0.61	4.62[+]
9	C	None	20	2.08	0.54	0.54
10	D	None	8	0	4.38[+]	6.00[+]

* A, IMS Instrument Daily Clean (5 oz per gallon of water); B, Healthco General Purpose Cleaner (1 part with 10 parts of water); C, L & R General Purpose Cleaner (1 part with 10 parts of water); D, Health-Sonics Multipurpose Ultrasonic Solution (1 part with 40 parts of water).
+ Represents total kill of the inoculum added.
# Contaminant present in used cleaning solution masked growth of test bacteria.
(Courtesy of Miller CH, Riggen SD, Sheldrake MA, et al: *Am J Dent* 6:27–31, 1993.)

ments are typically processed throughout the day, accumulation of microorganisms in the cleaning solution is a potential concern. Whether bacterial buildup occurs during ultrasonic cleaning in the dental office was examined.

Methods.—Ten dental offices participated in the study. Each office was requested to ultrasonically clean their instruments using 1 batch of their normal cleaning solution throughout the day. A quantitative analysis was then performed on each of the 4 solutions used to determine the levels of bacterial contamination and antibacterial activity against *Staphylococcus aureus* and *Pseudomonas aeruginosa*. The second phase of the study comprised an analysis for minimal inhibitory concentration, minimal bacteriocidal concentration, and killing time against *S. aureus, P. aeruginosa*, and *Salmonella choleraesuis*, using fresh, unused batches of each of the 4 cleaning solutions.

Results.—In the used solutions, levels of bacterial contamination ranged from 0 to 10,000 CFU/mL (table). In addition, each of the 4 cleaning solutions demonstrated varying levels of activity against the 2 test bacteria. During the second phase, 3 of the 4 solutions had some antibacterial activity against all 3 test bacteria. However, more than 10 minutes were required to kill all 3. The remaining solution exhibited high antibacterial activity and kill times of less than 1 minute. A repeat test of this solution was conducted in 17 dental offices, and they confirmed its antimicrobial activity during use.

Conclusion.—Some ultrasonic cleaning solutions can become contaminated with bacteria during use. The use of an antimicrobial cleaning solution may aid in minimizing this potential problem. It is important to routinely wear gloves, masks, and protective eyewear and clothing when processing contaminated instruments.

▶ The recommendations of this well-designed research report by one of the nation's leading experts emphasizes the need to maintain personal vigilance even when performing routine office procedures. Masking and using protective eyewear may seem unnecessary during instrument cleanup, but the results of this investigation argue otherwise. If you are using ultrasonic cleaning in your office, you may want to consider the cleaning solution manufactured by Health-Sonics. It exhibited high antimicrobial activity and kill times of less than 1 minute against the test bacteria.—L.H. Meskin, D.D.S., Ph.D.

A Clinical Method to Determine the Effectiveness of Dental Handpiece Sterilization
Cox MR, Carpenter RD, Goodman HS
J Md State Dent Assoc 36:26–28, 1993   105-94-1–17

Introduction.—The risk of transmission of infectious diseases via non-sterile dental instruments has led to a call for regulations on the sterilization of handpieces. There is now little evidence that the internal mechanism of the autoclaved dental handpiece is actually free of micro-organisms. In a pilot study, a clinical method was presented for determining the sterilization status of the internal mechanism of the dental handpiece after process in a steam autoclave.

Methods.—The study was conducted in a single private dental practice during a 5-day period. Standard operating procedures consisted of flushing, discharging, cleaning, and steam-heat autoclaving the fiberoptic high-speed handpieces before routine dental procedures. The unit-attached antiretraction valve of the autoclaved dental handpiece was activated immediately before each use by running water through the handpiece for 30 seconds and then discharging the water into a sink. On each study day, water samples were collected from the dental-unit water tubing, a sink in the dental operatory, and from an employee room sink.

Results.—As expected, the postoperative, contaminated handpieces tested positive for bacterial growth in every trial. However, contamination was also observed in 50% of the 22 tested preoperative, sterilized handpieces in which an air-water aerosol spray was discharged preoperatively. On days 4 and 5, when the handpieces were exposed to air only, none of the sterilized handpieces tested positive for bacterial growth. Sterilized handpiece cultures were contaminated by *Pseudomonas pseudoalcaligenes* and *Pseudomonas paucimobilus*; only *P. pseudoalcaligenes* was found in the tap water cultures.

Conclusion.—Sterilization of the handpiece in an autoclave does not guarantee that the device is free of micro-organisms. The dental unit water system was the source of contamination in this study. Current infection control protocols may be inadequate, because antiretraction valves do not prevent micro-organisms already existing in the water system from entering the dental handpiece. *Pseudomonas* micro-organisms may present risks for patients with AIDS, the frail elderly, and other medically compromised individuals.

▶ This study reveals the importance of looking at all components of a process before making a clinical decision. The authors of this paper have clearly demonstrated that heat sterilization alone will not ensure a micro-organism–free dental handpiece. If the dental-unit water lines (DUWLs) connected to the handpiece are contaminated, no amount of heat sterilization will prevent the handpiece from acting as a potentially infectious vehicle. Most DUWLs are contaminated. A recent research investigation of 150 dental operatories demonstrated that 72% of DUWL samples contained bacterial samples that would "qualify them as unfit for human consumption" (1). Flushing of handpieces for 2 minutes only reduced bacterial counts to approximately a third of the original contaminated level. With handpiece sterilization apparently compromised by the DUWL, the practitioner will want to receive further information on the control of these contaminated water lines.—L.H. Meskin, D.D.S., Ph.D.

Reference

1. Williams JF, et al: *J Am Dent Assoc* 124 (10):59, 1993.

Miscellaneous

Documenting Medication Use in Adult Dental Patients: 1987-1991

Miller CS, Kaplan AL, Guest GF, Cottone JA (Univ of Kentucky, Lexington; Univ of Texas Health Sciences Ctr, San Antonio)
J Am Dent Assoc 123(11):41–48, 1992   105-94-1-18

Background.—To provide quality care, dentists must understand the pharmocology of commonly used drugs and drug use patterns. The extent and patterns of drug use were investigated in a large, geographically diverse population of dental patients.

Methods.—The records of 5,002 adult patients were reviewed. All had received comprehensive dental care in the doctorial clinics of 2 university colleges of dentistry between 1987 and 1991.

Findings.—Forty-two percent of the patients surveyed reported taking a total of 3,418 drugs, including 329 different products. Drug use increased by almost 4 times with age, from .41 drugs among patients 18–33 years old to 1.57 drugs in patients older than 80 years. Women took 68.9% of all drugs used. The most commonly used drugs were hormones, including birth control pills. The most common drugs taken by men were analgesics. Anti-infective drugs comprised 5.4% of medications taken. Most common were penicillin and combination topical anti-infectives and erythromycin.

Conclusion.—The number, rates, and patterns of drug use documented in this study are comparable to those in previous studies. Women took more medicines than men, confirming that women are more likely to take drugs for an illness, and women are more likely than are men to take drugs for a longer time after direct physician care ends.

▶ This survey of use of medication by individuals seeking dental care should emphasize the importance of the dentist's pretreatment analysis of the drug-related questions in the patient's health history. Two concerns must be addressed by the dentist who is treating patients who are taking medication. First, are there dentally related side effects? Second, is there the possiblity of adverse reaction to a dentally administered drug? For example, Prozac, a very popular antidepressant drug, may cause enlargement of the salivary gland and ulceration of the mucous membranes, and dentally administered antibiotics may reduce the effectiveness of birth control pills. Obviously, to maintain a high level of care, dentists must continually review and update their pharmaceutical knowledge.—L.H. Meskin, D.D.S., Ph.D.

Guidelines for a Scientific Presentation
Rieder CE (Univ of Southern California, Los Angeles)
J Prosthet Dent 68:702–707, 1992   105-94-1–19

Purpose.—Guidelines for preparing an effective audiovisually assisted scientific presentation were provided.

Preliminary Steps.—The speaker must first determine the objective of the presentation and choose a subject, then consider the audience for which the presentation is intended. If the speaker chooses a projected presentation, a storyboard should be developed to help visualize the composition and sequence of each planned slide. Information on projection format, slide format, slide composition, graphics, slide colors, slide text size, slide quality, pacing of the presentation, and the correct use of audiovisual equipment is provided. Advice is also given on the presentation itself, including the need for rehearsal, the judicious use of humor, the control of anxiety, what to wear, and delivery technique.

▶ If you think you will ever be called on to make a scientific presentation, obtain a copy of the entire article by writing the author or using Mosby's Document Express (1-800-55-MOSBY). The article systematically describes every facet of preparation necessary to successfully assist the inexperienced dental professional who wishes to give a scientific presentation. Even if you do not anticipate being a presenter, this article belongs in your "just in case" file.—L.H. Meskin, D.D.S., Ph.D.

Understanding the Value of Teeth to Older Adults: Influences on the Quality of Life
Strauss RP, Hunt RJ (Univ of North Carolina, Chapel Hill)
J Am Dent Assoc 124(1):105–110, 1993   105-94-1–20

Background.—As the proportion of older American adults continues to grow, dentists are increasingly focusing attention on the needs and concerns of this population. To enhance the approaches and strategies used by dental health professionals who work with elderly individuals, it is important to understand their perceptions and value of teeth. More than 1,000 elderly adults were surveyed to determine how teeth affect the quality of their lives.

Patients and Methods.—A total of 818 dentate and 200 endentulous adults aged 65 years or older were studied. All participants were randomly chosen from a larger parent survey comprising 4,000 elderly adults from 5 contiguous North Carolina counties. Each participant was

The "Good Effects" of Teeth or Dentures in Older Adults

Perceived effect of teeth or dentures	N	Responding by type of effect %		
		Good	Bad	No Effect
Apperance to others (how you look to others)	845	46	15	40
Facial appearance (how your face looks to you)	880	44	13	43
Enjoyment of eating	902	43	19	38
Chewing and biting	903	42	30	28
Eating	908	42	25	33
Feeling comfortable	899	38	19	44
Living a long life	761	36	4	60
Having confidence	888	32	10	58
Speech	890	32	12	56
Enjoyment of life	893	31	5	63
General health	866	31	7	62
Smiling and laughing	896	31	11	58
Foods you choose to eat	901	28	21	51
General happiness	891	26	3	71
Social life	883	24	4	73
Sex appeal	766	21	5	75
Attendance at activities	884	19	2	79
Success at work	698	19	1	80
Kissing	782	18	4	78
Romantic relationships	754	17	3	81
Tasting	885	16	11	74
Appetite	896	14	5	81
Breath	869	14	17	69
Weight	861	9	6	85
Moods	879	9	4	88

Note: Perceived effect of teeth or dentures among older adults in North Carolina: rank ordered by positive effect.
(Courtesy of Strauss RP, Hunt RJ: *J Am Dent Assoc* 124(1):105-110, 1993.)

interviewed and examined by a trained dentist-interviewer. The 25-question interview was designed to elicit perceptions concerning the impact of teeth on relationships, eating, and health. Possible responses included good, bad, or no effect.

Results.—Participants most often reported that teeth enhanced appearance to others and oneself, eating and eating enjoyment, and chewing or biting. In addition, teeth had a positive influence on comfort, confidence, speech, enjoyment, and longevity of life. Other than breath, participant responses were more positive than negative for all 25 items (table). Between 19% and 30% of the participants stated that teeth had a negative impact on an eating-related item, including eating in general, chewing and biting, and enjoyment of eating. In addition, 11% indicated a negative effect from teeth on taste. In 13% to 15%, facial appearance was negatively affected by teeth.

Conclusion.—Elderly participants expressed concerns that teeth could detract from eating, comfort, breath, appearance, and speech. Approaches designed to provide assurance that negative effects in these areas will be avoided with dental care will most likely prove helpful when treating the elderly patient.

▶ Treatment planning for the dental patient requires both marketing and educational skills. Success in the treatment planning process, as measured by patient acceptance, involves an understanding of the patient's values and perceptions. This research contribution gives the dentist vital information about older adults. With the population of elderly individuals exceeding 30 million and projected to increase dramatically during the next 3 decades, this group will take on added importance to the dental professional. Today, even without any dental insurance to offset the cost of dental care, the elderly make more dental visits on the average than all but one age group. And when they make a visit, they spend more than the average expenditure for a dental visit. With more of these older adults retaining their teeth, plus the promise of some national dental health insurance coverage in the future, the information contained in articles such as this should become part of the dentist's practice management armamentarium.—L.H. Meskin, D.D.S., Ph.D.

2 Dental Education

Introduction

Although heartened by the increasing quality and number of applicants, dental schools find themselves buffeted by increasing costs and decreased revenues. Tuition increases are not the answer. Student debt now averages more than $100,000 per graduating senior at private dental schools, and 48% of all graduating seniors owe more than $50,000. This debt is of serious concern, because professional options available to new graduates may become limited or at least constrained as individuals attempt to repay their educational costs. Those involved in dental education must find mechanisms to lessen this student debt. In that regard, this year's report by the Institute of Medicine on the future of dental education is eagerly awaited. Also, a part of dental education's future equation is the proposed national health-care reform, which may give dental schools a greater role in the delivery of services, especially to patients with special needs. Cost containment, innovations in curriculum, licensure issues, and the impact of the increasing number of female dental graduates promise to make this an interesting year for dental education.

Lawrence H. Meskin, D.D.S., Ph.D.

CPR Requirements for Dental Schools and State Licensure
Mehrali MC, Gerbert B, Wycoff S (Brookdale Hosp, Brooklyn, NY; Univ of California, San Francisco)
J Dent Educ 57:27–28, 1993   105-94-2-1

Background.—Dentists may face a life-threatening emergency at some point in their career. The cardiopulmonary resuscitation (CPR) requirements of dental schools, state licensing agencies, and the Regional Board Testing Agencies were investigated.

Methods and Findings.—Three surveys were sent to all 55 U.S. dental schools, all 53 state and territorial dental licensing agencies, and the 4 large regional testing agencies. Fifty-four schools required CPR certification for graduation. In the remaining school, CPR was a prerequisite for clinical participation. Thirty percent of the dental schools recertified their students annually, as recommended. Another 30% recertified students biannually. The remaining 40% certified students only once. Eighty-seven percent of the schools certified students by the end of their

41

second year. Fifty-one percent of the licensing agencies indicated that CPR certification was a requirement for dental licensure, and all testing agencies required CPR as a requisite for participating in the dental licensing examination.

Conclusion.—All U.S. dental schools now require their students to be certified in CPR at some point in their education. State dental licensing procedures should be upgraded by mandating recertification annually.

▶ Dental schools have set the standard by requiring all students to be certified in CPR. Clinical faculty in dental schools are also required to hold a current CPR certification if they wish to continue their clinical instruction. Although 18 states do not require CPR for licensure or relicensure, dentists practicing in these regions should be aware that they may be held liable if an incident occurs in their office and they do not hold a current CPR certificate. The packaging information on local anesthetic addresses this issue by stating that if dentists are not proficient in CPR, they should refrain from administering local anesthetic. Good office procedure calls for the office team to review its CPR skills every 6 months. How well would your dental team function if you were experiencing emergency?—L.H. Meskin, D.D.S., Ph.D.

A Nine Year Follow-Up Survey of Medical Emergency Education in Dental Schools

Clark MS, Fryer GE Jr (Univ of Colorado, Denver)
J Dent Educ 57:363–365, 1993   105-94-2-2

Background.—The Commission on Dental Accreditation has called for all graduates to be competent in preventing and handling medical emergencies. Guidelines for curriculum on the management of such emergencies have been published. However, no accreditation requirements have been established, leaving curriculum responsibilities to the institutions. The status of programs of medical emergency education in U.S. dental schools was determined in a 9-year follow-up survey.

Requirement for Routinely Taking the Vital Signs (1983 vs. 1992)

Vital Sign	1983		1992	
	n	%	n	%
Blood Pressure	42	76	33	65
Respiration	27	49	17	33
Pulse	36	66	26	51
Temperature	13	24	8	16

Note: 55 schools responded to the 1983 survey, and 51 schools responded to the 1992 survey.
(Courtesy of Clark MS, Fryer GE Jr: *J Dent Educ* 57:363-365, 1993.)

Methods.—A questionnaire was mailed to the deans of all U.S. dental schools. The faculty member responsible for medical emergency instruction was to complete the survey. The response rate was 93%. Survey results were compared with those of a comparable survey done in 1983.

Findings.—Thirty-nine percent of the schools had a separate course for medical emergency instruction. At least 10 hours of medical emergency training were provided by 56% of the schools in 1983 and by 92% currently. The most common teaching method was lecture. The amount of training related to certain specific aspects of medical emergencies is about the same now as it was in 1983. The earlier survey had revealed that vital signs were not being taken routinely. These functions are routinely performed in fewer schools now than in 1983 (table). Simulated emergency drills without prior student knowledge are being performed in about one fifth of the schools, comparable to the earlier proportion.

Conclusion.—The number of schools providing less than 10 hours of medical emergency training has declined in the past 9 years. However, routine measurement of vital signs during clinical visits has diminished. The frequency of medical emergencies in dental offices underscores the need to take vital signs to determine patient risk.

▶ How frequently do medical emergencies occur in the dental office? A 2-state study of practicing dentists indicated that 1,605 dentists experienced 16,826 emergency encounters during a 10-year period (1). Five percent of these incidents required the dentist to provide CPR. Most emergencies occur during or just after administration of local anesthesia (55%), or during treatment (23%) The recognition and management of emergency situation require the dentist and his or her office team to constantly upgrade their skills. Since 1983, dental schools appear to have increased their emphasis on emergency medicine procedures in their dental training programs. However, it was disturbing to note that fewer schools still require the taking of vital signs on a routine basis. Future practice patterns are often formed during the dental school experience; failure to stress the importance of basic medical observation could lead to compromises in patient safety.—L.H. Meskin, D.D.S., Ph.D.

Reference

1. Fast TB, et al: *J Am Dent Assoc* 112 (4):499, 1986.

Women Dentists: 1992 and Beyond
Niessen LC (Baylor College of Dentistry, Dallas)
J Dent Educ 56:555–560, 1992   105-94-2–3

Background.—In 1920, when dentists were trained through apprenticeships, 3% were women. By 1960, when formal dental school education was the norm, less than 1% of dentists in the work force were women. This proportion remained the same until the late 1970s, when the number of women in dental school rose dramatically. There has been a substantial increase in the number of female dentists from the 1980s to the present.

Implications.—About 35% of current dental students are women. There is some evidence that women practice dentistry differently from men. Female dentists are less likely to be married or have many children. Private dental practice may provide an opportunity to examine how women integrate family and career.

Practice Ownership.—A greater proportion of practice owners or co-owners are men. Solo practice owners are more likely to be men. A recent survey showed that 89% of male dentists are practice owners, compared with 68% of female dentists. On average, male dentists are older than female dentists; thus, some differences may be because of age.

Dental Practice Patterns.—On average, female dentists work slightly fewer weeks per year and slightly fewer hours per week. They spend slightly more time with each patient, resulting in fewer patients seen per year on average. Women were more likely to see more patients from minority groups, handicapped patients, low-income patients, and patients receiving public assistance for dental care. The mean procedure fees differed little between women and men. After controlling for age, practice ownership, and hours worked per week, female dentists earn significantly less income than male dentists do. Most disturbing about the wage gap is that a large number of female dentists are employed as associates by other dentists.

Education.—Female dentists are applying to postdoctoral training programs in the same percentages as men. However, 50% of applicants to pediatric dentistry specialty programs are women; only 10% are applicants to oral and maxillofacial surgery programs. Sixteen percent of faculty in dental schools are female, and 35% of students are female.

Conclusion.—The dental profession has an ethical and moral responsibility to ensure that all members of the dental team, including assistants, reach their personal potential. Past misunderstandings and abuses among team members are not consistent with the notion of dentistry as a humanist profession.

▶ The author of this provocative essay on women in dentistry leaves little doubt in the reader's mind that women dentists will continue to have a marked impact on the future direction of the dental profession. Constituting just over 3% of dental first-year enrollees in 1971, women now constitute 40% of dental school graduating classes. These gains, coupled with increased retirements of predominantly older male dentists, are estimated to push the percentage of practicing female dentists to approximately 16% of all dentists by the year 2000. Although many of the barriers to full participation have been removed, there is a noticeable lack of women in leadership roles in dentistry. Records show that 2% of male and 1.4% of female dentists are politically active—a 30% difference. This disparity is accentuated when the younger dentists are compared: 40% fewer women than men under age 39 years are active. With two thirds of all women dentists clustered in this lower age bracket, continuation of their low particpation rate will result in a dearth of future leaders and a diminishing of attention to the needs of the female dentists. Considering the emphasis now placed on women's health, it would be unfortunate if the study of occupational health and safety of women in dentistry suffered from a lack of leaders who would place high priority on this subject.—L.H. Meskin, D.D.S., Ph.D.

Sexual Advances by Patients in Dental Practice: Implications for the Dental and Dental Hygiene Curricula
Chiodo GT, Tolle SW, Labby D (Oregon Health Sciences Univ, Portland)
J Dent Educ 56:617–624, 1992   105-94-2-4

Background.—Sexual harassment in the work place has recently become the focus of much national attention. The occurrence of patient-initiated sexual advances, recently considered in the medical and nursing literature, has not been studied in dentistry. One survey of dental hygienists found that 12.5% had been sexually harassed on the job. A more recent survey of medical students found that 26% of female students had been the object of patient-initiated advances. An anonymous survey was done to determine the frequency of patient-initiated sexual advances toward dental professionals.

Methods.—Three hundred dentists and 300 dental hygienists in Oregon were surveyed. Completed questionnnaires were returned by 83% and 78%, respectively. The 16-item questionnnaire elicited information on occurrence and on methods of dealing with sexual advances by patients.

Findings.—During a 5-year period, as many as 44% of providers experienced verbal advances and as many as 23% experienced one or more physical advances (table). These incidents were a significant source of concern for many dental professionals. The most common approach to dealing with such advances was to maintain a serious, professional, or business-like demeanor in the office at all times. In addition to answering the survey questions, a substantial number of dentists and hygienists wrote that although patient-initiated advances do occur in practice, it is more common for male dentists to make advances toward female staff.

Conclusion.—Patient-initiated sexual advances in dental practice occur with sufficient frequency to cause significant emotional discomfort. Dental and dental hygiene students would benefit from discussion of this issue in their professional training. A 3-step intervention model endorsed in the nursing and medical literature includes assessing patient

Incidence of Patient Advances Toward Dental Professionals in the Past 5 Years

	Dentists (n=248)*		Dental Hygienists (n=235)‡		Significance §
	Percentage of Providers Reporting at least 1 Advance	Number of Advances Received	Percentage of Providers Reporting at least 1 Advance	Number of Advances Received	X^2
Verbal Advances from Male	7.7% (19)*		44% (104)		83.2
Mean		2.7		4.9	
Range		0 to 10		0 to 25	
SD		1.015		3.950	
Verbal Advances from Female	23% (57)		1.7% (4)		47.6
Mean		4.6		1.3	
Range		0 to 50		0 to 2	
SD		4.048		.172	

Physical Advances from Male	3.6% (9) [†]	23% (53)	36.9
Mean	2.5	3.2	
Range	0 to 9	0 to 20	
SD	.664	2.138	
Physical Advances from Female	11% (27)	0.4 %(1)	22.3
Mean	2.3	5.0	
Range	0 to 5	0 to 5	
SD	.973	.326	

* 11 reported by female dentists
† 4 reported by female dentists
‡ Totals vary because not all respondents answered all questions.
§ For all categories: $df = 1, P < .001$.
(Courtesy of Chiodo GT, Tolle SW, Labby D: *J Dent Educ* 56:617–624, 1992.)

and provider behavior before the advance, assessing the environment, and developing a range of strategies for dealing with patient advances.

▶ In this retrospective study, dentists and hygienists were asked to recall examples of patient-generated verbal and physical abuse of a sexual nature occurring during a 5-year period. Memory recall probably understates the frequency of these events, so the number and type of incidents may be substantially underreported. Indeed, in a situation where manipulations in and around the oral cavity are coupled with the close proximity of the health provider, the high frequency of perceived sexual abuse should not be unexpected. The authors' suggestion that dental and dental hygiene students receive professional training to handle this type of event has great merit. However, such training should not be limited to students of dentistry. Continued education offered as a public service to the profession would be welcomed. All practitioners are at risk, and some incidents, if inappropriately handled, could permanently impact the dental practice and its employees.—L.H. Meskin, D.D.S., Ph.D.

The Effect of Instruction on Dentists' Motivation to Manage Fearful Patients
Tay K-M, Winn W, Milgrom P, Hann J, Smith T, Weinstein P (Univ of Washington, Seattle; Univ of British Columbia, Canada; Univ of Kentucky, Lexington)
J Dent Educ 57:444–448, 1993   105-94-2–5

Introduction.—Fear of dental treatment is a common problem. Behavioral and pharmacologic approaches have been used to help fearful patients accept treatment, and increasing attention is now being given to the value of behavioral sciences in the dental curriculum. The effect of behavioral education on dentists' efforts to manage fearful patients was assessed.

Methods.—Surveys were mailed to the 1988 and 1989 graduates of the University of Washington (UW), the University of Kentucky (UK), and the Univeristy of British Columbia (UBC). Behavioral approaches were taught at UW and UK; a pharmacologic approach was taught at UBC. Responses were received from 164 of the 204 graduates; analysis was limited to the 121 general practitioners who practiced more than 20 hours a week. Some UBC graduates who received continuing dental education in behavioral management were combined with the UW/UK group.

Results.—Dentists who had received behavioral science instruction in fear management recognized a higher proportion of fearful patients in their practice than did dentists trained in pharmacologic approaches. At initial visits, graduates of UW and UK made efforts to identify the barriers that hindered fearful patients from receiving care. Dentists who had received instruction on the psychological aspects of fear and anxiety did

Average Scores for the Effort Variables by Type of Instruction

	Behavioral instruction received	
	yes	no
Provide training (range 0-3)	0.9 (1.0)	0.7 (0.8)
Address fear in health questionnaire (range: 0 - 5)	1.5 (1.7)	1.9 (2.1)
Address fear in initial interview (range: 3 - 18)	12.9 (3.3)	12.3 (3.4)
Address fear during initial contact (range: 2 - 12)	6.3 (2.7)	5.2 (2.3)
Practice active listening (range: 3 - 18)	16.2 (1.8)	16.4 (1.8)
Increase patient's perceived control (range: 5 - 30)	26.9 (3.0)	26.3 (3.5)
Efforts taken to teach coping skills (range: 3 - 18)	8.5 (3.4)	8.2 (3.5)

Note: For all effort variables, a higher score indicates greater efforts taken to treat fearful patients.
(Courtesy of Tay K-M, Winn W, Milgrom P, et al: *J Dent Educ* 57:444-448, 1993.)

not, for the most part, report greater efforts toward management of fearful patients (table). The UW and UK graduates were more likely than were UBC graduates to perceive the costs of treating fearful patients as being great.

Conclusion.—The behavioral approach to caring for fearful patients can be effective when taught at the predoctoral or continuing education level. There is a need, however, for the student dentist to be progressively exposed to difficult patients. Clinical faculty should emphasize the impact of the behavioral approach on practice and its value in promoting community dental health.

▶ Reducing concerns of fearful dental patients often results in a more cooperative patient, thus reducing treatment time. Although the behavioral approach to fear management may initially appear to be superior to a pharmacologic regimen, students trained in the behavioral approach perceived the costs to be greater. Unless the dental fees for procedures performed for fearful patients are allowed to reflect increased practitioner effort, it is doubtful if the behavioral approach to fear reduction will gain many supporters.—L.H. Meskin, D.,D.S., Ph.D.

3 Pediatric Dentistry

Introduction

Prior informed consent by parents affects their acceptance of the many treatment modalities offered for their children, independent of the parents' social status. Audio orientation influences one's visual perceptions. A child's reluctant or negative behavior may not be associated with the fears of the unknown or of being hurt. Active patient-doctor interaction is recommended. Both parental expectation of a negative reaction from the child and the child's anxiety with meeting unfamiliar people have strong predictive value for behavior-management problems. Pretreatment consultations should be considered. Studies of long-term memory in children who were physically restrained during dental care do not seem to demonstrate negative after effects.

The wide variation in the use of sedation with children seems less dependent on the type of patient and more so on the particular practitioner or educator.

The presence of alveolar bone loss in otherwise healthy children with primary and/or permanent teeth has a racial predilection; it is seen more in black children than in white children. However, good periodontal review should be done in all children, independent of race.

A retrospective biopsy analysis of children and adolescents as old as 20 years of age suggests that, by far, the most common lesions studied were inflammatory and reactive lesions, with the mucus extravasation phenomenon being the most common.

The volume and concentration of local anesthesia given to children vary among practitioners. A respective review of technique and amount is suggested.

G. Fräns Currier, D.D.S., M.S.D., M.Ed.

Behavior

The Influence of Social Status and Prior Explanation on Parental Attitudes Toward Behavior Management Techniques
Havelka C, McTigue D, Wilson S, Odom J (Ohio State Univ, Columbus)
Pediatr Dent 14:376–381, 1992   105-94-3–1

Background. —A variety of behavior management techniques are used in pediatric dentistry. In deciding which technique to use, dentists consider parents' preferences as well as their own. Whether parental social status affects dentists' preferences regarding behavior management techniques used in the treatment of children was investigated.

Methods.—Two private practices and 1 institutional site participated in the study. A total of 122 parents completed a questionnaire, rating 8 commonly used behavior management techniques in pediatric dentistry. The methods rated were the tell-show-do method, nitrous oxide/oxygen, the Papoose Board, voice control, hand-over-mouth oral premedication, active restraint, and general anesthesia. Half of the parents saw these 8 methods demonstrated on a videotape that contained explanations of each. The other parents saw the same methods on videotape but without explanations. Degree of acceptability was marked on a visual analogue scale ranging from 1 to 99. In analyzing the findings, parents were divided into "high" and "low" social status groups.

Findings.—There were significant differences for hand-over-mouth and general anesthesia between the mean scores of the groups hearing and not hearing explanations on the videotapes for both high and low social status groups. Parents not hearing explanations were less accepting of each technique, except for general anesthesia in the low social status group, which was more accepting. The hand-over-mouth, general anesthesia, Papoose Board, and oral premedication techniques were judged to be the least acceptable. Great variation was noted in parental acceptance of individual techniques.

Conclusion.—Significant differences between high and low social status groups' acceptance of individual techniques were found in few cases. The high social status group was more accepting of active restraint and tell-show-do than the low group but less accepting of Papoose Board and general anesthesia. Because parental acceptance of the various techniques greatly differs, it is very important to get informed consent, regardless of social status.

▶ This study contains much information for analysis. It emphasizes that prior parental consent is essential for physical or chemical restraint. Voice inflection and the tell-show-do method are such common, universal methods that they are part of standard care for all children.

The physical restraints (active restraint, papoose board, and hand-over-mouth) should be considered separately from the chemical restraints (inhalation of nitrous oxide/oxygen, oral medication, and general anesthesia).

There are differences in perceptions between high and low social status groups and between those receiving verbal explanation and those who did not. There was a mild trend for the parents in high social status groups to be less accepting of techniques. However, using generalized and nonspecific approaches to consent or basing consent on an assumption of social status seems unwise.

The least acceptable technique is the hand-over-mouth method. The child, if recalcitrant, should probably be returned to the parent before the use of hand-over-mouth, or at least a time-out should be taken. Most dental schools have discontinued teaching this technique, at least at the predoctoral level.

In most cases, a verbal explanation of a video presentation is thought to be superior than a video presentation without explanation. An individualized, personal approach is commonly taught before the more difficult approaches. However, in the low social status group in this study, an explanation actually worsened acceptability for nitrous oxide, oral premedication, and general anesthesia and had little effect on voice control and active restraint. Prior explanation given to the high social group had no worsening effect on acceptability, except for general anesthesia and the hand-over-mouth technique, a difference that was statistically significant.

One should be continually impressed with individual variability and adopt a universal approach for prior explanation and consent to cover all types of children and their parents or guardians.—G.F. Currier, D.D.S., M.S.D., M.Ed.

The Roles of Requests and Promises in Child Patient Management
Pinkham JR (Univ of Iowa, Iowa City)
J Dent Child 60:169–174, 1993   105-94-3-2

Background.—Pediatric dentists have long understood the importance of educating a child about what to expect from a dental appointment while simultaneously assuring the child that everything will be fine. For more than 70 years, the 2 primary behavior modification techniques used by pediatric dentists have been the preappointment experience and tell-show-do. Other "old" techniques are listed in the table. The usefulness of these methods in managing noncooperating and misbehaving children was examined.

Discussion.—Although it is not denied that there are real fears associated with dental treatment for children, it is easy to use fear as a catchall, when other explanations are plausible. Fear can be a predictor of noncooperation by the child. However, noncooperation is often found in children who are familiar with dentistry and know that the treatment will not hurt them. It is suggested that a pediatric dentist use aggressive techniques to make the child respond to requests for cooperation. The assertive management of children by the dentist should not be viewed as punishment, but only as a technique to get the child to learn to cooperate.

▶ Behavior management in pediatric dentistry preceded the prevention movement by almost 50 years, and now the recommended age for the first dental visit has been moved from 3 years of age to 1 year.

The 3 categories of behavior management to emerge since World War I are:

1. Desensitization: elimination or at least reduction of emotions and/or fears of the unknown. Preappointment experience and the tell-

---

"Old" Techniques That Predicted Successful
Dentistry-for-Children Movement

* 1.   Preappointment experience

* 2.   Tell, show, do

* * 3.   Voice control

* * 4.   Hand-over-mouth

* * 5.   Towel techniques

* * 6.   Physical restraint

* * * 7.   Praise, communications, etc.

* * * 8.   Gifts

*   Desensitization

* *   Flooding

* * *   Reinforcement

(Courtesy of Pinkham JR: *J Dent Child* 60:169–174, 1993.)

---

show-do method are historically the 2 primary desensitization techniques used.

2.   Flooding: a student/teacher relationship in which the student is allowed great freedom in picking behaviors until he/she picks the
wrong behavior and is then intercepted to redirect it into a more
appropriate behavior. This is an assertive approach, ranging from
voice control and physical restraint (holding the child's hand during
injection) to the papoose board and hand-over-mouth.

3.   Reinforcement (positive): rewarding the child verbally or with prizes.
Pinkham describes 4 types of misbehaving children (attention-get-
ting) or the 4 misdirected goals of childhood:

Attention: "I'm not outstanding, but at least I will not be overlooked."
Power: "I may not be a winner, but at least I can show people that
they cannot make me do what they want."
Revenge (retaliation): "People do not care for me, but at least I can
do things to strike back when I am hurt."

Inadequacy: "I will not be able to measure up, but at least if I do nothing people may let me alone."
The child's aversion to adult authority seems more commonplace today than in the past. Association of assertive management techniques with punishment, anger, or pain is an inaccurate analysis. It is a promise from the child to the dentist to cooperate, nothing more and nothing less.—G.F. Currier, D.D.S., M.S.D., M.Ed.

Prediction of Behavior-Management Problems in 3-Year-Old Children
Holst A, Hallonsten A-L, Schröder U, Ek L, Edlund K (Blekinge County Council, Karlskrona, Sweden; Inst for Postgraduate Dental Education, Jönköping, Sweden; Univ of Lund, Malmö, Sweden; et al)
Scand J Dent Res 101:110–114, 1993   105-94-3-3

Introduction.—Non-dental background variables may have a greater influence on the behavior of children at a dental visit than does any previous negative experience of dental treatment. The power of such non-dental background factors was examined to predict behavior-management problems in 3-year-old children.

Methods.—The subjects were 273 children who represented city, town, and rural areas of Sweden. The group included 128 boys and 145 girls. None had any previous dental experience. Before the child's first dental visit, the parent was interviewed by telephone. A 23-item questionnaire covered items related to health status, personality factors, and environmental conditions. All participating dentists and dental assistants were briefed so that examinations would be standardized. The degree of the child's acceptance was rated as negative, reluctant, or positive (Table 1).

Results.—Nine children who were tired, hungry, or ill at the examination were excluded from analysis. Successful examinations were possible with 76% of the subjects. Negative reactions occurred in 11% and reluctant acceptance in 13% (Table 2). Regardless of background factors, the child's willingness to sit alone in the dental chair was a valuable predictor of positive acceptance (Table 3). Boys and girls did not differ significantly in background variables or behavior in the dental situation. Logistic regression analysis found 2 interview variables with statistically significant predictive power: the parent's expectation of a negative reaction from the child and the child's anxiety when meeting unfamiliar people.

Conclusion.—Because it is important that both parent and child have a positive attitude about the dental setting, parents should have a preappointment interview with the dentist before taking their young child for his or her first visit. Children who are mature and not anxious about

TABLE 1.—Ratings of Levels of Acceptance and Influence on Treatment

Rating	Categories of behavior	Level of Acceptance	Influence on treatment
1	Active physical resistance, protests, screaming; no cooperation	No or negative	Treatment cannot be carried out without physical restraint or undue delay. Hands raised and interference with treatment.
2	Signs of resistance such as strained muscles. Reserved attitude. No answers; following directions with your cooperation.	Reluctant	Raised hands but no interference with treatment, which can be carried out without undue delay.
3	Relaxing, calm eyes, talking, and showing interest in the procedures. Good cooperation.	Positive	Treatment can be carried out immediately (after proper information.)

(Courtesy of Holst A, Hallonsten A-L, Schröder U, et al: *Scand J Dent Res* 101:110–114, 1993.)

meeting new people are more likely to sit alone in the chair and accept the entire examination.

▶ Nondental factors have had a greater influence on dental behavior from early childhood to adolescence than have earlier negative experiences asso-

TABLE 2.—Number and Percentage of Children With Acceptance 1, 2, or 3 at Different "Steps"

	Acceptance						Missing observations
	1		2		3		
	no.	(%)	no.	(%)	no.	(%)	
1. Enter treatment room	9	(3.5)	31	(12.0)	218	(84.5)	6
2. Mirror in mouth	27	(10.5)	37	(14.3)	194	(75.2)	6
3. Probe on fingernail and tooth surface	26	(10.2)	36	(14.1)	194	(75.8)	8
4. Air-blower on hand and in mouth	29	(11.3)	38	(14.8)	189	(73.8)	8
5. Lie or sit in operating chair	18	(7.0)	41	(16.0)	197	(77.0)	8
6. Examination	28	(10.9)	34	(13.2)	195	(75.9)	7

$n = 264$.
(Courtesy of Holst A, Hallonsten A-L, Schröder U, et al: *Scand J Dent Res* 101:110–114, 1993.)

ciated with dental treatment, for example, a problem with a visit to the physician, dental fear experienced by the parent(s), and anxiety in meeting unfamiliar people. In this study, 2 interview variables had statistically significant predictive power for 3-year-old children with no past dental experience: parental expectation of a negative reaction from the child and the child's anxiety in meeting unfamiliar persons.

TABLE 3.—Prediction of Dental Behavior by the Variable "Sitting or Not Sitting Alone in Dental Chair"

Predictor	Behavior at Examination		Predictive value for
	Negative	Positive	
Sitting in the dental chair			
Not alone	46	58	Positive test (PV +) 46/104 = 0.44
Alone	8	127	Negative test (PV-) 127/135 = 0.94
	Sensitivity 46/54 = 0.85	Specificity 127/185 = 0.69	

(Courtesy of Holst A, Hallonsten A-L, Schröder U, et al: *Scand J Dent Res* 101:110–114, 1993.)

Whether a child would sit alone in the dental chair was found to be a valuable predictor, irrespective of background factors. Sensitivity was .85; specificity, .69; positive predictive value, .44; and negative predictive value, .94.

The problem with studies that use chronologic age is the lack of correlation between this age and mental or emotional ages. Three-year-old children who are noncompliant or reluctant to visit the dentist may have a developmental milestone that is delayed but within the range of normal. Separation anxiety still may be too strong; this is usually seen in 9- to 30-month-old children.

There was no difference between the dental assistant and the dentist regarding the effect of systematic behavior shaping.—G.F. Currier, D.D.S., M.S.D., M.Ed.

Dental Attitudes and Memories: A Study of the Effects of Hand Over Mouth/Restraint
Barton DH, Hatcher E, Potter R, Henderson HZ (Indiana Univ, Indianapolis)
Pediatr Dent 15:13–19, 1993   105-94-3–4

Background.—Nonpharmacologic behavior management techniques in pediatric dentistry, such as the hand-over-mouth (HOM) method and physical restraint, allow dentists to treat children without the potential risk that drugs entail. However, the long-term effects of methods such as HOM and physical restraint have not been established definitively. Whether the number and severity of generalized fears and dental fears differed between patients who did and those who did not have HOM and/or physical restraint during dental treatment in childhood was studied.

Methods.—Patient records from a children's clinic in a dental school and a private pediatric dental practice were reviewed, and patients who had had HOM and/or restraint were identified. Sixty-one patients who had had HOM and/or restraints and 61 who had not were interviewed.

Findings.—The 2 groups did not differ significantly in generalized fears or specific dental fears. There also were no differences between how the 2 groups felt about visiting the dental office. There were no significant differences in negative or positive responses between groups when 3 different formats were used to question the subjects about their early dental memories. However, more than 2 times as many subjects experiencing HOM and/or restraint than comparison subjects described negative experiences in a physician's office or hospital, a difference that was significant (Tables 1 and 2).

Conclusion.—Children apparently do not remember and are not affected by early experiences with HOM and/or physical restraint in the dental office. Practitioners using such techniques in an appropriate way and with parental consent should not be uncomfortable about this decision.

▶ This 7-year follow-up study of children who underwent HOM restraint in dental offices did not demonstrate any adverse effects resulting from the experience. When compared with others, no differences in generalized or dental fears were shown.

In the HOM/restraint group, 46% of the subjects reported traumatic experiences in a physician's office or hospital, compared with only 21% in the comparison group.

TABLE 1.—Generalized and Dental Fears

		Comparison			HOM/Restraint	
	Y	S	N	Y	S	N
1. The dark	2	12	47	2	11	48
2. Sudden loud noises	16	29	16	9	26	26
3. Being left alone	13	17	31	12	17	32
4. Thunder and lightning	4	16	41	4	12	45
5. Snakes	20	10	31	27	13	21
6. Dogs and cats	1	12	48	5	9	47
7. Places haven't been to before	9	28	24	8	17	36
8. Water	3	3	55	4	2	55
9. Masks	2	9	50	3	5	53
10. Scary movies	13	20	28	11	22	28
11. The dentist	3	8	50	2	5	54
12. What the dentist will do to your teeth	11	23	27	8	18	35
13. The dentist might scold you for not doing a good job	3	5	53	6	11	44
14. Other people in the dental office	1	3	57	8	2	51
15. The needle	23	12	26	33	7	21
16. The sound of the drill	13	11	37	17	9	35
17. Losing a tooth	15	8	38	15	1	45
18. Choking	15	10	36	17	10	34

Abbreviations: Y, yes; S, sometimes; N, no.
(Courtesy of Barton DH, Hatcher E, Potter R, et al: *Pediatr Dent* 15:13–19, 1993.)

Almost all of the children who reported an adverse visit to a physician's office could remember the experience but not the traumatic dental episode. Why? More study is needed to determine this relationship.

If one is going to argue against HOM/physical restraint, citing development of long-term adverse sequelae from it, one will be strongly challenged and will have to use a different argument.—G.F. Currier, D.D.S., M.S.D., M.Ed.

TABLE 2.—Reported Negative Experiences by Age and Gender

	<3 years	*4–6 years*	*7–9 years*	*10–12 years*	*> 13 years*	*Total*
Male	8	1	3	6	4	22
Female	4	6	12	7	13	42

Note: Values are combined responses from 3 different questions used to elicit memories of negative dental experiences.
(Courtesy of Barton DH, Hatcher E, Potter R, et al: *Pediatr Dent* 15:13–19, 1993.)

Pharmacology

Project USAP the Use of Sedative Agents in Pediatric Dentistry: 1991 Update
Houpt M (UMD–New Jersey Dental School, Newark)
Pediatr Dent 15:36–40, 1993   105-94-3-5

Background.—Conscious sedation, deep sedation, or general anesthesia are sometimes necessary when treating patients who are very young or severely mentally handicapped who cannot communicate sufficiently and who have severe behavioral problems. Sedation practices vary widely. A national survey was done to update information on the sedation practices of pediatric dentists.

Methods.—All 2,532 members of the American Academy of Pediatric Dentistry (AAPD) were sent questionnaires regarding their use of sedation; 1,497 members responded. Another survey was sent to the directors of all 55 postdoctoral training programs in pediatric dentistry; 46 responded.

Findings.—Both surveys showed wide variation in the use of sedation among training programs and among practitioners. Heavier use of sedation was generally unrelated to the percentage of handicapped patients receiving sedation and to the type of training. Practitioners using sedation frequently, defined as more than once a day, tended to be located in the southern, southeastern, and western parts of the country and to have been in specialty practice for more than 10 years (Tables 1 and 2).

Conclusion.—The wide differences in sedation use probably reflect differences in the biases of individual practitioners and educators. There is a need for research to enable better determination of when a child should be sedated for dental treatment and of which regimen should be used.

▶ Approximately 50% of the pediatric dentists surveyed used nitrous oxide alone for fewer than 10% of their patients, and two thirds indicated that they used nitrous oxide less than 25% of the time. Most practitioners used little, if any, other sedation. In 86% of the respondents, sedation was used

TABLE 1.—Frequency of Use of Sedative Agents

	Total Sample N = 1497	Sample Using Sedative Drugs Other Than N₂O		
		> 1/3 months N = 1043	> 1/day N = 173	> 2/day N = 57
Per cent of patients sedated only with nitrous oxide				
0	18	10	10	12
1–5	26	26	15	14
6–10	13	15	13	14
11–25	14	17	18	12
26–50	12	14	19	23
> 50	17	18	25	25
Per cent of patients sedated with other sedative agents				
0	26	0	0	0
1–5	50	69	30	15
6–10	13	17	27	23
11–25	7	9	23	32
26–50	3	4	14	23
> 50	1	1	5	7
Per cent of sedated patients (other than N₂O) who were handicapped				
	—	12	7	7
Per cent of patients sedated (other than N₂O) who were ages:				
0–2 years	—	34	21	20
3	—	38	39	38
4–5	—	19	29	29
6–10	—	6	9	10
> 10 years	—	3	2	3

Note: Values shown are percent of sample.
(Courtesy of Houpt M: Pediatr Dent 15:36–40, 1993.)

for 10% or fewer of their patients. Of the remaining 14% who were heavy users (more than 2 times per day) about one third sedated fewer than 10% of their patients, whereas two thirds did more.

During the past 2 years, 31% had decreased their use of sedation compared with 57% who had not changed. The 5 major reasons cited were increased management skills, fewer patients who needed it, increased use of general anesthesia, compliance with the new AAPD guidelines, and increased cost or regulation from insurance companies and state legislatures.

About one third of the sedations were administered by only 57 practitioners who used sedative agents other than nitrous oxide twice a day, whereas almost two thirds of the sedations were administered by only 12% of the practitioners (173) who used sedation on the average of more than once each day.

TABLE 2.—Mean Number of Sedations Performed by Each Student Each Year in Postgraduate Training Programs Using Particular Sedative Agents

	Number for Each 1st Year Student			Number for Each 2nd Year Student		
	Range	All Programs	Programs Using Agent	Range	All Programs	Programs Using Agent
a. Hydroxyzine (Atarax or Vistaril) alone	0–40	2	8 (15)*	0–80	4	11 (15)
b. Hydroxyzine and N_2O	0–60	4	9 (19)	0–99	5	11 (21)
c. Chloral hydrate (Noctec) alone	0–20	1	7 (9)	0–25	2	11 (8)
d. Chloral hydrate and N_2O	0–20	2	6 (15)	0–35	3	10 (16)
e. Chloral hydrate and promethazine (Phenergan) alone	0–10	0	6 (2)	0–10	0	6 (2)
f. Chloral hydrate, promethazine, and N_2O	0–48	1	15 (4)	0–30	2	13 (6)
g. Chloral hydrate and hydroxyzine (alone)	0–40	3	11 (11)	0–40	3	10 (13)
h. Chloral hydrate, hydroxyzine, and N_2O	0–45	7	15 (23)	0–45	10	19 (24)
i. Meperidine (Demerol) alone	0–15	1	5 (5)	0–20	1	6 (6)
j. Meperidine with N_2O	0–10	0	5 (4)	0–30	1	7 (7)
k. Meperidine and promethazine	0–20	1	6 (8)	0–99	4	19 (9)
l. Meperidine, promethazine, and N_2O	0–35	4	11 (16)	0–60	6	46 (18)
m. Diazepam (oral valium) alone	0–20	2	5 (23)	0–20	4	7 (24)
n. Diazepam (oral) and N_2O	0–50	4	7 (28)	0–99	7	10 (31)
o. Other	0–35	3	8 (18)	0–25	4	6 (19)
Total (Average number for each student each year)	0–105	Mean = 35 Median = 27		0–335	Mean = 56 Median = 36	

*Number in parentheses equals number of programs in which agent was used.
(Courtesy of Houpt M: Pediatr Dent 15:36–40, 1993.)

The most commonly used drug combination was Noctec (choral hydrate) and Atarax (hydroxyzine) supplemented with nitrous oxide. However, most of the individual teaching programs (28 of 46) used oral diazepam (Valium) supplemented with nitrous oxide.

In 1985, 6% of the practitioners surveyed used sedative agents other than nitrous oxide twice daily during a 3-month period. However, by 1991, this number was reduced to 3% of respondents. Although most educational programs have continued using sedation other than nitrous oxide with the same frequency as in 1985, programs that were heavy users of sedation have substantially reduced their frequency of drug use. Guidelines, regulations, and costs have taken their toll in the pharmacologic management in dentistry for children.—G.F. Currier, D.D.S., M.S.D., M.Ed.

A Survey of Local Anesthetic Usage in Pediatric Patients by Florida Dentists
Cheatham BD, Primosch RE, Courts FJ (Univ of Florida, Gainesville)
J Dent Child 59:401–407, 1992   105-94-3-6

Background.—Dentistry must continuously survey and monitor its routine practice so that a justifiable range of standardized care becomes acceptable practice. The safe and effective local anesthetic dose for children is one such concern. One hundred seventeen Florida dentists were surveyed about their practice habits regarding local anesthetic use in children.

Findings.—Ninety-six percent of the respondents used an amide local anesthetic, with 69% using 2% lidocaine with 1:100,000 epinephrine. Opinions varied as to recommended maximum dosage, usually reported as number of cartridges, and was not highly influenced by the child's weight or age (table). Thus, smaller children received larger doses and

Range and Mean Dose (Mg) and Dosage (Mg/Kg) for the Recommended Maximum Anesthetic Delivered to Children

Dose	Weight of the child		
	13 kg	20 kg	35 kg
Mean	69.9 mg	96.5 mg	135 mg
	(5.4 mg/kg)	(4.8 mg/kg)	(3.8 mg/kg)
Range	12 - 252 mg	18 - 252 mg	36 - 252 mg
	(0.9 - 19.3 mg/kg)	(0.9 - 12.6 mg/kg)	(1 - 7.2 mg/kg)

(Courtesy of Cheatham BD, Primosch RE, Courts FJ: *J Dent Child* 59:401-407, 1992.)

larger children received smaller doses, in terms of dose per weight. Seventy-seven percent of respondents would use periodontal ligament (PDL) injection only as a supplemental technique. Fifty-seven percent used a special pressure syringe for PDL injections, and two thirds of those using PDL injection said they would use a vasoconstrictor along with the local anesthetic. Just 30% of respondents used bilateral inferior alveolar nerve blocks, many of them with a 30-gauge needle. Failure rate with this technique was 15% to 20%. Eighty-four percent of the dentists believed that .9–1.8 mL of local anesthetic should be given as the initial volume. Nearly one third gave a full cartridge as the initial volume.

Conclusion.—Many dentists giving local anesthetics to their pediatric patients give a higher than necessary dose. Many practitioners give a maximum dose that is higher than recommended. There is a need for alternative techniques of local anesthesia that can reduce the chances of local anesthetic toxicity, particularly volume and concentration reductions. Dosage may also be reduced by selective use of PDL injections and mandibular infiltrations.

▶ Adverse reactions to local anesthetics are well documented in pediatric dental patients. Approximately 2.5% to 10% of patients experience adverse local anesthetic reactions. Many times, the potential complications of local anesthetics, such as convulsive reactions, are overlooked in discussions of the complications of sedative agents.

The overwhelming choice for anesthesia (69%) was an amide local anesthetic, 2% lidocaine with 1/100,000 epinephrine. The maximum recommended dose of lidocaine in children is 4.4 to 7 mg/kg (2 to 3 mg/lb). In this study, for an inferior alveolar block, 60% of dentists used a 27-gauge needle, and nearly 40% used a 30-gauge needle. The use of half a Carpule for an initial load, rather than a full 1.8-cc Carpule, should be considered in children.

Problems remain for those who give inferior alveolar blocks to children. If one uses only an intraoral tactile approach to the ascending ramus referencing to the occlusal plane, unacceptable failure rates may occur. The mandibular canal is located about two thirds of the way back on the ascending ramus at its shallowest depth, or the closest distance between the thumb and finger of the same hand. It is independent of the occlusal plane and can be found in infants and adults, regardless of whether they have teeth present. The depth of the ascending ramus is as difficult to identify visually, because it is vertical, without bimanual, intraoral-extraoral tactile sites. One should consider neurologic growth centers and capsular matrices in finding the nerve.—G.F. Currier, D.D.S., M.S.D., M.Ed.

Disease Occurrence

Destructive Periodontal Disease in Healthy Children

Cogen RB, Wright JT, Tate AL (Univ of Alabama, Birmingham; Univ of North Carolina, Chapel Hill; Huntsville, Ala)
J Periodontol 63:761–765, 1992   105-94-3-7

Background.—Juvenile periodontitis (JP) is a condition in which advanced alveolar bone loss occurs in otherwise healthy adolescents. Three mechanisms appear to be involved in the etiology of JP: microbiology, heredity, and defects in polymorphonuclear leukocytes (PMN). It has been widely assumed that the condition rarely affects the primary deciduous dentition, but evidence of JP may appear many years before the onset of puberty.

Methods.—During a 5-year period, 4,757 children who were patients at a children's hospital dental clinic had radiographic surveys suitable for diagnosing of JP. Criteria for diagnosis included age 15 years or younger, negative medical history, and radiographic evidence of arc-shaped alveolar bone loss. Two examiners confirmed JP in the permanent dentition; 3 examiners had to concur that bone loss was present in primary and transitional dentitions.

Results.—The study group was one third white and two thirds black, reflecting the general patient population of the clinic. The prevalence of JP was .3% among white subjects (4 girls and 1 boy) and 1.5% among black subjects (24 girls and 23 boys), a statistically significant difference. Among the black children with radiographs of transitional dentition, 85.7% showed evidence of bone loss; of those with radiographs of the primary dentition, 71.4% had discernible alveolar bone loss.

Conclusion.—The presence of JP in the prepubertal years and in the primary as well as the permanent dentition was confirmed. Otherwise healthy children are affected, and the condition is much more prevalent in black children. Diligent periodontal evaluation is needed for all children.

▶ Certain terms that were acceptable 50 years ago are given little support today. The term "mixed" (as in mixed dentition) is from segregationist America; the term "transitional" is preferred. The use of "primary" instead of "deciduous" and "childhood," or "children" instead of "juvenile" are other terms we should adopt. Also, "JP" should be "CP."

It is essential for all practitioners to observe any alveolar bone loss around the primary and permanent teeth from the primary dentition, through the transitional, and up to the young permanent dentition. This should become easier with reduction in caries and an appreciation of the differences between normal exfoliation and pathologic bone loss.

There are reasonable familial tendencies other than species specificity (black and female) with this disorder of childhood periodontitis; these include

PMN leukocyte dysfunction and a strong association with gram-negative anaerobic rods, especially Aa (*Actinobacillus actinomycetemcomitans*).

Alveolar bone loss in children is more common than has been reported in the literature. More documentation from practitioners is needed.—G.F. Currier, D.D.S., M.S.D., M.Ed.

A Review of Pediatric Oral Biopsies From a Surgical Pathology Service in a Dental School

Das S, Das AK (Univ of Illinois, Chicago)
Pediatr Dent 15:208–211, 1993   105-94-3-8

Introduction.—There have been few surveys of oral lesions in children. A review was undertaken of the results of oral biopsies from patients younger than 20 years old treated in the biopsy service at a university hospital from 1978 through 1988.

Methods.—During the study, 19,379 oral biopsies involving patients of all ages were done; data from 2,370 patients younger than 20 years of age were examined. Data were divided according to patient age (10 years and younger and 11–20 years of age) and race (white, black, and Hispanic). The lesions were divided into 4 categories: inflammatory and reactive, cystic, neoplastic, and other anomalies.

Results.—Private practitioners had sent in 73.9% of the biopsy specimens. The older age group accounted for 75% of the cases. Fifty-seven percent of biopsies were from whites, 26% were from blacks, and 17% were from Hispanics. The most common biopsied sites were the periodontium (20.7%) and the lips (17.8%). Two thirds of the lesions were classified as inflammatory/reactive. In this category, mucus extravasation phenomenon and fibrous hyperplasia were the most common lesions. Neoplastic lesions accounted for 11.2% of the total; papilloma was the most prevalent in this category. Cystic lesions were identified in 10.7% of cases. In 9.07% of the biopsy specimens the tissue was normal (table).

Conclusion.—Some lesions, especially in the inflammatory/reactive category, were more common in the first decade of life. The incidence of neoplasms, however, was greater in older children. The 7 most commonly occurring lesions were the same for both age groups. Mucus extravasation phenomenon headed the list in both younger and older patients, but the sequence differed for the remaining 6 lesions. An apparent higher occurrence of certain lesions among whites may be related to their greater likelihood of receiving surgical care.

▶ During an 11-year period at a dental school in Chicago, almost 20,000 oral biopsies were done, with approximately 12% of them performed in patients younger than 20 years of age. Children 0 to 10 years of age accounted for one fourth of the 2,370 biopsies; three fourths of the biopsies were done in children in the 11- to 20-year-old age group.

Oral Lesions and Their Prevalence

Age Group Number of Biopsies	Whites		Blacks		Hispanic		Total 2370	% of Total
	0–10 288	11–20 1034	0–10 205	11–20 432	0–10 162	11–20 249		
Categories of Lesions								
I. Inflammatory/reactive	201	763	155	263	107	178	1567	66.1
Mucus extravasation phenomenon	58	147	15	18	17	19	274	11.6
Periapical granuloma/abscess	5	145	6	33	2	25	216	9.2
Periapical cyst	10	107	12	50	4	11	194	8.2
Fibrous hyperplasia	26	77	22	36	21	23	206	8.8
Peripheral ossifying fibroma	6	9	6	9	4	5	39	1.6
Pyogenic granuloma	10	33	8	11	3	9	74	3.1
Gingivitis/periodontitis	28	44	19	21	7	13	132	5.5
Nonspecific inflammation	32	46	19	32	11	21	161	6.7
Remaining lesions	26	55	48	53	37	52	271	11.4
II. Cystic lesions	27	140	4	50	12	21	161	10.7
Dentigerous	10	77	—	24	5	6	122	5.2
Traumatic bone*	2	5	—	2	1	—	10	0.3
Epidermoid	2	12	—	1	1	1	16	0.7
Aneurysmal bone*	2	1	—	1	1	—	5	0.2
Other odontogenic	10	43	4	23	2	11	93	3.9
Remaining cysts	1	2	—	—	2	3	8	0.3

III. Neoplastic lesions	34	132	32	57	13	21	288	11.6
Papilloma	8	39	9	7	13	4	70	2.1
Odontoma	5	22	5	12	1	3	70	2.0
Neurofibroma/neuroma	4	7	1	2	1	1	16	0.7
Hemangioma	1	5	1	3	1	1	12	0.5
Peripheral odontofibroma	3	20	2	6	1	4	36	1.5
Nevus	2	5	—	2	—	1	10	0.4
Other neoplasms	11	24	13	24	5	8	85	3.5
IV. Other oral anomalies	13	26	7	12	5	7	70	2.56
Supernumerary teeth	2	2	—	—	2	—	6	0.2
Remaining lesions	8	17	7	10	3	6	51	2.25
Normal tissue	16	88	11	53	25	22	215	9.07

* Not true cysts, but included after Regezi and Sciubba.
(Courtesy of Das S, Das AK: *Pediatr Dent* 15:208–211, 1993.)

The mucocele (mucus extravasation phenomenon) was the most common lesion, showing a predilection for the lower lip. The incidence of the lesion in all racial groups increased in the second decade. This study found a ratio of 6:1 in white compared with black patients and 5:1 in white compared with Hispanic patients. Periapical granuloma/abscess was the next most commonly encountered lesion, and the majority of these lesions were found in the maxillary anterior region. The next most common lesion in this category, periapical cyst, was the most common cyst in the study. Fibrous hyperplasia (fibrous scar, fibroma, or fibrous hyperplasia) was the next most common group in the inflammatory/reactive category (66% in the 11- to 20-year-old age group). The most prevalent cystic lesion was the dentigerous cyst, which was usually found in the mandibular molar area and had a higher occurrence in the 11- to 20-year-old age group. The most prevalent neoplasm, papilloma, was usually found on the buccal mucosa and, sometimes, on the palate. It was followed by odontoma, which was the most common odontogenic neoplasm.

According to the table, the most common lesions in the first decade (0- to 10-year-olds) were mucocele (90 cases), nonspecific inflammation (62), fibrous hyperplasia (fibrous scar, fibroma; 69), gingivitis/periodontitis (54), periapical cyst (26), pyogenic granuloma (21), dentigerous cyst (15), and periapical granuloma/abscess (13). In the second decade (11- to 20-year-olds), the most common lesions were periapical granuloma/abscess (203), mucocele (184), periapical cyst (168), fibrous hyperplasia (fibrous scar, fibroma; 136), dentigerous cyst (107), nonspecific inflammation (99), gingivitis/periodontitis (78), and pyogenic granuloma (53).—G.F. Currier, D.D.S., M.S.D., M.Ed.

4 Growth and Development

Introduction

The consideration of genetics vs. the environment in human growth and development is a never-ending story with an ever-expanding area of new knowledge using proper twin analysis, especially if one includes prenatal development.

Cranial and facial parameters, whether soft or hard tissues, need to be reviewed relative to age, gender, and race for accurate comparisons. Anomalies of the teeth should be considered with familial patterns to determine the extent of the disorder.

Orientation to soft tissue influences on the developing occlusion remains more difficult to analyze than the hard tissues, such as the bones and teeth. The maxillary incisor crown-root axis, or angulation, can be altered as a result of the pathway of eruption, as seen in various types of malocclusions, especially class III and class II division 2 patterns.

G. Fräns Currier, D.D.S., M.S.D., M.Ed.

Palate

The Use of Twins in Dentofacial Genetic Research

Lauweryns I, Carels C, Vlietinck R (Katholieke Universiteit Leuven, Belgium)
Am J Orthod Dentofacial Orthop 103:33–38, 1993   105-94-4-1

Introduction.—During the past 2 decades, there have been a number of advances in the use of twins in genetic research. The technique of analysis has been refined, and major differences have been found in development, growth, and behavior in twin families compared with nontwin families. Development of the twin half-sib method, using the children of monozygotic (MZ) twins, is another innovation. The dental characteristics of twins were reviewed.

Occlusal and Dentofacial Structure.—The results of early twin research suggested that genetic factors were a more important influence on occlusal traits than were nongenetic factors. More recent research, however, found that even dizygotic (DZ) twins were occlusally not identical. Environment appears to play a large role in malocclusions, which have been linked to the impact of modernization.

Dental Characteristics.—Tooth structure and tooth dimensions appear to be affected by both genetic and environmental factors. A wider range of genetic factors were found to influence the mandibular rather than the maxillary teeth. There is a higher incidence of certain congenital anomalies in twins, particularly in MZ twins, when compared with singletons. Maternal factors predisposing to twinning appear to be associated with those that lead to midline neurologic defects. Twins and their close relatives have been found to have an excess of nonright-handedness and fusion malformations.

Functional Components of the Face.—Predominantly hereditary factors are active in the very early stages of fetal development. Genetic information for facial growth appears to be primarily situated in the neuromuscular system and soft tissues. The structure of individual bones in the craniofacial complex is thought to be influenced by rather rigid hereditary forces. However, in general, little is known regarding the heritability and the mode of inheritance of muscular components. New and standardized methods of investigation are needed.

▶ The frequency of MZ twins is 3.5 to 4 per 1,000, and it is the same in all races and at all maternal ages. Dizygotic twinning rates vary from 3.5 to 18 per 1,000, increase with maternal age, and show large racial variations. Dizygotic twinning rates are genetically determined, whereas MZ rates are not. The inheritance of DZ twinning is confined to the female line; an increased twinning rate is found among relatives of mothers but not fathers.

To determine zygosity at birth, gender, placental morphometry, protein enzyme analyses, histocompatability tests, and dermatoglyphs can be used. Individual facial bones (not their spatial arrangements), dental arch width, and dental arch depth or length have strong genetic tendencies. The teeth have powerful genetic patterns, but such patterns are much less powerful in the occlusion, especially the anterior region. The genetic determination of the maxillary and mandibular teeth are independent of each other, with the mandibular teeth being influenced more genetically.

Mirror imaging should be considered in MZ twinning; the twins are mirror images of each other, not duplicates. Therefore, the left anomaly in one would be the right one in the other. One should consider the genetic information for facial growth not from skeletal or dental tissues, but from the neuromuscular system and the soft tissues. A functional matrix orientation is helpful here, but further research is certainly needed.

It is important to divide genetic patterns into those that are species specific, such as the congenital absence of second premolars in humans, and those that are familial tendencies, such as when a mother and daughter might have smaller-sized laterals. One still finds second premolar absence in one MZ twin but not in the other. It is the pattern of species specificity overriding familial tendency.—G.F. Currier, D.D.S., M.S.D., M.Ed.

The Development and Morphology of the Incisive Fissure and the Transverse Palatine Suture in the Human Fetal Palate

Njio BJ, Kjær I (Univ of Copenhagen)
J Craniofac Genet Dev Biol 13:24–34, 1993   105-94-4-2

Background.—Knowledge of normal development in the human palate is a prerequisite for understanding pathologic palatal development. However, no descriptions of the development of the incisive fissure and transverse palatine suture exist in the literature. The macroscopic and microscopic development of these oral features was examined.

Methods.—Ninety-six fetal specimens, with gestational ages of 9 to 24 weeks, were examined. Maxillary ossification in these samples ranged from MAX IV to MAX VII (Fig 4-1). To compare these values with general development parameters, general skeletal maturation and crown rump length were also recorded (Fig 4-2). Macroscopic analysis, using vertical and lateral radiographs, and histologic staining were performed on all specimens.

Results.—The incisive fissure was radiographically characterized by bony outgrowths of the nasopalatine duct along the anterior border during MAX V and bony outgrowths from the canine area along the posterior border during MAX VI. MAX VII was characterized by a pronounced midpalatal suture with parallel fissure borders in a lateroposterior position. Midsagittal cuts revealed a C-shaped anterior fissure opening. Histologic examination confirmed the above features. The central layer of the fissure was composed of loose connective tissue, whereas the bony surfaces consisted of alternating osteoblasts and osteoclasts. The transverse palatine suture was first observed during MAX V development. The suture was seen as a narrow radiolucent area between

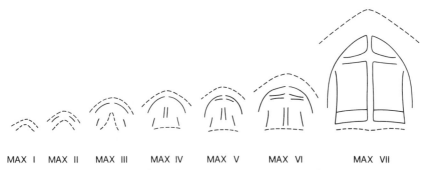

MAX I   MAX II   MAX III   MAX IV   MAX V   MAX VI   MAX VII

Fig 4–1.—Schematic drawing of maxillary stages, showing the location of osseous tissue in the developing human maxilla. The developmental sequence is divided in stages from MAX I to VII. The formation of the incisive fissure and the transverse palatine suture takes place during MAX V, VI, and VII. (Courtesy of Njio BJ, Kjær I: *J Craniofac Genet Dev Biol* 13:24–34, 1993.)

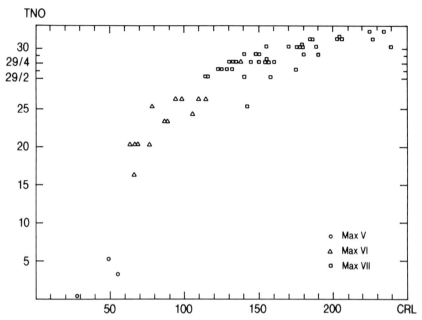

Fig 4–2.—Distribution of the material according to crown rump length (CRL), general skeletal maturation (TNO), and maxillary skeletal maturation (MAX). The data shown are from 57 fetuses. (Courtesy of Njio BJ, Kjær I: *J Craniofac Genet Dev Biol* 13:24–34, 1993.)

the cranial palatine contour and the caudal maxillary contour. Histologic examination revealed metachromatic connective tissue between bony edges.

Comparisons between the 2 structures revealed pronounced differences. When seen vertically, the incisive fissure had a curved posterolateral aspect, whereas the transverse palatine suture had a straight course perpendicular to the midsagittal suture. Sagittal sections revealed a C-shaped incisive fissure, whereas the palatine suture had a distinct oblique orientation.

Conclusion.—The incisive fissure and transverse palatine suture differ in several important aspects, which may reflect the different developmental roles. The lateral union of the incisive fissure precludes anteroposterior growth. However, the accumulation of osteoblasts and osteoclasts suggests that it may influence developing dentition and anterior maxillary bone. Conversely, the transverse palatine suture appears to be responsible for anteroposterior palatal development.

▶ This study of human fetal material is rare and includes analysis of radiographic, macroscopic, and microscopic features of the palate. There are numerous differences between the incisive fissure (premaxillary-maxillary junction) and the transverse palatine suture (palatomaxillary suture or the overlapping of the maxillary bone from the palatal bone).

The incisive fissure is not a real suture, because it does not completely separate the upper jaw at any stage during normal development; the premaxilla appears as a separate bone in primates but not in humans. The edges of this fissure laterally unite with no anteroposterior growth function and affect the anterior maxillary dentition. However, the palatomaxillary suture can affect sagittal growth of the palate.

The days of the premaxillary-maxillary suture are over. There are 2 maxillae with 2 anterior fissures that happen to have no effect on orthopedic therapy but are an orthodontic consideration in the cleft alveolus.—G.F. Currier, D.D.S., M.S.D., M.Ed.

Cranial Base

A Comparative and Correlational Study of the Cranial Base in North American Blacks
D'Aloisio D, Pangrazio-Kulbersh V (Univ of Detroit, Mich)
Am J Orthod Dentofacial Orthop 102:449–455, 1992   105-94-4-3

Purpose.—Although the cephalometric differences between blacks and whites have been well studied, the anterior cranial base length, angulation, and flexure of the American black adult have never been characterized. The cranial bases of blacks and whites were compared, and the portion of the variation in the black craniofacial skeleton that can be explained by the variation in cranial base length was determined.

Methods.—The lateral cephalograms of 42 black men with an average age of 25.6 years and 58 black women with an average age of 31.5 years were traced, analyzed, and compared with values of white subjects obtained from the *Atlas of Growth in the Aging Craniofacial Skeleton.* All patients were native-born North American blacks undergoing orthodontic treatment. Descriptive statistics were calculated from the observed values for each measurement.

Results.—A comparison of black and white cranial base measurements revealed that the cranial base in blacks is significantly shorter than it is in whites (Tables 1 and 2). There was a strong biological relationship between the cranial base length in blacks and their denture bases. Correlations of the vertical measurements demonstrated a high degree of variability between men and women.

Conclusion.—Cephalometric differences between blacks and whites are not simply anatomical for parameters that use the sella nasion as their reference plane. Therefore, the cranial base length in blacks should not be manipulated to match it to standards for whites.

▶ The Frankfort horizontal plane is essentially the same in whites and blacks. This is not true for the cranial base. The adult cranial base is about 2–3 mm shorter in females compared with males and in blacks compared with whites. However, the standard deviations in the samples are about the same value or larger. The angulation of sella nasion to Frankfort horizontal is about 2 de-

TABLE 1.—Craniofacial Skeletal and Dental Measurements in North American Black Adults

Measurements	$\overline{X}$	SD	x	SD	t	p
Cranial base						
Length (SN)	73.7	3.8	71.0	3.2	3.73	***
Angulation (SN-FH)	9.1	3.4	9.6	4.2	0.72	ns
Flexure (N-S-BA)	131.6	5.8	132.5	6.3	0.72	ns
Maxillary position						
SNA	84.3	4.1	86.4	5.4	−2.18	*
Maxillary length (CO-A pt)	98.7	5.6	95.4	5.7	2.81	**
Mandibular position						
SNB	80.0	4.7	80.5	5.0	−0.49	ns
Mandibular length (CO-Gn)	130.9	7.3	122.9	7.0	5.46	***
AP relationship						
ANB	4.2	3.0	5.9	3.2	−2.53	*
Witts	0.4	5.9	1.5	4.8	−1.0	ns
Max-mand differential	32.2	6.0	27.4	5.3	4.13	***
Vertical relation						
SN-Go-Gn	38.2	5.8	36.6	7.0	1.28	ns
FMA	29.0	5.8	27.2	6.7	1.42	ns
ANS-ME	80.3	6.2	75.6	6.7	3.66	***
I position						
I to NA (angle)	24.2	8.0	25.1	8.6	−0.59	ns
I to NA (distance)	7.0	3.6	6.9	3.3	0.16	ns
I to A pt	8.5	4.3	9.3	3.6	−0.95	ns
I to ANS-PNS	116.1	8.7	117.5	8.9	−0.79	ns
Ī position						
Ī to NB (angle)	31.8	6.2	37.4	8.5	−3.75	***
Ī to NB (distance)	10.2	3.7	11.1	4.5	−1.07	ns
Ī to A-Po	7.1	3.4	7.6	4.0	−0.61	ns
IMPA	93.1	6.9	99.9	8.7	−4.26	***
Palatal plane						
ANS-PNS to SN	7.3	3.7	6.1	4.1	1.48	ns
ANS-PNS to FH	1.4	4.0	3.8	3.9	−3.09	***
Occlusal plane						
Downs-SN	14.2	5.6	14.7	4.1	−0.47	ns
Downs-FH	5.4	4.9	5.2	3.2	0.26	ns

Note: *P < .05; **P < .01; ***P < .001.
(Courtesy of D'Aloisio D, Pangrazio-Kulbersh V: Am J Orthod Dentofacial Orthop 102:449-455, 1992.)

grees to 3 degrees more in blacks than in whites, and cranial base flexure (N-S-Ba) is 2.5–3.5 degrees larger in blacks than in whites. Females have a mildly greater cranial base angle. However, the standard deviations are larger than these differences. The average cranial base in blacks is shorter, steeper, and flatter than that in whites. The length of anterior cranial base showed a

TABLE 2.—Cranial Base Comparison Between White and
Black Adult Subjects

Group	X	SD	t	p
SN length				
White male	75.7	3.3	3.23	***
White female	73.4	2.6		
Black male	73.7	3.8	3.73	***
Black female	71.0	3.2		
White male	75.7	3.3	2.84	***
Black male	73.7	3.8		
White female	73.4	2.6	3.71	***
Black female	71.0	3.2		
Angulation (SN FH)				
White male	6.1	3.2	1.99	*
White female	7.8	3.9		
Black male	9.1	3.4	0.72	NS
Black female	9.6	4.2		
White male	6.1	3.2	4.46	***
Black male	9.1	3.4		
White female	7.8	3.9	1.93	NS
Black female	9.6	4.2		
Flexure (S-N-Ba)				
White male	127.9	5.3	1.55	NS
White female	129.8	5.3		
Black male	131.6	5.8	0.72	NS
Black female	132.5	6.3		
White male	127.9	5.3	3.3	***
Black male	131.6	5.8		
White female	129.8	5.3	2.04	*
Black female	132.5	6.3		

Note: *$P < .05$; ***$P < .001$.
(Courtesy of D'Aloisio D, Pangrazio-Kulbersh V: *Am J Orthod Dentofacial Orthop* 102:449–455, 1992.)

strong correlation with the length of the maxilla and mandible in both males and females. This was not true for the cranial base angulation and the maxillary and mandibular lengths. The vertical plane did not correlate well between males and females, nor did the high variability of incisor position with the cranial base.

One should analyze cases considering variations in age, race, and gender. To group everyone into a singular orientation, such as an adult, and then to use mean data only, is not an acceptable standard of contemporary care in America.—G.F. Currier, D.D.S., M.S.D., M.Ed.

General

Normalization of Incisor Position After Adenoidectomy

Linder-Aronson S, Woodside DG, Hellsing E, Emerson W (Karolinska Institutet, Huddinge, Sweden; Univ of Toronto; Univ of Loma Linda, Calif)
Am J Orthod Dentofacial Orthop 103:412–427, 1993   105-94-4-4

Introduction.—Some developmental crowding relates to changes in the neuromuscular environment rather than to discrepancies in tooth-jaw size or interarch tooth-size ratio. Whether alteration in the neuromuscular environment could improve incisor position in children who had undergone adenoidectomy was determined.

Methods.—The subjects were 38 children who had converted from mouth to nose breathing after adenoidectomy was performed to relieve severe nasal obstruction. An additional 37 children, all of whom had a clear airway and no history of nasal obstruction, served as controls. The groups were matched for age and sex. Incisor inclination and position in both jaws were examined at baseline and 5 years later, when the children were approximately 12 to 14 years of age. Variables examined included gender, change in the sagittal size of the nasopharyngeal airway, change in airflow, and change in mandibular growth direction.

Results.—The sagittal size of the nasopharyngeal airway increased significantly in the adenoidectomy group vs. controls, allowing these children to reach normal values. The main change was a significantly increased labial inclination of the incisors in the adenoidectomy group. For both sexes, all variables that measure the labiolingual position of the mandibular incisors confirmed a significant labial incisor positioning. Two regressors, female sex and increase in the sagittal size of the nasopharynx, were found in stepwise regression analysis to account for 41% to 44% of the incisor proclination after adenoidectomy. Arch width and length increased significantly in male adenoidectomy patients; female adenoidectomy patients experienced a significantly greater horizontal mandibular growth than female controls.

Conclusion.—Adenoidectomy and a change from mouth to nose breathing are associated with a significant labial positioning of the incisor teeth. However, because responses are variable, adenoidectomy cannot be routinely recommended as a prophylactic orthodontic procedure.

▶ This longitudinal study was from middle childhood (7½ years in boys and 8½ years in girls) to adolescence (12½ years in boys and 13½ years in girls). Environmental factors have a profound effect on the anterior occlusion, as demonstrated in this study, in which the effect was related to airway (Scammon's general curve of growth or the sigmoid or S curve) compared with arch perimeter-tooth mass discrepancies.

The increase in the size of the nasopharyngeal airway was chiefly responsible for labial positioning, and this was more pronounced in girls. Individual variability, however, is so large that adenoidectomy cannot be recommended as a prophylactic orthodontic procedure. In orthodontics, labial positioning of anterior teeth usually is not a major goal for most children seeking orthodontic therapy, except those with anterior crossbite.—G.F. Currier, D.D.S., M.S.D., M.Ed.

Maxillary Incisor Crown-Root Relationships in Different Angle Malocclusions
Harris EF, Hassankiadeh S, Harris JT (State Univ of New York, Stony Brook)
Am J Orthod Dentofacial Orthop 103:48–53, 1993   105-94-4–5

Background.—The angulation of the roots of anterior teeth to their crowns is a subject of particular interest in orthodontics. The crown-root relationships of maxillary incisors for 3 major types of malocclusion were studied to determine whether crown-root angulation puts the root at risk of apical resorption during orthodontic treatment and to identify cephalometric predictors of angulation.

Methods.—The records of 79 patients who had completed orthodontic treatment for Angle's class I, II, and III malocclusion were retrospectively reviewed. Each cephalogram was examined under low magnification, and the long axes of the crown and the root of the more visible maxillary central incisor were traced. The collum angle was measured to the nearest .5 degree as the deflection of the long axis of the root from that of the crown. A 5-grade scale was used to assess the degree of external apical root resorption of the more visible maxillary central incisor.

Results.—Patients with class III malocclusions, particularly those with severe incisor underjet, had significantly increased collum angles. After full-banded orthodontic treatment, 99% of cases showed distinct apical root resorption. However, root resorption was not significantly associated with the crown-root angle either before or after orthodontic treatment. Cephalometric predictors of the amount of deflection of the crown-to-root axis were localized to intertooth relationships. It is proposed that the crown is torqued lingually during eruption, especially when constrained within the mandibular arcade. In contrast, the formative root is not affected by the altered eruptive path of the crown and will mineralize in its normal orientation.

Conclusion.—Deflected crown-root angles may limit the degree to which incisors can be torqued without damaging the root and the cortical plate.

▶ Almost all the cases presented had some apical root resorption. One should expect this with corrective orthodontic therapy. The average pretreatment collum angle was 6 degrees (± 7 degrees) in class I and class II division 1 cases and 12 degrees (± 6 degrees) in class III cases.

Overjet was the single best predictor of upper incisor collum angle (in this study, overjet as underjet) with moderate-to-severe class III malocclusions in which the maxillary incisors were trapped and constrained by the prognathic mandible.

This crown-root flexure, which shows remarkable lingual root angulation with normal crown positioning, is also seen in class II division 2 malocclusions for the permanent central incisors in the maxillary arch. That is why it is so difficult to get adequate torque on these teeth. This is also true for class III underbites. There are also problems in incisor intrusion or extrusion because of this increased angulation.—G.F. Currier, D.D.S., M.S.D., M.Ed.

Secondary Retention of Permanent Molars: A Report of Five Families
Raghoebar GM, Ten Kate LP, Hazenberg CAM, Boering G, Vissink A (Univ Hosp Groningen, The Netherlands; Univ of Groningen, The Netherlands)
J Dent 20:277–282, 1992   105-94-4-6

Introduction.—Because the reason for secondary retention, the incompletion of tooth eruption, remains unclear, family pedigrees have come under scrutiny to determine the etiology of this condition. The amount of secondary retention found in the first-degree relatives of 53 patients with this dental condition affecting the permanent molars was reported.

Methods.—During a 5-year period, 52 individuals (mean age, 18 years) who demonstrated secondary retention of the permanent molars participated in the study. The parents and siblings of the 52 patients underwent screening for secondary retention of the molars; complete dental information was obtained in 39 families.

Results.—Five families demonstrated secondary retention of the molars, including 3 mothers, 2 fathers, and 3 of 7 siblings. Transmission among the 5 families had occurred female to female, female to male, and male to female. The frequency of families with parental secondary retention was 13% among this study population. In family 1, the father and 1 daughter had 3 retained molars; the daughter also had an impacted maxillary canine (Fig 4–3). In family 2, the father and 2 children were affected. Family 3 included the affected mother and both members of an identical female twin pair (Fig 4–4). In family 4, the mother and son showed secondary retention (Fig 4–5). In family 5, the mother, a son, and a daughter retained molars. The lod scores for the HLA linkage with the secondary retention were related to the blood group system P, which increased at a recombination fraction of 5%.

Conclusion.—Secondary retention of the permanent molars occurs as a heterogeneous condition related to the inheritance of an abnormal autosomal dominant gene. Because of the genetic nature of this occurrence, the dentist should assess the relatives of all probands, especially very young patients who can avoid future pathology by early treatment.

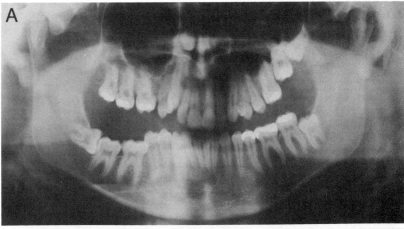

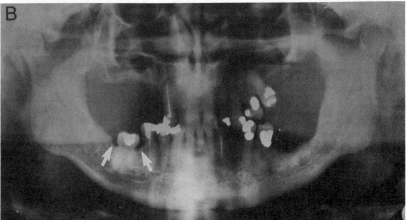

Fig 4–3.—A, dental panoramic tomograph of a girl, 15 years, with secondary retention of the maxillary left second molar. The mandibular first and second molars on the right side are also affected. Note the amalgam restoration in the maxillary left second molar, indicating that the molar had emerged into the oral cavity. **B,** dental panoramic tomograph of her father, 52, who had secondary retention of the right mandibular first molar. Note the decreased margin of the alveolar bone in the area of the affected first molar *(arrow).* (Courtesy of Raghoebar GM, Ten Kate LP, Hazenberg CAM, et al: *J Dent* 20:277–282, 1992.)

▶ One should consider familial patterns with all tooth anomalies, whether they are anomalies of number (congenital absence or supernumerary), size and shape (gemination or fusion, small or conical-shaped lateral incisors), structure and texture (amelogenesis imperfecta, dentinogenesis imperfecta, or cementogenesis imperfecta), or eruption and position (ectopic eruption, ankylosis, transposition, or impaction).

Ankylosis of the primary molar is almost 10 times more common than that of the permanent tooth. The lower molar is more commonly affected than is the upper molar, by 2 to 1. All ankylosed permanent molars become major

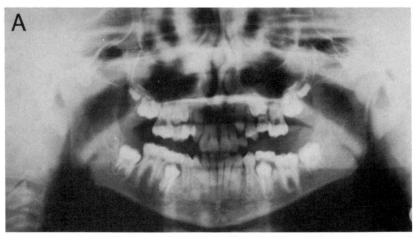

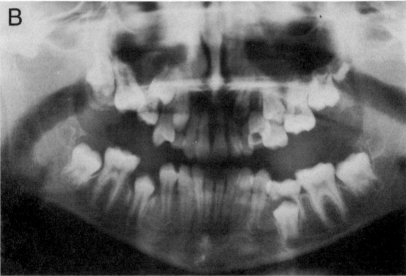

Fig 4–4.—A, dental panoramic tomograph of a girl, 11 years, with secondary retention of the maxillary second deciduous molar and mandibular first permanent molar on the left side. **B,** dental panoramic tomograph of her twin sister showing secondary retention of the mandibular left second deciduous molar, and the maxillary second deciduous molar and first permanent molar on the right side. (Courtesy of Raghoebar GM, Ten Kate LP, Hazenberg CAM, et al: *J Dent* 20:277–282, 1992.)

occlusal problems that need to be addressed or at least monitored early for accurate diagnosis. These teeth cannot be moved orthodontically, and their removal is needed in planned occlusal orientation. These can be autosomal problems that have a strong possibility of having familial tendencies.—G.F. Currier, D.D.S., M.S.D., M.Ed.

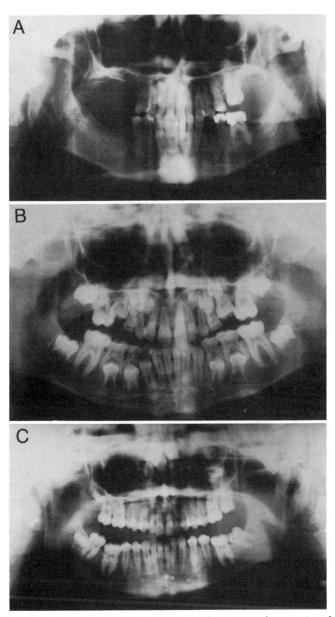

Fig 4–5.—A, dental panoramic tomograph of a mother, showing secondary retention of the maxillary left first molar. **B,** dental panoramic tomograph of her 10-year-old son, showing secondary retention of the maxillary second deciduous molars. **C,** dental panoramic tomograph of the son 4 years later, showing secondary retention of the mandibular first permanent molars. (Courtesy of Raghoebar GM, Ten Kate LP, Hazenberg CAM, et al: *J Dent* 20:277–282, 1992.)

5 Orthodontics

Evaluation

Current orthodontic evaluation of patients necessitates facial analysis in conjunction with occlusal descriptions. They do not correlate well. Considerations of various chin and nose positions alter acceptable compromises with the lips and, therefore, the teeth. Age, gender, and ethnicity must be considered for sound orthodontic treatment planning.

A reliable method of constructing the nasolabial angle in the analysis of the soft tissue profile has been established. However, this angle is independent of the underlying skeletal relationships.

Initial orthodontic evaluation of children during early transitional dentition can be done by the family dentist, with problems primarily related to sagittal occlusal problems (class II), posterior crossbite, and clinical anterior crowding.

Supernumerary succedaneous anterior teeth are almost always found in the maxilla, but they often do not have early clinical symptoms. Depending on the timing of removal of these teeth, either during the primary dentition or during the early transitional dentition, panoramic radiographic evaluation (or the equivalent) done between the ages of 5 and 8 years is recommended for all children and should be supplemented with any appropriate anterior films for determining accurate tooth positioning.

Missing maxillary permanent incisors are difficult cases to treat esthetically and functionally. If the patient is missing a maxillary permanent central incisor, the case is even more complex. Replacement of a maxillary lateral incisor for a maxillary central or the transplantation of a maxillary premolar that is rotated 90 degrees for a maxillary central presents major functional, esthetic, and periodontal problems.

As the population ages from childhood to adolescence to youth, there is an increased frequency of clinical symptoms, such as joint sounds, jaw fatigue, clenching, and headache, but there is no increased demand for treatment of these TMJ disorder problems. Those studies that attempt to correlate these symptoms with orthodontic care present problems for the long term because of these developmental changes. Fixed edgewise orthodontic appliances with class II elastics (a force vector from mandibular posterior to maxillary anterior in correction of class II malocclusions) in the short term do not have any adverse effect on TMJ disorder.

A major concern in orthodontic management of adolescents beyond the growth spurt with skeletal class II malocclusions is the ability to treat them either with orthodontic therapy alone or in conjunction with orthognathic surgery. Those helpful, differential parameters that suggest surgery include marked overjet (more than 10 mm), more severe mandibular retrognathia, and increased anterior vertical face height.

G. Fräns Currier, D.D.S., M.S.D., M.Ed..

Perceptions of a Balanced Facial Profile
Czarnecki ST, Nanda RS, Currier GF (Univ of Oklahoma, Oklahoma City)
Am J Orthod Dentofac Orthop 104:180–187, 1993   105-94-5-1

Introduction.—The position of the teeth in relation to the skeletal components has been the basic consideration among orthodontists attempting to achieve a balanced facial profile. Now that the importance of an overall facial balance is widely accepted, a constructed androgynous profile for establishing objective criteria for facial aesthetics was derived.

Methods.—After an ideal skeletal and soft tissue facial profile had been developed, various profiles were constructed to illustrate different shapes of the nose, lips, and chin (Fig 5-1). There were 6 series of profiles, each consisting of 7 profiles with changes in facial angle and angle of convexity (Fig 5-2). The profiles and a questionnaire were mailed to 1,300 members of the dental profession. They were asked to rank each series of profiles, in order of preference, from 1 (best) to 7 (worst). The facial silhouettes were designed to be androgynous, although 2 pages in the survey were described as male and 2 as female.

Results.—A total of 545 correctly completed surveys were returned for analysis. Preferred nose and chin configurations were close to or slightly larger than the constructed ideal. Gender differences, however, were noted in regard to lip position. Respondents preferred comparatively retruded lip contours for males (Fig 5-3). For both females (Fig 5-4) and males (Fig 5-5), the least favored chin contours were retrusive. A slightly more pronounced chin was favored for males as compared with females (Fig 5-6). Although more lip protrusion was acceptable in either sex when a large nose or a large chin was present, 3 times more lip protrusion was allowed with a large chin than with a large nose.

Conclusion.—Rigid adherence to standard average dental and skeletal parameters should be avoided when planning orthodontic treatment. Clinicians who treat malocclusions to the face can benefit from observing the favored variations in nose, lip, and chin relationships. It is also necessary to consider gender and ethnic variations and the changes in facial contour anticipated with growth.

Please subjectively rank order each row of seven
Young Adult White **Male** profiles.

Each profile should have a number (1 - 7) assigned. **No ties.**
Number **1** would be your favorite.
Number **7** would be your least favorite.

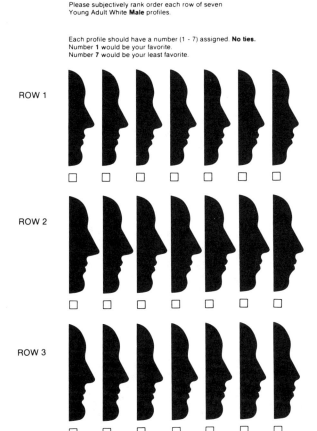

ROW 1

ROW 2

ROW 3

Fig 5–1.—Androgynous profile relative to lip changes **(row 1)**, lip changes plus 6 mm nose increase **(row 2)**, and lip changes plus 6-mm chin increase **(row 3)**, along with a static forehead contour and static facial vertical dimension. (Courtesy of Czarnecki ST, Nanda RS, Currier GF: *Am J Orthod Dentofac Orthop* 104:180–187, 1993.)

▶ When using lateral cephalometric radiography, it is essential that the soft tissue profile be visible, including the nose. Using only teeth and bones in the film, without evaluating the soft tissue thicknesses and profile or drape, leads to orthodontic treatment planes that will exclude balanced facial profiles with excellently treated occlusions.

Intraoral and extraoral standardized photographs should be used with the cephalometric film in evaluating the patient. Photographs without radiographic film of the profile do not allow adequate evaluation of the actual tooth-bone-soft tissue interaction because the skeletal patterns cannot be reliably assessed.

It is necessary to separate genders in any facial analysis. However, it is essential that one also consider age with the amount of growth left in addition

YOUNG ADULT WHITE MALE

Please subjectively rank order each row of seven
Young Adult White **Male** profiles.

Each profile should have a number (1 - 7) assigned. **No ties.**
Number **1** would be your favorite.
Number **7** would be your least favorite.

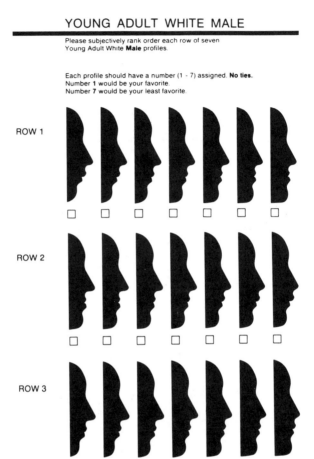

ROW 1

ROW 2

ROW 3

Fig 5–2.—Changes in facial angle and angle of convexity, separately and combined to produce different facial types. All profiles demonstrate static facial vertical dimension, static nose size, and forehead contour. (Courtesy of Czarnecki ST, Nanda RS, Currier GF: *Am J Orthod Dentofac Orthop* 104:180–187, 1993.)

to the racial or ethnic characteristics of various groups in our pluralistic society. For example, children have more convex profiles (sagittal), but they also have short face syndrome. The profile analysis in this study does not apply to African-Americans or Asians.

It is more acceptable for males to have more retrusive lips and females more protrusive lips. If the nose or chin is more prominent, more lip protrusion is acceptable, especially with a larger nose. Retrusive profiles are universally the least acceptable for both genders. A singular androgynous profile for any facial or ethnic group is not possible. One must factor in age and gender to the sample one is evaluating.—G.F. Currier, D.D.S., M.S.D., M.Ed.

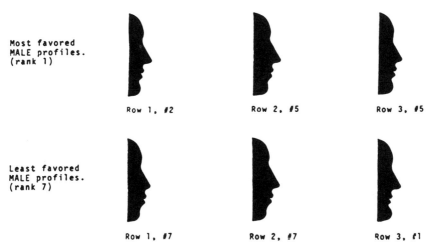

Fig 5–3.—Most favored and least favored male profiles regarding lip contour. (Courtesy of Czarnecki ST, Nanda RS, Currier GF: *Am J Orthod Dentofac Orthop* 104:180–187, 1993.)

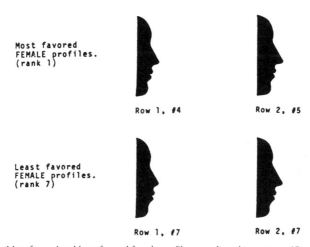

Fig 5–4.—Most favored and least favored female profiles regarding chin contour. (Courtesy of Czarnecki ST, Nanda RS, Currier GF: *Am J Orthod Dentofac Orthop* 104:180–187, 1993.)

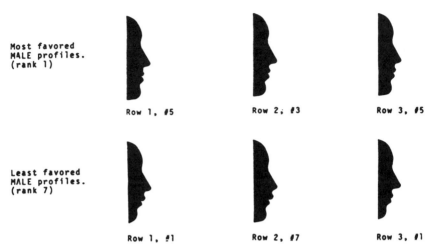

Most favored
MALE profiles.
(rank 1)

Row 1, #5   Row 2, #3   Row 3, #5

Least favored
MALE profiles.
(rank 7)

Row 1, #1   Row 2, #7   Row 3, #1

Fig 5–5.—Most favored and least favored male profiles regarding chin contour. (Courtesy of Czarnecki ST, Nanda RS, Currier GF: *Am J Orthod Dentofac Orthop* 104:180-187, 1993.)

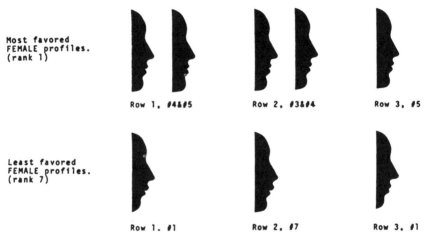

Most favored
FEMALE profiles.
(rank 1)

Row 1, #4&#5   Row 2, #3&#4   Row 3, #5

Least favored
FEMALE profiles.
(rank 7)

Row 1. #1   Row 2, #7   Row 3, #1

Fig 5–6.—Most favored and least favored female profiles, showing more pronounced chin than preferred in males. (Czarnecki ST, Nanda RS, Currier GF: *Am J Orthod Dentofac Orthop* 104:180-187, 1993.)

An Evaluation of the Nasolabial Angle and the Relative Inclinations of the Nose and Upper Lip

Fitzgerald JP, Nanda RS, Currier GF (Univ of Oklahoma, Oklahoma City)

Am J Orthod Dentofacial Orthop 102:328–334, 1992   105-94-5-2

Background.—The nasolabial angle, which is formed by a line from the lower border of the nose to a line representing the inclination of the upper lip, is a commonly used soft tissue parameter in orthodontic diagnosis. However, because of this region's structural variability, no uniform method of drawing the nasolabial angle currently exists. A study was undertaken to develop a standard, reproducible method for measuring the nasolabial angle and its components.

Methods.—The cephalometric radiographs of 104 adults aged 22–32 years were studied. All participants had class I occlusions with good facial balance. Radiographs were traced on matte acetate paper, and 9 reference points were located and entered into a computer digitizer system. With the exception of the nasolabial parameters, 6 skeletal angular measurements were recorded, including facial angle, angle of convexity, ANB angle, SGn/FH, SGn/Sn, and FMA. The new, reproducible method of drawing the nasolabial angle was then designed, using a 3-step approach. The posterior columella point (the most posterior point of the lower border of the nose) was first located, onto which a tangent was drawn to the lower border of the nose. From this point, a line was drawn to the labrale superius. This proved a reliable technique for constructing the nasolabial angle. The posteroinferior angle, created by the intersection of the Frankfort horizontal plane with the line drawn tangent to the lower border of the nose, provided a representative inclination of the nose. Finally, the anteroinferior angle, created by the intersection of the Frankfort horizontal plane with the line drawn from the posterior columella point tangent to labrale superius yielded a representative inclination of the upper lip.

Results.—The mean and standard deviations from the study sample of 104 adults were 18 degrees ± 7 degrees for the lower border of the nose to Frankfort horizontal plane angle; 98 degrees ± 5 degrees for the upper lip to Frankfort horizontal plane angle; and 114 degrees ± 10 degrees for the nasolabial angle. No statistically significant differences were noted between men and women. Individual measurements of soft tissue profile landmarks using 15 selected cephalometric radiographs were completed by 4 orthodontists and compared. The proposed method of nasolabial angle construction was consistent and reproducible by the same and by different orthodontists. No significant relationship between the soft tissue profile of the nasolabial region and the underlying skeletal relationships was noted.

Conclusion.—This new method provides both a reliable and reproducible means of constructing the nasolabial angle.

▶ The nasolabial angle is an important consideration in the placement of the incisors in the face. It can now be reliably drawn. The value of 114 degrees ± 10 degrees is for white adults with balanced faces. Children and those with sagittal or vertical skeletal variations, large or small noses, and different racial types will have values other than the ones found here.

This angle could not be correlated to the underlying skeletal framework, i.e., posterior vertical face height (FMA), overall directional growth (Y-axis to FH or to SN), and anterior sagittovertical relations as seen in facial angle (NPog/FH), ANB, and angle of convexity (NAPog). The soft tissues of the facial integument are independent of the thickness and size from the underlying facial skeleton.—G.F. Currier, D.D.S., M.S.D., M.Ed.

Early Screening for Orthodontic Treatment: Differences in Assessments Made by a Consultant Orthodontist and Three Public Health Dentists
Pietilä T, Pietilä I, Väätäjä P (Univ of Turku, Finland; Health Centre of Varkaus, Finland; Health Centre of Tampere, Finland)
Community Dent Oral Epidemiol 20:208–213, 1992   105-94-5-3

Introduction.—Dental health has improved among Finnish children and has promoted an increase in the early screening for orthodontic treatment. However, no common screening method or index has been developed for the country's health centers. The differences in functional and occlusal aspects of the young patients' teeth and their need for orthodontics were studied.

Methods.—Three hundred primary school children, aged 7 to 8 years, participated in the study; 39 either were excluded or dropped out over time. An orthodontist and 3 dentists examined the children for specific occlusal deviations, functional deviations, and craniomandibular disorders (Tables 1–3). After this examination, the child's need for, the timing of, and the complexity of treatment were evaluated (Table 4). The agreement and disagreement between the orthodontist and dentists represented the sensitivity, specificity, and predictive value for the examination.

Results.—The orthodontist believed that a class II malocclusion constituted the most frequent primary indication for treatment, followed by posterior crossbite and crowding. The dentists concurred with the class II malocclusion diagnosis, followed by crowding and posterior crossbite (Table 5). False positive findings, in which only the dentists believed treatment was needed, occurred in 16 children (6%). The orthodontist

TABLE 1.—Components of Occlusal Deviations

1. Frontal crossbite (at least one tooth in crossbite)
2. Lateral crossbite (at least one tooth in crossbite)
3. Lateral scissors-bite (at least one tooth in scissors-bite)
4. Open bite (overbite <0 mm, Björk et al. (32))
5. Deep bite (overbite >5 mm, Björk et al. (32) or mandibular incisors in contact with palate)
6. Crowding (missing space at least half the breadth of lateral incisor)
7. Missing permanent tooth (delayed eruption compared with the corresponding contralateral tooth, negative finding at palpation or in roentgenogram)
8. Supernumerary tooth (found clinically or in roentgenogram)
9. Trauma (history of trauma reported by child or scar in area around lips or chin)
10. Some other deviation

(Courtesy of Pietilä T , Pietilä I, Väätäjä P; *Community Dent Oral Epidemiol* 20:208-213, 1992.)

TABLE 2.—Components of Functional Deviations

1. Faulty position of lower lip
2. Mouth breathing (observed by examiner or reported by child)
3. Oral habits (chiefly thumb sucking)
4. Speech disorders (observed by examiner or history of speech therapy reported by child)

(Courtesy of Pietilä T, Pietilä I, Väätäjä P: *Community Dent Oral Epidemiol* 20:208-213, 1992.)

TABLE 3.—Signs and Symptoms of Craniomandibular Disorder

1. TMJ-sounds (observed without stethoscope or reported by child)
2. Deviations in maximal opening
3. Spontaneous pain in the TMJ area (reported by child)
4. Pain on palpation in the TMJ area
5. Maximal opening less than 37 mm, Ingervall (33)
6. Bruxism (observed by examiner or reported by child)

Abbreviation: TMJ, temporomandibular joint.
(Courtesy of Pietilä T, Pietilä I, Väätäjä P: *Community Dent Oral Epidemiol* 20:208-213, 1992.)

TABLE 4.—Evaluation Form for Determining Need, Timing, and Complexity of Treatment

1. Does the child need orthodontic treatment? (no, yes, don't know)
2. If in need of treatment, state reasons. (one to three reasons in order of importance)
3. Does the child need a more thorough examination by an orthodontist? (no, yes, don't know)
4. If the examination is needed, state reasons. (one to three reasons in order of importance)
5. If necessary, when should the treatment begin? (immediately, within a year, in 1-2 yr, later, don't know)
6. If necessary, who should carry out the treatment? (dentist independently, dentist with help of orthodontist, orthodontist, university clinic, don't know)

(Courtesy of Pietilä T, Pietilä I, Väätäjä P: *Community Dent Oral Epidemiol* 20:208-213, 1992.)

TABLE 5.—Distribution of Primary
Treatment Indications

| | Examiners | |
| | Dentists | Ortho-
dontist |
Indications	n	n
C II occlusion with some additional problem*	50	51
Lateral crossbite	20	20
Crowding	35	16
Frontal crossbite	3	5
Deep bite	7	4
Missing permanent tooth	4	2
Sign or symptom of CMD	–	2
Lateral scissors-bite	1	1
Open bite	7	1
Trauma	2	–
Other indications	8	9
	137	111

* Faulty lip position or overjet > 5 mm, etc.
Abbreviation: CMD, craniomandibular disease.
(Courtesy of Pietilä T, Pietilä I, Väätäjä P:
Community Dent Oral Epidemiol 20:208–213, 1992.)

would have started treatment later than the dentists would have in 44 children and earlier in 20 (Table 6). The orthodontist judged the treatment more complex in 36 youngsters and simpler in 16 cases than did the dentists (Table 7).

Conclusion.—It is more economical for dentists to screen young children for early orthodontic requirements than it is for orthodontists. The dentist should become familiar with the appropriate examinations for

TABLE 6.—Comparison of Dentists' and Orthodontists' Assessments of Treatment Timing

	Dentists				
Orthodontists	Immediately	Within a year	In 1–2 yr	Later	Total
Immediately	**48**	7	1	–	56
Within a year	22	**7**	8	1	38
In 1–2 years	13	8	**7**	3	31
Later	1	–	–	–	1
Total	84	22	16	4	126

Kappa statistic, .18; *t*-value, 3.14.
Note: Agreement shown in bold type.
(Courtesy of Pietilä T, Pietilä , Väätäjä P: *Community Dent Oral Epidemiol* 20:208–213, 1992.)

TABLE 7.—Comparison of Dentists' and Orthodontists' Assessments of
Treatment Complexity

Orthodontists	Dentists				
	Dentist alone	Dentist + orthod	Orthod	Univ. clinic	Total
Dentist alone	**1**	7	–	–	8
Dentist + orthod	–	**60**	9	–	69
Orthod	–	36	**18**	–	54
Univ. clinic	–	–	–	**1**	1
Total	1	103	27	1	132

Kappa statistic, .22; *t* value, 3.37.
Note: Agreement shown in bold type.
(Courtesy of Pietilä T, Pietilä I, Väätäjä P: *Community Dent Oral Epidemiol* 20:208–213, 1992.)

growing and developing children and practice the skills necessary for orthodontic diagnosis.

▶ The early transitional dentition, as seen at the beginning of middle childhood (8 to 10 years of age), is an important period of orthodontic evaluation. Crossbites, clinical anterior crowding, and class II malocclusions are the predominant problems that need to be addressed. The indications for treatment can be rather easily solved with cooperation of the general practitioner and the specialist. In assessing need, sensitivity (children who truly need treatment) ranged from .86 to .97; specificity (children who did not need treatment) ranged from .72 to .92. However, timing of intervention and the complexity of treatment were divergent between the groups. The general practitioners wanted earlier treatment but usually underestimated the complexity compared with the orthodontist.

This type of public health screening could be slightly improved at 8 to 9 years of age rather than 7 to 8 years. The permanent lateral incisors are erupting, and there is the beginning of the cognitive change away from egocentric to the more concrete operations stage. Some of the crowding problems could have been improved, and if treatment is needed, the child is usually a bit more cooperative during the second or third grade.—G.F. Currier, D.D.S., M.S.D., M.Ed.

Anterior Maxillary Supernumerary Teeth: A Clinical and Radiographic Study
von Arx T (Kantonsspital, Lucerne, Switzerland)
Aust Dent J 37:189–195, 1992   105-94-5–4

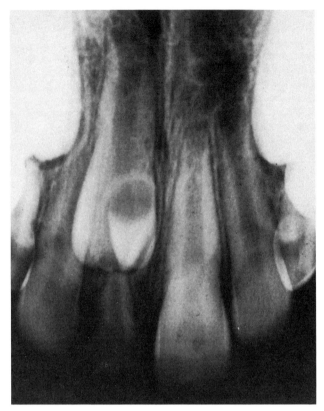

Fig 5–7.—Persistence of a deciduous central incisor and retention of the permanent central incisor caused by a mesiodens. (Courtesy of von Arx T: *Aust Dent J* 37:189-195, 1992.)

Background.—In patients with supernumerary teeth (mesiodentes), clinical symptoms are rare, although delayed eruption and alignment disturbances of the permanent maxillary incisors can occur (Fig 5-7). The number, direction, and location of supernumerary teeth and their effects on adjacent teeth can be determined via clinical and radiographic examination. The clinical and radiographic characteristics associated with anterior supernumerary teeth were determined in a large series of patients.

Patients.—The records and radiographs of 90 patients with a diagnosis of 113 anterior maxillary supernumerary teeth were evaluated. There were 65 male and 25 female patients, yielding a gender ratio of 2.6-1. Most of the study population ranged from age 6 to 10 years.

Results.—Seventy patients had 1 supernumerary tooth, 18 had 2 mesiodentes, and 2 had multiple occurrences with either 3 or 4 mesiodentes, respectively. Clinical symptoms were seen in only 2 cases. Complete and partial eruptions were rare, occurring in just 5 and 2 patients, respectively. The most frequently seen direction of the long axis of the mesio-

Position of Mesiodens

Position	No.*
Normal (non-inverted)	50 (44)
Inverted	42 (37)
Horizontal-transverse	12 (11)
Horizontal-sagittal	9 (8)
Total	113 (100)

* Percentage in parenthesis.
(Courtesy of von Arx T: *Aust Dent J* 37:189–195, 1992.)

dens was a normal, or noninverted position, occurring in 50 patients (table). Most of the 113 mesiodentes were located palatal to the dental arch (Fig 5–8). Three patients had dentigerous cyst formations, and 8 patients had complete ossification of the pericoronal space with resorption of the mesiodentes crown. In 39 and 24 cases, respectively, retention and malposition of the adjacent permanent incisors were seen.

Conclusion.—In this patient population, complete and partial eruptions were very uncommon. Therefore, the importance of radiographs in locating premaxillary supernumerary teeth is emphasized. All children should undergo radiographic screening at age 6 in order to detect supernumerary anterior teeth.

▶ The timing of obtaining anterior maxillary radiographs to assist in diagnosis of supernumerary teeth should be done according to one's approach to removal of these teeth. If one removes these succedaneous supernumeraries in the late primary dentition (5 years of age), radiographs should be taken then. If one removes them in the early transitional dentition (7 to 8 years of age), which is nearer the timing of the normal eruption of the maxillary permanent central incisors, the radiographs should be taken at that time.

For all children 5 to 8 years of age, a radiographic evaluation that includes the anterior segments, independent of any gross or obvious adverse findings,

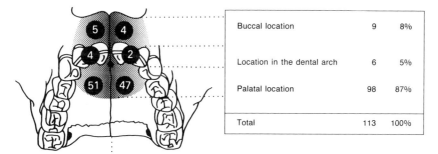

Buccal location	9	8%
Location in the dental arch	6	5%
Palatal location	98	87%
Total	113	100%

Fig 5–8.—Location of 113 supernumerary maxillary anterior teeth in relation to the dental arch. (Courtesy of von Arx T: *Aust Dent J* 37:189–195, 1992.)

is essential. Anterior supernumerary teeth are more common in boys than in girls (ratio, at least 2:1). Succedaneous supernumerary teeth usually do not erupt and are overwhelmingly found on the palatal side; this is just the opposite for primary supernumerary teeth, which usually erupt into the arch without any problems. Supernumerary primary teeth are, however, much more rare than the succedaneous ones.

The classic signs of maxillary anterior supernumerary teeth in the child 6 to 8 years of age are asymmetric eruption or positioning of permanent incisors (or both) compared with the more normal, contralateral tooth.—G.F. Currier, D.D.S., M.S.D., M.Ed.

Orthodontic Closure and Transplantation in the Treatment of Missing Anterior Teeth: An Overview
Stenvik A, Zachrisson BU (Univ of Oslo, Norway)
Endodont Dent Traumatol 9:45–52, 1993   105-94-5-5

Introduction.—Young patients with missing incisors can be treated with orthodontic closure or autotransplantation of teeth. Because these alternative methods have different indications, the choice should be

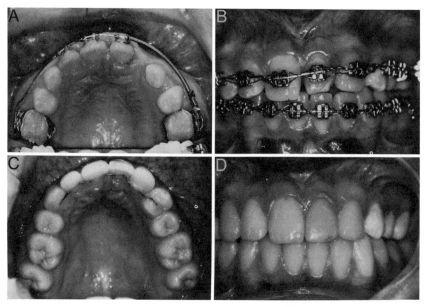

Fig 5–9.—Early loss of maxillary left central incisor. The left lateral is moved toward the midline, and the deciduous canine is extracted to allow for mesial eruption of the permanent canine (**A**). A second period of orthodontic treatment follows premolar eruption when posterior teeth are brought forward and tooth positions are adjusted (**B**). A bonded lingual retainer holds the six anterior teeth together (**C**). The final result (**D**) shows good midline coordination and esthetics. (Courtesy of Stenvik A, Zachrisson BU: *Endodont Dent Traumatol* 9:45–52, 1993.)

Principles for Treatment in the Early Mixed Dentition When Upper Central
Incisor Is Missing

1. Move lateral to midline immediately upon loss of central
2. Extract upper second deciduous molars early to guide first permanent molars mesially
3. Deciduous canine is extracted depending upon the eruption path of the permanent canine
4. Final treatment period in the early permanent dentition

(Courtesy of Stenvik A, Zachrisson BU: *Endodont Dent Traumatol* 9:45–52, 1993.)

---

based on a comprehensive, individualized evaluation. The issues involved
in developing a treatment plan for missing anterior teeth were discussed.

Orthodontic Closure.—Some things to consider in the decision to
proceed with orthodontic closure are the number of teeth lost, occlusal
status, facial morphology and growth pattern, the size and shape of the
other teeth, and the need for orthodontic treatment. Typical indications
for orthodontic closure when an upper incisor is missing include overjet;
proclined incisors; crowding; large laterals; and small, white canines. The
patient should be young and have the need and desire for orthodontic
treatment, and the other teeth should be healthy. Treatment in the early
transitional dentition (Fig 5–9) may be necessary when teeth are lost at a
very young age (table).

Autotransplantation.—The factors to consider in the choice of anterior transplants are recipient area, space conditions, morphology and
size of the donor tooth, positioning of the transplant, anterior occlusion,
and transformation of the grafted tooth to incisor morphology. First priority should be given to the graft with the best prognosis (Fig 5–10). Although upper premolars are normally too narrow to make good central
incisors, they may be compatible if incisors are narrow (Fig 5–11).

Conclusion.—Treatment planning for young patients with missing incisors should involve identification of alternative procedures, prediction
of the relative odds for success with each option, and evaluation of the
relative cost/risk/benefit ratios. Both biological factors and cultural considerations will affect the treatment plan. Combined orthodontics and
transplantation may be indicated in some patients.

► Congenital absence or small-sized, conical-shaped maxillary permanent
lateral incisors present esthetic and periodontal problems. The mandibular
permanent central incisor is the one that is commonly absent congenitally;
the lower midline suture fuses at 1 year after birth. However, the maxillary
permanent central incisor is rarely absent, except as a result of trauma. Its
loss presents major problems. Early loss prevents normal vertical alveolar

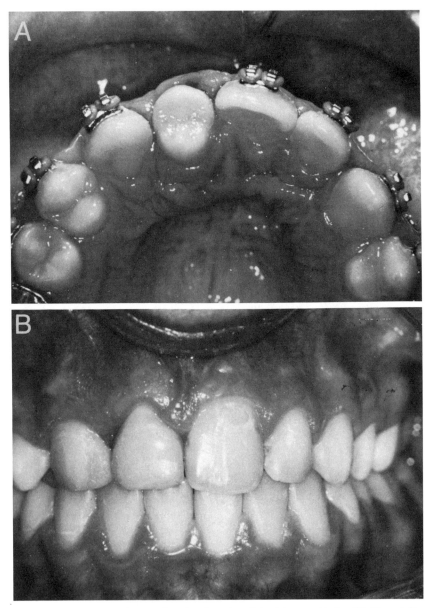

Fig 5–10.—Lower premolar transplanted to the region of the right central incisor **(A).** After grinding and composite buildup **(B),** the esthetic result is not optimal, primarily because of the reduced mesiodistal width along the gingival margin. (Courtesy of Stenvik A, Zachrisson BU: *Endodont Dent Traumatol* 9:45-52, 1993.)

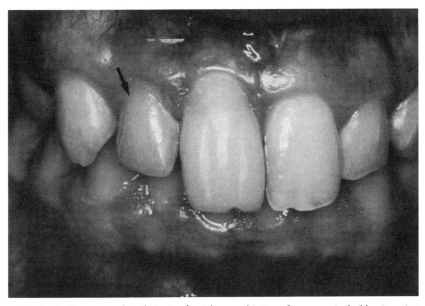

Fig 5–11.—Upper premolar substituting for right central incisor after composite buildup in patient with narrow incisors. The graft is in supraposition (*arrow*) because the deep bite otherwise would have conflicted with the palatal cusp. (Courtesy of Stenvik A, Zachrisson BU: *Endodont Dent Traumatol* 9:45-52, 1993.)

bone growth with subsequent bony defect; therefore, these teeth need to be replanted even if the 5-year prognosis is not very bright.

Two unique treatment plans are presented in this study: asymmetric extraction to compensate for the lost maxillary permanent central incisor with removal of the first premolar or the lateral incisor on the other side, depending on the molar relationship, or transplantation of the first premolar for the central incisor with a 6- to 9-month postponement of any orthodontic movement on that tooth.

The authors state that several undesirable factors occur and reduce an optimal aesthetic result:

1. Midline Deviation
2. Spacing reopening
3. Improperaxial inclinations
4. Unaesthetic crowns
5. Crown height discrepancies
6. Inadequate canine grinding
7. Premolar rotation

When the time comes for treatment planning, details and problems should be emphasized for the various alternatives. It is important that the patient and parents acquire a realistic expectation of the treatment outcome.—G.F. Currier, D.D.S., M.S.D., M.Ed.

Changes in Subjective Symptoms of Craniomandibular Disorders in Children and Adolescents During a 10-Year Period

Magnusson T, Carlsson GE, Egermark I (Inst for Postgraduate Dental Education, Jönköping, Sweden; Univ of Göteborg, Sweden)
J Orofac Pain 7:76–82, 1993   105-94-5-6

Objective.—Signs and symptoms of craniomandibular disorder (CMD) are prevalent, but there is no consensus about the role of various etiologic factors or on their long-term development. Children and adolescents first evaluated at age 7 to 15 years were followed up and studied again 10 years later. Ninety-five subjects aged 17 years were available for final follow-up, as were 95 aged 21 years and 103 aged 25 years.

Findings.—Temporomandibular joint sounds became significantly more frequent in all age groups (table, Fig 5–12). Reported jaw fatigue also increased during the 10-year interval. Only those aged 21 years reported more frequent problems in mouth opening. Awareness of tooth clenching while awake had become more frequent in all age groups and nocturnal bruxing increased in the 2 older groups. More than one fourth of the persons in each age group reported having headaches at least once a month at final follow-up (Fig 5–13). Most symptoms were reported significantly more often by women than by men. Seven men and 12 women, 6.5% of the entire series, had sought treatment for symptoms of CMD. Two thirds of them reported having improved. Occlusal splint therapy was the most frequent management.

Conclusion.—Symptoms of CMD are fairly prevalent in the general population, and they tend to become more frequent in young adult life. A high prevalence of occasional symptoms, however, does not translate into a high need or demand for treatment.

▶ This 10-year longitudinal study of the signs and symptoms of CMD or TMJ in 3 different age groups (7–17 years, 11–21 years, and 15–25 years of age) presents information that shows the adverse environmental or maturational influences from childhood through youth.

At the 10-year follow-up, reports of TMJ sounds, jaw fatigue, difficulty in mouth opening, or any combination of these symptoms had increased in all 3 age groups. Awareness of tooth clenching during the waking hours also increased in all 3 age groups, whereas nocturnal bruxism increased only in the 2 older groups. Reports of TMJ sounds, intermittent locking of the jaw, jaw fatigue, difficulties in jaw opening, and headaches were significantly more common in women than in men. The correlations found between the different symptoms that were registered clearly illustrate that patients who exhibit one symptom of dysfunction are likely to have other symptoms. This emphasizes that patients with CMD are often polysymptomatic.

The use of subjective reports on CMD symptoms in estimating treatment need has been seriously questioned because the sensitivity of the method, i.e., the probability of correctly identifying a disease, is poor. The demand for

Frequency (in %) of Reported Symptoms and Orofacial Parafunctions in Patients Surveyed at Ages 7, 11, and 15 Years and Again 10 Years Later

	7 y	17 y	11 y	21 y	15 y	25 y
1. TMJ sounds						
Frequent	0	7	0	8	2	12
Occasional	6	26	12	27	21	22
2. Jaw fatigue						
Frequent	0	1	0	4	0	2
Occasional	5	14	6	14	5	14
3. Difficulties in mouth opening						
Frequent	0	2	0	3	0	3
Occasional	8	4	6	13	6	6
4. Pain or fatigue in the jaws or face during chewing, for example of chewing gum						
Frequent	3	13	8	12	11	11
Occasional	33	46	61	53	54	56
5. One or more of the symptoms 1–3						
Frequent	0	9	0	11	2	12
Occasional	17	33	20	33	23	34
6. One or more of the symptoms 1–4						
Frequent	3	19	8	17	13	19
Occasional	40	49	63	57	57	58
7. Tooth clenching						
Frequent	3	7	1	10	1	13
Occasional	9	27	10	38	10	32
8. Bruxing						
Frequent	4	6	1	12	1	12
Occasional	15	18	13	16	14	26
9. 7 and/or 8						
Frequent	6	11	1	16	1	15
Occasional	18	29	18	34	16	39
10. Nail, lip, cheek, tongue biting or biting on foreign objects						
Frequent	4	22	27	17	30	16
Occasional	36	47	45	37	48	35
11. 9 and/or 10						
Frequent	19	32	27	28	31	27
Occasional	39	46	48	44	51	49

(Courtesy of Magnusson T, Carlsson GE, Egermark I: *J Orofac Pain* 7:76–82, 1993.)

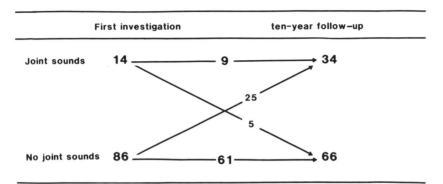

Fig 5–12.—Changes in joint sounds (in %) in 276 children and adolescents during 10-year period. (Courtesy of Magnusson T, Carlsson GE, Egermark I: *J Orofac Pain* 7:76–82, 1993.)

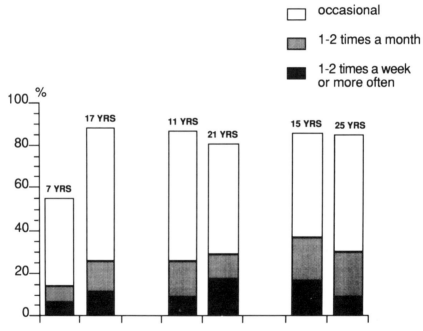

Fig 5–13.—Prevalence (in %) of headache in 293 subjects in 3 different age groups (7, 11, and 15 years) followed for 10 years. (Courtesy of Magnusson T, Carlsson GE, Egermark I: *J Orofac Pain* 7:76–82, 1993.)

CMD treatment in children and youth is low. High prevalences of occasional CMD symptoms do not equal either need or demand for treatment.—G.F. Currier, D.D.S., M.S.D., M.Ed.

Class II Elastics and Extractions and Temporomandibular Disorders: A Longitudinal Prospective Study
O'Reilly MT, Rinchuse DJ, Close J (Univ of Pittsburgh, Pa)
Am J Orthod Dentofacial Orthop 103:459–463, 1993   105-94-5-7

Objective.—There is some anecdotal evidence to suggest that orthodontic treatment with premolar extractions and class II elastics causes TMJ disorders. A study was undertaken to determine whether patients treated with class II elastics and extractions have a greater incidence of signs and symptoms of TMJ disorder than do nonorthodontically treated controls.

Patients.—Sixty patients with a mean age of 15.3 years at the start of treatment and 60 age-matched untreated controls were enrolled in the study. All patients underwent straight wire mechanotherapy, including extractions and class II elastics. Muscle tenderness was assessed by palpation of selected sites (Fig 5–14). Joint sounds were assessed by auscultation, palpation, and patient self-report. Range of mandibular movement was measured during active opening, maximum protrusion, and lateral movements. Patients were examined at baseline, twice during orthodontic treatment, and 2 months after treatment.

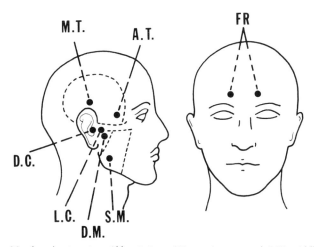

Fig 5–14.—Muscle palpation sites: *Abbreviations: AT*, anterior temporal; *MT*, middle temporal; *SM*, superficial masseter; *DM*, deep masseter; *LC*, lateral to capsule; *DC*, dorsal to capsule; *FR*, frontal. (Courtesy of O'Reilly MT, Rinchuse DJ, Close J: *Am J Orthod Dentofacial Orthop* 103:459–463, 1993.)

Results of Pain Measurement at Muscle Palpation Sites

Sites	Time 1 Pretreatment		Time 2 (8-10 months)		Time 3 (12-16 months)		Time 4 (2 months after treatment)	
	E	U	E	U	E	U	E	U
AT	1.0	1.0	1.11 ± 0.06	1.03 ± 0.02	1.06 ± 0.03	1.06 ± 0.03	1.06 ± 0.04	1.11 ± 0.04
MT	1.0	1.0	1.21 ± 0.06	1.13 ± 0.04	1.25 ± 0.05	1.21 ± 0.05	1.23 ± 0.06	1.30 ± 0.06
SM	1.0	1.0	1.26 ± 0.05	1.35 ± 0.06	1.26 ± 0.05	1.38 ± 0.06	1.38 ± 0.08	1.20 ± 0.05
DM	1.0	1.0	1.28 ± 0.05	1.20 ± 0.05	1.31 ± 0.06	1.23 ± 0.05	1.41 ± 0.08	1.21 ± 0.05
LC*	1.0	1.0	1.40 ± 0.05	1.01 ± 0.01	1.35 ± 0.06	1.06 ± 0.03	1.28 ± 0.07	1.10 ± 0.03
DC	1.0	1.0	1.11 ± 0.05	1.01 ± 0.01	1.18 ± 0.05	1.03 ± 0.02	1.18 ± 0.05	1.10 ± 0.03
FR	1.0	1.0	1.0 ± 0.06	1.01 ± 0.01	1.01 ± 0.01	1.05 ± 0.02	1.11 ± 0.04	1.08 ± 0.03

Abbreviations: E, experimental group; U, untreated group. For site abbreviations, see **Figure 5-14.**
Note: Pain scale: 1, no pain; 2, mild; 3, moderate; 4, severe.
* $P < .005$.
(Courtesy of O'Reilly MT, Rinchuse DJ, Close J: Am J Orthod Dentofacial Orthop 103:459-463, 1993.)

Results.—The only significant finding was that 40% of the patients who were pain-free at baseline reported mild pain on palpation lateral to the TMJ capsule when examined after 8–10 months of treatment. The remaining 60% of patients were pain free (table).

Conclusion.—Extractions and class II elastics have little or no effect on TMJ signs and symptoms.

▶ Class II elastics and extractions were considered together a single variable in this study of adolescents. The only significant finding was mild pain on palpation lateral to the TMJ capsule at the 8- to 10-month period during orthodontic treatment in 40% of the treated patients. This change could have been caused by space closure mechanics in the extraction patients, altered awareness, or referred pain from the intraoral mechanics. Pretorqued, preangulated edgewise appliances involving extractions and class II elastics have little or no effect on TMJ signs and symptoms.—G.F. Currier, D.D.S., M.S.D., M.Ed.

Surgical Versus Orthodontic Correction of Skeletal Class II Malocclusion in Adolescents: Effects and Indications
Proffit WR, Phillips C, Tulloch JFC, Medland PH (Univ of North Carolina, Chapel Hill)
Int J Adult Orthod Orthognath Surg 7:209-220, 1992   105-94-5-8

Background.—Adolescents with a skeletal class II malocclusion who are beyond the growth spurt require either orthodontic repositioning of the teeth to correct the occlusion or orthognathic surgery to correct the maxillomandibular relationship. Because few guidelines are available to help select the optimal treatment, the treatment outcomes for class II malocclusion in a large group of adolescents were reviewed.

Patients.—The study population consisted of 40 class II patients with a mean age of 15.2 years at the start of treatment who had a successful outcome after orthognathic surgery, 40 patients with a mean age of 13.9 years who had been treated successfully with orthodontics alone, and 21 patients with a mean age of 12.7 years whose orthodontic treatment was considered a failure and who were offered further surgical treatment. Ten patients accepted and all had a successful outcome. Pretreatment and posttreatment lateral cephalometric radiographs were digitized and the changes in cephalometric landmarks were calculated.

Results.—Unsuccessfully treated orthodontic patients initially had greater overjet, a more severe mandibular deficiency, and greater anterior facial height than did successfully treated patients. Analysis of the data revealed that orthognathic surgery is likely to be required in class II patients beyond the growth spurt if the overjet is greater than 10 mm, especially if the distance from the pogonion (Pog) to the nasion perpendicular (NPerp) is 18 mm or greater, if the mandibular body length is less than 70 mm, or if the facial height is greater than 125 mm.

Conclusion.—The size of the overjet, distance from Pog to NPerp, mandibular body length, and facial height are important indicators in planning treatment for class II adolescents beyond the growth spurt.

▶ The unsuccessfully treated orthodontic patients differed from the successfully treated patients in 2 major ways. They had more severe class II problems initially and less dental change during treatment, especially less reaction of the maxillary permanent incisors.

Four indications for surgical management (sagittal split with or without maxillary impaction and with or without augmented genioplasty) for class II division 1 malocclusions are:

1. Overjet greater than 10 mm. Less sagittal growth and less maxillary incisor retraction were factors in orthodontic failures.

2. Pogonion to nasion perpendicular distance greater than 18 mm (or amount of chin behind the true vertical). The pretreatment mean for successfully treated cases was about 13 mm.

3. Gonion to pogonion distance less than 70 mm. The successfully treated orthodontic patients had significantly longer mandibles than did the unsuccessfully treated patients.

4. Facial height greater than 125 mm. Many of the unsuccessfully treated patients had a steep mandibular plane angle. Usually, orthodontic camouflage is not successful treatment for vertical maxillary excess.

A final factor that should be considered in choosing between orthodontic camouflage and surgery is the probability of growth, especially vertical growth, during treatment. In the successfully treated orthodontic patients, even though the treatment mechanics were extrusive, there was enough vertical growth to prevent backward rotation of the mandible during treatment. In the unsuccessfully treated group, the maxillomandibular relationship often worsened during treatment because of the mandible rotating downward and backward, i.e., vertical growth was less than dental extrusion.—G.F. Currier, D.D.S., M.S.D., M.Ed.

Treatment

INTRODUCTION

The use of an orthopedic protraction face mask for maxillary deficiencies should be considered in cases of true maxillary deficiency, evaluating both the sagittal and vertical planes. Surgically repaired patients with cleft lip, alveolus, and palate are excellent candidates because of the iatrogenic nature of the problem.

The limits of an edgewise appliance necessitates orientation in the third order (torque) for the incisor segment with either the moment of a couple or the moment of a force. The moment of a couple as seen in bypass wires, utility arches, or torquing arches alters the center of rotation by placement of the bend in the wire in the area between the molars and the incisors. The moment of a force is very effective in the base arch wire to gain facial crown/lingual root incisor rotation.

The prescriptions that are used for contemporary edgewise appliances still cannot replace poor or inconsistent bracket placement or the inherent differences between the centers of resistance and rotation. The problems of the freedom of the arch wire in the arch wire slot of the bracket must be addressed as well as the force diminution, or decay, that occurs. Stiffer, fuller wires can help here.

Even though fully banded/bonded edgewise appliances with either stainless steel arch wires or nickel-titanium arch wires corrode in a salivary environment, releasing nickel and chromium, the amount is significantly below the mean dietary intake.

There are 3 different types of external root resorption: surface (self-limiting, small outline areas), transient and progressive inflammatory (dentinal tubule involvement), and replacement (bone replacement that can lead to ankylosis). Most root resorption in orthodontics is seen at the apices of maxillary teeth as a surface phenomenon with a transitory inflammatory process. Pretreatment long cone, periapical radiographs, using the paralleling technique, are essential in prognostication. Familial tendencies, specific individual susceptibility with any presence before therapy, application of intrusive or heavier forces, and increased age should be precautionary signs for potential problems. Obvious root resorption can be seen in up to 10% of patients who have had no orthodontic treatment. These patterns are usually associated with compromised tooth support as seen with loss of adjacent tooth support, the presence of fewer teeth, and decreased bony anchorage for the roots.

G. Fräns Currier, D.D.S., M.S.D., M.Ed.

Orthopedic Protraction of the Upper Jaw in Cleft Lip and Palate Patients During the Deciduous and Mixed Dentition Periods in Comparison With Normal Growth and Development

Tindlund RS, Rygh P, Bøe OE (Univ of Bergen, Norway)
Cleft Palate Craniofac J 30:182–194, 1993   105-94-5–9

Introduction.—In some patients with cleft lip and palate (CLP), growth deficiencies of the middle face may develop. An analysis was made of the potential of an interceptive orthodontic treatment phase involving protraction in patients with CLP who experienced underdevelopment of the upper jaw after cleft repair.

Methods.—Researchers compared outcomes in patients with CLP who had undergone protraction treatment with the normal growth and development in noncleft children. All children treated for CLP at the study institution were examined at 4 and 6 years of age for growth disturbances. Protraction was started in 108 patients with anterior crossbite; 10 children did not complete the treatment. The study group consisted of 65 boys and 33 girls. Treatment was begun at a mean age of 6 years, 11

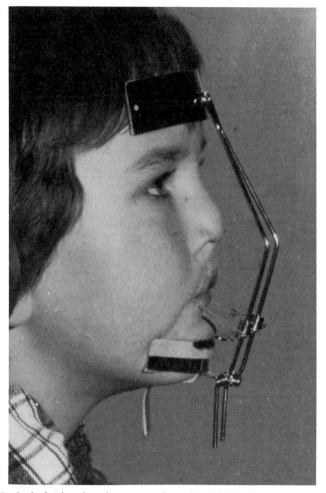

Fig 5–15.—In the facial mask used, protraction forward and slightly downward is provided by elastics from intraoral hooks in the canine region. (Courtesy of Tindlund RS, Rygh P, Bøe OE: *Cleft Palate Craniofac J* 30:182–194, 1993.)

months. A face mask, worn primarily at night, was used to accomplish protraction (Fig 5-15). Forty-one noncleft children matched by age and sex with the CLP subjects served as controls. Cephalograms were obtained for all subjects. The patients with CLP and controls differed considerably in facial morphology at baseline.

Results.—The goal of treatment was to achieve favorable occlusion with positive overjet and overbite (Figs 5-16 and 5-17). The mean duration of protraction to achieve positive overjet was 13 months. Facial appearance usually improved quite early in treatment (Fig 5-18), motivating the children to be cooperative in using the protraction device. The CLP

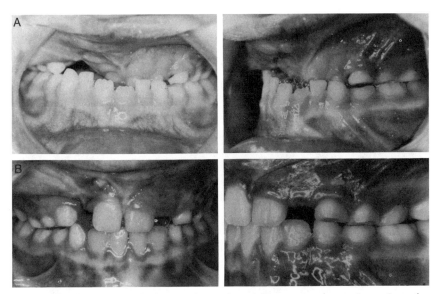

Fig 5–16.—Protraction treatment to correct anterior crossbite was started at age 5 years 3 months and lasted 11 months. The maxillary incisors erupted spontaneously to normal occlusion without active frontal tipping. **A left and right** show before and **B left and right** after protraction. (Courtesy of Tindlund RS, Rygh P, Bøe OE: *Cleft Palate Craniofac J* 30:182–194, 1993.)

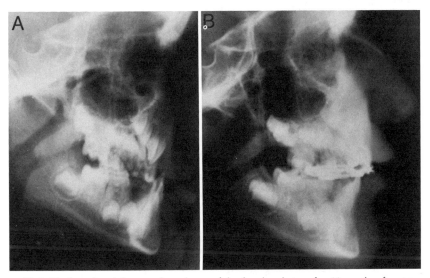

Fig 5–17.—Lateral cephalograms show change of the dental occlusion after 11 months of protraction in the same patient depicted in Figure 5–16. **A** was taken before and **B** after protraction. (Courtesy of Tindlund RS, Rygh P, Bøe OE: *Cleft Palate Craniofac J* 30:182–194, 1993.)

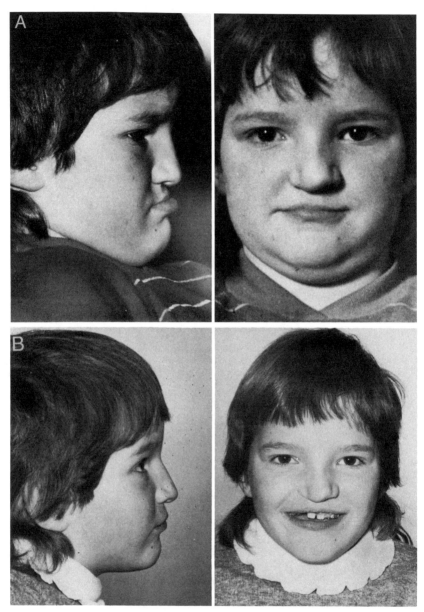

Fig 5–18.—Characteristic improvement of facial appearance by interceptive orthodontic treatment in the deciduous and early mixed dentition. The patient is the same one depicted in Figures 5-16 and 5-17. **A left and right** show patient before and **B left and right** show patient after 11 months of protraction. (Courtesy of Tindlund RS, Rygh P, Bøe OE: *Cleft Palate Craniofac J* 30:182–194, 1993.)

patients achieved normalization of the sagittal maxillomandibular relationship, with a more anterior position of the upper jaw and a more posterior position of the lower jaw. All cases were retained after protraction with a fixed palatal arch.

Conclusion.—Early orthopedic protraction of the upper jaw in patients with CLP normalizes maxillomandibular discrepancies and creates a better basis for conventional orthodontic treatment during the permanent dentition period. Similar treatment can be applied to noncleft patients with anterior crossbite caused by maxillary underdevelopment in the late primary/early transitional dentition.

▶ This longitudinal study with a follow-up of at least 5 years for nearly 100 patients with cleft palate/alveolus lip was started in the late primary or early transitional dentition and lasted for a mean of nearly 1 year with the orthopedic protraction (range, 3 months to 5 years). Except in some extreme cases, however, favorable occlusions were established within 3–24 months of treatment.

The initial appliance was either a 4-tooth banded quadhelix (if posterior crossbite) or a 4-tooth banded maxillary lingual arch. The primary second molars and the primary canines were banded. The face mask was applied to the canine with 350 g per side, or 700 g total, for half-time wear.

The cranial base seemed not to be affected by treatment. The SNA increased an average of 1 degree, with the posterior border of the maxilla moving anterior about .3 mm and the anterior border, 1.3 mm. The maxilla dropped vertically, and the mandible dropped vertically and posteriorly.

The data were not presented in a chart that provided pre-, interim, and postcomparisons; data were presented on cleft vs. normal groups. By doing this, it was rather difficult to compare changes within the cleft group or within the normal group. The use of the different labels for the references used in the United States made the information difficult to extrapolate. Greater standardization between Europe and North America is needed.

It seems unfortunate this iatrogenic dentofacial anomaly is still surgically labeled as cleft lip vs. cleft palate, whereas the cleft alveolus is a major void in orientation. It shows poor understanding of the problem and the solution. The surgical repair of these children is by far the most important factor for the growing child with restricted maxillary trans-sagittovertical problems of the dentofacial complex. However, because the sequelae for patients with cleft palate/alveolus is so marked, the surgical approach needs reevaluation. Orthodontic treatment of surgically created skeleto-dental problems should also be reevaluated. There is a need to reorient what can be loosely called the cleft team away from surgery.—G.F. Currier, D.D.S., M.S.D., M.Ed.

Moments With the Edgewise Appliance: Incisor Torque Control

Isaacson RJ, Lindauer SJ, Rubenstein LK (Virginia Commonwealth Univ, Richmond)
Am J Orthod Dentofacial Orthop 103:428–438, 1993   105-94-5-10

Background.—Because of limitations of bracket-to-bracket mechanics and the poorly defined reciprocal actions inherently produced, traditional edgewise orthodontic mechanics are significantly restricted in their ability to provide incisor torque control. To date, clinical investigations undertaken to examine this issue have been largely empirical. In

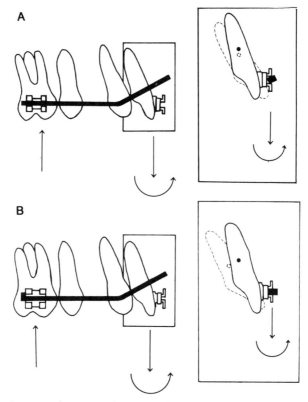

Fig 5–19.—A, actions of torquing arch not cinched. The larger incisor moment of the couple produces rotation with the center of the rotation coincident with the center of resistance. The equilibrium forces are extrusive at the incisor and intrusive at the molar, which tends to produce extrusion of the incisor center of resistance, as shown. Clinically, no overbite increase may be seen because of rotation of the incisal edge. *Solid lines* show pretreatment and *dotted lines* show post treatment. Centers of resistance for the incisors were arbitrarily positioned and carried forward. **B,** net actions of a cinched torquing arch. The incisor crown feels the greater moment of the couple but it is restrained from facial movement by the cinch. The incisor root is free to respond to the lingual force. Restraint of the incisor crown by the wire is transmitted to the molar crown as a mesial force, the "rowboat" effect. The vertical equilibrium forces are unchanged from uncinched situation. (Courtesy of Isaacson RJ, Lindauer SJ, Rubenstein LK: *Am J Orthod Dentofacial Orthop* 103:428–438, 1993.)

A

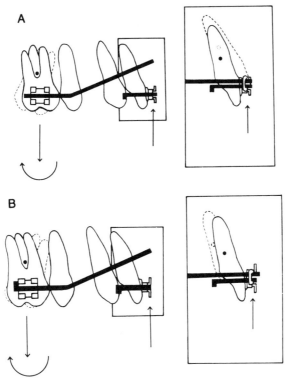

B

Fig 5–20.—**A,** actions of base arch not cinched and tied at incisor with no incisor couple. The moment of the molar couple is crown distal/root mesial rotation, and the center of rotation will be coincident with the center of resistance. The equilibrium forces are intrusive at the incisors and extrusive at the molars, and produce intrusion of the incisor center of resistance. When a rectangular wire is also inserted into the incisor bracket (as in a utility arch), depending on the moments created when the wire is inserted, the moments at the incisor bracket can be in the same or opposite direction with additive or subtracting equilibrium forces. **B,** net actions of cinched base arch. The molar crown feels the greater moment of the couple but is restrained from distal movement by the cinch. The molar root is free to respond to the mesial force. The restraint of the molar crown by the wire is transmitted to the incisor crown as a lingual force, the reverse "rowboat" effect. The vertical equilibrium forces are unchanged from the uncinched situation. (Courtesy of Isaacson RJ, Lindauer SJ, Rubenstein LK: *Am J Orthod Dentofacial Orthop* 103:428-438, 1993.)

this report, the fundamental mechanics used in developing incisor torque are described.

Discussion.—According to mechanical science, all incisor torque control mechanisms must act through 1 of 2 basic principles, including the moment of a couple or the moment of a force. The torquing arch, a modification of the conventional edgewise system, includes a large moment to rotate incisors in a crown facial/root lingual direction and simultaneous equilibrium forces to extrude incisors and intrude molars (Fig 5-19). The base arch also uses the moment of a force to rotate incisors in a crown facial/root lingual direction. However, it includes a large moment to rotate molars in a crown distal/root mesial direction, and simultaneous equilibrium forces to intrude incisors and extrude molars (Fig 5–20). Torquing arches and base arches can also rotate molars in a faciolingual direction, augment or curtail posterior anchorage, and increase or preserve arch perimeter.

Conclusion.—Clinicians involved in contemporary orthodontic care must have an awareness and effective control of the force systems created by orthodontic appliances.

▶ There are 3 orders of bends in orthodontics: first order in the horizontal (sagittal or transverse planes), second order in the vertical (vertical), and the third order as a torque or twist in the wire or bracket. With edgewise third-order mechanics, a rectangular wire engages a rectangular bracket to create a pair of equal and opposite parallel forces, which is called a couple. This couple has a tendency to rotate (rotating influence is a moment), and this tendency is measured as the magnitude of the force times the distance between the forces (measured in gram-millimeters).

A couple moves the center of rotation of the tooth, but not the center of resistance. A variation in edgewise mechanics is seen with Burstone's segmented arch, the utility arch, the intrusion or extrusion arch, or the bypass arch. Groups of teeth act as a single unit against another group. The incisor to molar areas are affected, not the premolar-canine segments. If forces are equal, a torquing arch activated for incisor facial crown torque or rotation (or lingual root torque) has equilibrium forces that have incisor extrusion and molar intrusion. With unequal moments, the brackets with the greater moment will act.

A moment of a force is always created if a force is applied to a tooth but not directed through the center of resistance. The moment of a force is measured as the magnitude of the force multiplied by the perpendicular distance between the line of the force vector and the center of the tooth. Most orthodontic forces create moments (rotations), because these forces are not able to act directly through the center of resistance. The tooth's center of rotation is somewhere between the centers of resistance and infinity, with the exact location determined by the moment-to-force ratio.

Although the torquing arch places the couples with the greatest moment at the incisor brackets, a base arch has its activation near the molar that produces a large couple and a greater moment at the molar tube. Compare Figures 5–19 and 5–20. Incisor faciolingual rotational forces are developed by the moments of a couple or a force. This difference makes possible incisor facial crown/lingual root forces with moment a couple (open bite reduction) or intrusive forces with moment of a force (deep bite opening).

The greater moment of the couple at the molar has concurrent intrusive forces on the incisors and extrusive forces on the molars in both cinched and uncinched systems. The arch perimeter changes are a function of cinching or not cinching. If the molar is uncinched, the arch perimeter will increase. Transpalatal bars to the molars help prevent the torquing arch effect of facial molar crown movement or the base arch effect of lingual molar crown rotation.—G.F. Currier, D.D.S., M.S.D., M.Ed.

Straight Wire: The Next Generation
Creekmore TD, Kunik RL (Houston)
Am J Orthod Dentofacial Orthop 104:8–20, 1993   105-94-5–11

Introduction.—The results of treatment using preadjusted appliances and straight wires are frequently not as expected (Table 1). This may result from inaccurate bracket placement, variations in tooth structure, variations in maxillary/mandibular relationships (Fig 5–21), tissue rebound, and mechanical deficiencies of edgewise orthodontic appliances (Table 2). When all these factors have been taken into account, the clinician can individualize prescriptions for preadjusted orthodontic appliances.

Discussion.—The clinician can use the cephalogram and visual treatment objective to determine the desired position of the maxillary and mandibular incisors, as related to the maxillary/mandibular relationships. An incisor torque template may be used to measure torque angle of the labial surface of maxillary and mandibular incisors in terms of the arch wire plane. These problems may be addressed by a system that varies the orientation of the bracket arch wire slot relative to the labial surface of each tooth (Table 3). The problems of freedom between the arch wire and arch wire slot and force diminution, though unavoidable using current appliances, can be minimized by means of stiff arch wires of about the same size as the arch wire slots. Teeth may be delivered to the desired positions by adding or subtracting the amount of freedom plus the amount of force diminution inherent to the appliance to the torque, tip, rotation, and height parameters for each bracket. This will maximize efficiency in meeting the treatment goals.

Summary.—By recognizing and accounting for the reasons for failure of preadjusted appliances and straight wires, the dentist can make indi-

TABLE 1.—Prescriptions for Torque

Prescriptions for torques (degrees)

	Andrews	*Roth*	*Alexander*	*Hilgers*
Maxillary				
1/1	+7	+12	+14	+22
2/2	+3	+8	+8	+14
3/3	−7	−2	−3	+7
54/45	−7	−7	−7	−7
6/6	−9	−14	−10	−10
Mandibular				
21/12	−1	−1	−5	−1
3/3	−11	−11	−7	+7
4/4	−17	−17	−11	−11
5/5	−22	−22	−17	−22
6/6	−26	−30	−22	−27

Note: Prescriptions differ as much as 15 degrees for maxillary anterior teeth.
(Courtesy of Creekmore TD, Kunik RL: *Am J Orthod Dentofacial Orthop* 104:8–20, 1993.)

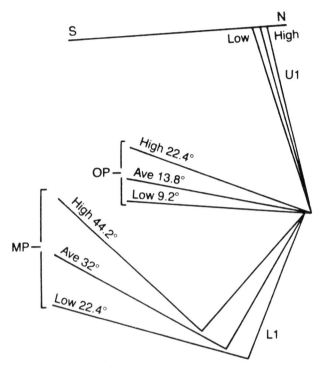

Fig 5-21.—Spatial relationships of the mandibular plane (MP), occlusal plane (OP), upper incisor (U1), and lower incisor (L1), superimposed on the caranial base. The values represent the mean inclinations. (From Creekmore TD, Kunik RL: Am J Orthod Dentofacial Orthop 104:8-20, 1993. Courtesy of Ross V, Isaacson RJ, Germane N, et al: Am J Orthod Dentofacial Orthop 98:422-429, 1990.)

vidual prescriptions for preadjusted appliances. Although this requires planning before the brackets are placed on the teeth as well as more training and laboratory time for auxiliary staff, important benefits are realized in quality control, simplicity of treatment, and reduction of treatment and chair time.

▶ Bonding has increased, not decreased, the demands for accurate placement of brackets. There is now infinite error. Brackets are placed on crowns that therefore are always placed away from the centers of resistance, which are approximately halfway down the roots or in the furcal areas of molars. There will be rotational effects on the teeth that need to be controlled.

Apical base variability necessitates different incisor angulations and torque. One should consider Steiner chevron compromises.

The freedom of movement of the arch wire in the bracket slot must factor in resistance as well as control, but whatever the slot sizes one uses, i.e., a .018 or .022 system, an appreciation of the lack of full expression of a prescription must be recognized with the smaller-sized wires. The term "freedom" is more an American term than is "play," which the authors use. Verti-

TABLE 2.—Amount of Torquing Play From Parallel

Arch wire size	Bracket slot size	
	0.018 × 0.025†	*0.022 × 0.028‡*
16 × 16§	12.5°	Rotates
16 × 22	11.8°	34.3°
17 × 22	7.3°	27.9°
17 × 25	5.9°	21.0°
18 × 18‖	5.5°	Rotates
18 × 22‖	3.8°	23.1°
18 × 25‖	3.1°	17.7°
19 × 25		12.8°
21 × 25		5.2°
215 × 28		2.9°

Note: The values are the amount the arch wire can rotate in the slot in either direction from a parallel position. Calculations are based on midrange values. Delivered labial or lingual root torque equals torque in the slot plus or minus play, respectively. Data courtesy of 3M/Unitek.
† .018 tolerances .0182 to .0192 midrange .0187.
‡ .022 tolerances .0220 to .0230 midrange .0225.
§ .016 × .016 dimension actually .01625 × .01625.
‖ .018 dimension actually .0178.
(Courtesy of Creekmore TD, Kunik RL: *Am J Orthod Dentofacial Orthop* 104:8-20, 1993.)

cal bracket placement on the molar-premolar segment changes more with the age of the patient than with the type of malocclusion; more anatomical crowns as clinical crowns allow a placement closer to the center of resistance with the adult. This is not possible with the child or adolescent because of the height of the gingiva on the crown.

Stiffer arch wires approximating the size of the arch wire slots help in more precise orientation with less force diminution.

The basic bracket height should be determined by the vertical height of the anatomical crown (1) (Table 4).

Bracket heights of 7/ at 3.5 mm, 6/ at 4 mm, and 5/ or 4/ at 4.5 mm are consistent with the average vertical anatomical crown data. The placement of 3/ at 5 mm for class I occlusions with canine rise varies on initial bracket placement, depending on the canine relationship. It is placed nearer the incisal edge if there is a need for class II correction. Because most malocclusions that need treatment are deep bite problems, there is a greater incisal placement of the brackets on the incisors, i.e., 4 mm for 1/ and 3.5 mm for 2/ (Table 5).

Bracket heights of /7 at 3 mm, /6 at 3.5 mm, and /5 or /4 at 4 mm are consistent with the average vertical crown height data. There basically is no change in bracket heights for the posterior segments in anterior deep bite or

TABLE 3.—Orientation of the Bracket Arch Wire
Bracket heights (mm)

	Deep bites	Standard	Open bites
Maxillary			
1/1	3.9	4.5	5.1
2/2	3.62	4.25	4.87
3/3	4.37	4.75	5.12
4/4	4.5	4.5	4.5
5/5	4.5	4.5	4.5
6/6	3.75	3.75	3.75
Mandibular			
21/12	3.37	4.0	4.62
3/3	3.87	4.25	4.62
4/4	4.0	4.0	4.0
5/5	3.75	3.75	3.75
6/6	3.5	3.5	3.5

Note: Standard bracket heights are determined by the orientation templates. Height adjustment spaces (shims) placed under the bracket holder or under the orientation templates position the brackets more incisally or gingivally, respectively, the thickness of the spacer.

(Courtesy of Creekmore TD, Kunik RL: *Am J Orthod Dentofacial Orthop* 104:8-20, 1993.)

TABLE 4.—Determination of Basic Bracket Height

Maxillary permanent central incisor: $10.5 \text{ mm} \times 1/2 = 5.25 \text{ mm}$

Maxillary permanent lateral incisor: $9.0 \text{ mm} \times 1/2 = 4.5 \text{ mm}$

Maxillary permanent canine: $10.0 \text{ mm} \times 1/2 = 5.0 \text{ mm}$

Maxillary premolar: $8.5 \text{ mm} \times 1/2 = 4.25 \text{ mm}$

Maxillary permanent first molar: $7.5 \text{ mm} \times 1/2 = 3.75 \text{ mm}$

Maxillary permanent second molar: $7.0 \text{ mm} \times 1/2 = 3.5 \text{ mm}$

(Courtesy of Kraus BS, Jordan RE, Abrams L: *Dental Anatomy and Occlusion.* Baltimore, Williams and Wilkins, 1969.)

TABLE 5.—Greater Incisal Placement of Brackets on Incisors

Mandibular permanent central incisor:	9.0 mm x 1/2 = 4.5 mm
Mandibular permanent lateral incisor:	9.5 mm x 1/2 = 4.75 mm
Mandibular permanent canine:	11.0 mm x 1/2 = 5.5 mm
Mandibular first premolar:	8.5 mm x 1/2 = 4.25 mm
Mandibular second premolar:	8.0 mm x 1/2 = 4.0 mm
Mandibular permanent first molar:	7.5 mm x 1/2 = 3.75 mm
Mandibular permanent second molar:	7.0 mm x 1/2 = 3.5 mm

(Courtesy of Kraus BS, Jordan RE, Abrams L: *Dental Anatomy and Occlusion.* Baltimore, Williams and Wilkins, 1969.)

open bite cases. Canine bracket positioning varies on the need for initial canine retraction in the maxilla, and the incisors are usually placed slightly more incisal at 3.5 mm for deep bite opening if needed.

Small amounts of bracket placement to compensate for original rotations or in extraction sites are now possible with bonding at 2-degree to 4-degree variations. Upsidedown and reversed maxillary lateral brackets can reverse normal lingual root torque to facial root torque for those extremely lingually placed lateral incisors.—G.F. Currier, D.D.S., M.S.D., M.Ed.

Reference

1. Kraus BS, et al: *Dental Anatomy and Occlusion.* Baltimore, Williams and Wilkins, 1969.

Biodegradation of Orthodontic Appliances: Part I. Biodegradation of Nickel and Chromium In Vitro
Barrett RD, Bishara SE, Quinn JK (Univ of Iowa, Iowa City)
Am J Orthod Dentofacial Orthop 103:8–14, 1993   105-94-5-12

Purpose.—Orthodontic appliances consisting of bands, brackets, and wires may contain nickel, chromium and titanium, exposing patients to metal corrosion products. Because the biodegradation of orthodontic appliances has not been well studied, the in vitro corrosion rates of a standard orthodontic appliance were investigated.

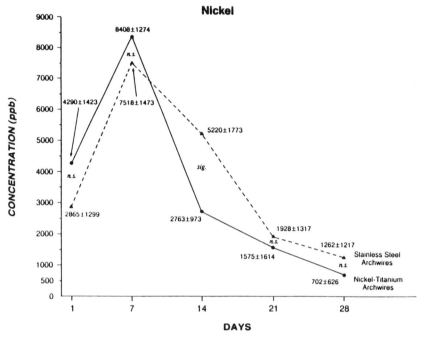

Fig 5–22.—Changes in nickel release rates for orthodontic appliances with stainless steel and nitrinol arch wires. (Courtesy of Barrett RD, Bishara SE, Quinn JK: et al: *Am J Orthod Dentofacial Orthop* 103:8–14, 1993.)

Methods.—Ten orthodontic appliances as used on a maxillary arch with a full complement of teeth were used for the study. Five sets of appliances were ligated to stainless steel arch wires, and the other 5 sets were ligated to nickel-titanium arch wires. The appliances were immersed in an artificial saliva medium and kept at 37°C for 4 weeks. The pH of the artificial saliva was held at 6.75, which is the pH value for human saliva. On days 1, 7, 14, 21, and 28 the artificial saliva solution was removed and replaced with a fresh solution. The removed solutions were analyzed for nickel and chromium content.

Findings.—None of the samples contained rust-colored precipitates, but about 10% of the brackets and bands had localized areas of rust-colored corrosion. The appliances released measurable amounts of nickel and chromium. The nickel release reached a maximum after about 1 week, then diminished with time (Fig 5-22), and the chromium release increased during the first 2 weeks and leveled off during the next 2 weeks (Fig 5-23). The nickel and chromium release rates from stainless steel arch wires did not differ significantly from the release rates from nickel-titanium arch wires. The average nickel release rate was 37 times greater than the average chromium release rate.

Conclusion.—Fully banded and bonded orthodontic appliances release measurable amounts of nickel and chromium when placed in arti-

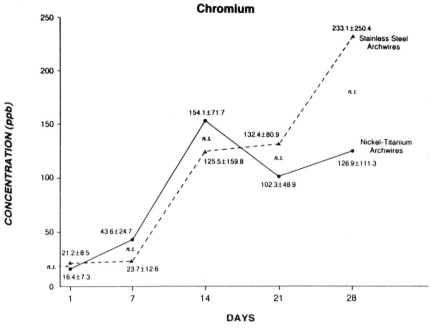

Fig 5–23.—Changes in chromium release rate for orthodontic appliances with stainless steel and nitrinol arch wires. (Courtesy of Barrett RD, Bishara SE, Quinn JK: et al: *Am J Orthod Dentofacial Orthop* 103:8–14, 1993.)

ficial saliva. How much of these corrosive products are actually absorbed by patients undergoing orthodontic treatment remains to be determined.

▶ Orthodontic bands, brackets, and wires are universally made of austenitic stainless steel containing approximately 18% chromium and 8% nickel. The nickel on the surface of the stainless steel quickly corrodes with the natural rate reduction. The total release of nickel during the 4-week period here averaged 13.05 μg/day. Even if doubled to simulate the equivalent release from a fully banded/bonded maxillary and mandibular appliance, the release rate of 16.1 μg/day is about one tenth of the reported average daily dietary intake of 200 to 300 μg/day.

Contrary to the nickel rate, the rate of chromium did not decrease after 7 days. The total release of chromium during the 4-week period averaged .35 μg/day. Doubling this figure to simulate orthodontic appliances placed in both arches would give a release rate of .7 μg/day. This is about .25% of the reported average daily intake of 280 μg/day for chromium.—G.F. Currier, D.D.S., M.S.D., M.Ed.

Biodegradation of Orthodontic Appliances: Part II. Changes in the Blood Level of Nickel

Bishara SE, Barrett RD, Selim MI (Univ of Iowa, Iowa City)
Am J Orthod Dentofacial Orthop 103:115–119, 1993   105-94-5-13

Background.—Nickel and chromium exposure can produce adverse effects. In addition to causing hypersensitivity, dermatitis, and asthma, compounds containing these metals have a carcinogenic and mutagenic potential. Assessing the adverse potential of orthodontic appliances involves determining the rate at which an appliance releases potentially harmful metal compounds in the mouth, the degree to which humans absorb these metal compounds, and the length of time the compounds are retained in the body.

Methods.—Whether orthodontic patients accumulate measurable levels of nickel in the blood during an initial course of orthodontic treatment was investigated. Serum was collected before orthodontic appliance placement, 2 months after placement, and 4–5 months after placement. The study subjects were 18 females and 13 males aged 12–38 years, with malocclusions requiring the use of a fully banded, bonded edgewise appliance.

Findings.—Patients with fully banded and bonded orthodontic appliances did not have significant or consistent increases in nickel blood levels during the first 4–5 months of orthodontic treatment. Orthodontic treatment using appliances made of alloys containing nickel-titanium did not significantly or consistently increase blood nickel levels.

Conclusion.—Orthodontic appliances corrode in the oral environment, releasing nickel and chromium, but in amounts significantly below the mean dietary intake. The biodegradation of orthodontic appliances during the initial 5 months of treatment does not consistently or significantly increase blood nickel levels.

▶ All of the blood levels of nickel found in these subjects were below the normal levels previously reported in the literature (2.4 ± .5 ppb, 4.8 ± 1.3 ppb, 6 ± 1 ppb, or 30 ± 19 ppb). The levels of chromium in frozen whole blood could not be determined with the equipment presently available at the commercial laboratory. The safety of current fixed orthodontic appliances relative to possible adverse heavy metal poisoning seems very acceptable.—G.F. Currier, D.D.S., M.S.D., M.Ed.

Root Resorption After Orthodontic Treatment: Part 1. Literature Review

Brezniak N, Wasserstein A (Tel Aviv Univ, Israel)
Am J Orthod Dentofacial Orthop 103:62–66, 1993   105-94-5-14

Roots Resorption Data From Published Articles

Study	Year	Patients Number	Average age range	No. of teeth	Teeth examined	Treatment type	Extractions and nonextractions	Source
Ketcham	1927	385	—	—	All	Fixed	—	PA
Ketcham	1929	500	—	—	All	Fixed	—	PA
Ketcham	1929	2012	—	—	All	NT	—	PA
Becks	1936	100	—	—	All	Unknown	—	PA
Becks	1939	72	—	—	All	NT	—	PA
Becks	1939	72	—	—	All	Unknown	—	PA
Rudolph	1936	439	10	—	All	LL	—	PA
Rudolph	1936	4560	7-70	—	All	NT	—	PA
Rudolph	1940	513	—	—	All	LL	—	PA
Hemley	1941	195	—	4959	All	Fixed	—	PA
Henry and Weinman	1951	15	16-58	261	All	NT	—	HIST
Massler and Malone	1954	708	12-49	13263	All	NT	—	PA
Massler and Malone	1954	81	12-19	2085	All	Unknown	—	PA
Massler and Perreault	1954	301	17	5844	All	NT	—	PA
Phillips	1955	69	—	1745	All	EW	48/21	PA
Phillips	1955	62	13:7	62	$\frac{1}{1}$	EW	44/18	CEPH
McLaughlin	1964	28	—	—	$\frac{1}{1}$	EW	—	PA
Deshields	1969	52	12:3	208	21/12	EW	—	CEPH

Abbreviations: RTS, roots; All, all teeth; I, maxillary central incisors; 21/12, maxillary incisors; PM, premolars; 3,5, canines and second premolars; 5/5, maxillary and mandibular incisors, canines, and premolars; Fixed, fixed appliances; NT, no treatment; LL, labiolingual; EW, edgewise; Begg, Begg; ACT, activator; INTR, intrusion; Varies, fixed and removable; SER, serial extraction; B/EW, Begg edgewise; PA, periapical; CEPH, lateral headfilm; HIST, histology; PANO, panoramic film.

(Courtesy of Brezniak N, Wasserstein A: Am J Orthod Dentofacial Orthop 103:62-66, 1993.)

Introduction.—Apical root resorption associated with orthodontic treatment has recently received considerable attention because of medicolegal considerations. Although numerous studies have been carried out to investigate the process and predictability of root resorption, its origins remain unclear. The literature on idiopathic apical root resorption was reviewed.

Review.—The first paper discussing root resorption of permanent teeth was published in 1856, and the first study to relate root resorption directly to orthodontic treatment was published in 1914. Since then, numerous studies have investigated the histologic, clinical, and physiologic aspects of root resorption after orthodontic treatment (table).

There are 3 types of external root resorption: surface resorption, inflammatory resorption, and replacement resorption. Inflammatory resorption is further subclassified into transient and progressive inflammatory resorption. Root resorption after orthodontic treatment is either surface resorption or transient inflammatory resorption. Replacement resorption after orthodontic treatment is very rare.

Root resorption is most often found at the apex, followed by mesial, buccal, distal, and lingual surfaces. It has been suggested that root resorption during orthodontic treatment occurs in the same areas where physiologic root resorption originates, but supporting data are not available.

▶ All patients who are to receive any tooth movement must be notified before therapy that apical root resorption should be planned for and that periapical radiographs will be needed. Those patients who do not wish to have radiographs or who believe the risk of resorption is too high should not receive orthodontic therapy. This risk is present for all patients to have at least small amounts of root resorption of some teeth. It is a matter of degree and pattern, not whether or not it will occur.—G.F. Currier, D.D.S., M.S.D., M.Ed.

Root Resorption After Orthodontic Treatment: Part 2. Literature Review

Brezniak N, Wasserstein A (Tel Aviv Univ, Israel)
Am J Orthod Dentofacial Orthop 103:138–146, 1993   105-94-5-15

Introduction.—The potential of permanent dentition to undergo significant external root resorption varies in persons and between different teeth in the same person. This variation may result from tooth structure, types of movement, the extent of orthodontic treatment duration, and mechanical factors. The biological and mechanical factors affecting root resorption were reviewed, and clinical considerations related to this process were discussed.

Biological Factors.—Individual susceptibility is thought to be a major factor determining root resorption potential. Resorption may also be related to genetic and systemic factors, increasing age, habits such as nail biting and tongue thrust, endodontic treatment, and the presence of root resorption before orthodontic treatment. Gender and nutritional status do not appear to be important factors. Some researchers found a relationship between greater density of alveolar bone and root resorption. Maxillary teeth appear to be more sensitive than do mandibular teeth.

Mechanical Factors.—Many studies have found the degree of root damage to be a function of the appliance used. Intrusion seems to be the type of orthodontic movement most detrimental to the roots involved. Higher stress may also cause more root resorption. Many investigators believe that a direct relationship exists between root resorption and the distance moved by the roots.

Clinical Diagnostic Aids.—Radiographic evidence of root resorption before orthodontic treatment is the most important diagnostic aid in predicting root resorption. The periapical paralleling technique offers the most accurate information. Periapical radiographs of the incisors should be taken at least every year after appliance placement.

Conclusion.—The root resorption phenomenon is both widespread and unpredictable. Functional capacity and the effective life of the tooth should not be affected. Patients should be advised that apical root shortening may be a consequence of orthodontic treatment. To avoid excessive resorption, treatment should begin as early as possible, and the orthodontic force should be intermittent and light. The objectives of treatment must take into consideration individual anatomical and physiologic limitations. Sequential root canal therapy with calcium hydroxide is advisable if root resorption continues after appliance removal or during retention.

▶ A panoramic radiograph is not sufficient in the pretreatment analysis of an orthodontic patient. Long-cone periapical films of the anterior teeth with the paralleling technique are essential. This is the region in which most of the apical root resorption occurs, either because of incisor retraction or apical displacement, especially with the maxillary incisors. Because of the high probability of anterior trauma, preexisting pulp canal changes, and possible root or crown microfractures, these periapical films are needed in the pretreatment evaluation.

The individual preexisting status is probably the best initial indicator of possible future problems. Genetic information or familial patterns certainly help; unusual endocrine problems should be addressed. Increasing age as well as prolonged treatment time should be considered. Narrow, tapered roots are not a good sign.

Root resorption associated with orthodontic treatment usually ceases after active tooth movement is stopped. Postorthodontic traumatic occlusion or habit-oriented mobility should be considered possible follow-up problems after therapy.—G.F. Currier, D.D.S., M.S.D., M.Ed

An Analysis of Causes of Apical Root Resorption in Patients Not Treated Orthodontically

Harris EF, Robinson QC, Woods MA (Univ of Tennessee, Memphis)
Quintessence Int 24:417–428, 1993   105-94-5–16

Background.—Most cases of external apical root resorption have no apparent cause, especially when root blunting from orthodontic treatment has been excluded. The frequency of apical root resorption in the permanent dentition of patients not orthodontically treated was investigated.

Methods.—Three hundred six patients, aged 14–84 years, who were treated at 1 center from 1986 through 1990 were studied. In addition to the frequency of apical root resorption, associations between the occurrence of external apical root resorption and number of missing teeth, periodontal probing depths, and alveolar crestal bone heights were assessed.

Findings.—Seven percent to 10% of the patients showed obvious apical resorption. The occurrence of resorption was strongly associated with tooth loss, increased periodontal probing depths, and decreased crestal bone heights.

Conclusion.—Root resorption is significantly more common in patients with compromised tooth support. Factors significantly predicting external apical root resorption include loss of stability from adjacent teeth, increased use of fewer remaining teeth, and loss of root anchorage in the bone.

▶ Noticeable external apical root resorption should be expected to be found in 1 of 10 patients, excluding any tooth movement, with 1% to 2% severe resorption, especially in the incisors. This 10% finding should be expected as idiopathic when trauma, endodontic therapy, infection, systemic disease, etc., have been eliminated.

In this study, age alone did not increase the tendency for root resorption. The common theme was that resorption seemed to stem from the loss of tooth stability, a mechanical stimulation (traumatic) rather than an inflammatory resorption. Those individuals with severe involvement of the periodontium and the most compromised occlusion, i.e., missing teeth, were at greatest risk for apical root resorption.—G.F. Currier, D.D.S., M.S.D., M.Ed.

6 Caries

Introduction

The use of the dental explorer in detecting pit and fissure caries has been challenged because of low sensitivity scores. In fact, the orientation of dental caries as a clinical symptom of a bacterial infection of specific causes necessitates treatment specificity and a collage of various adjunctive therapies.

The understanding of the caries process includes the association of organisms that produce a gel matrix of extracellular glucans, primarily from sucrose, and then larger bacterial populations through adhesion. Once the pH drops at the interface of the gel plaque and tooth surface, dissolution of the apatite phase occurs. However, nonsurgical healing should be considered. There are various definable risk factors and different disease states that include the earlier reversible disease, arrested caries, and the active/rapid disease. One should use the concept of demineralization/remineralization balance.

The current criteria for caries diagnosis need reevaluation as a result of large inconsistencies among dentists concerning where restoration or rerestoration is needed. A high positive predictive value becomes more important as the prevalence of caries declines.

The 4 basic techniques for detecting caries are visual examination, tactile examination, radiographic diagnosis, and transillumination. The tactile method has been emphasized more in North America than in Europe.

With the change in the nature of dental caries, new technologies for diagnosis of caries are needed. Sensitivity vs. specificity approaches are recommended. High-risk vs. low-risk factors, along with the assessment of lesion status and activity over time, should be helpful. Differentiation of static vs. remineralizing lesions should remain a challenge.

With the remarkable improvement in children's dental health in the past generation, focus has shifted to distribution of caries in various suspect populations as well as altering the fluoride dose at earlier ages. With the widespread use of fluoride dentifrices and water fluoridation, concern has been expressed about the continued use of dietary fluoride supplements and adult-sized toothpaste amounts compared with child-sized amounts because children tend to swallow toothpaste.

The acquisition of mutans streptococci is related to the presence of primary teeth, with most children colonized by 25 to 30 months of age. Transferability from maternal saliva should be considered. There also seems to be a variable salivary clearance pattern in the mouths of children, with the maxillary anterior facial region rather unfavorable, thus contributing to baby bottle syndrome or nursing bottle caries. As the child progresses into adolescence, the salivary flow rate increases with a rather stabilizing buffering effect, but with such individual variability that using single-point measures of the saliva to diagnose or predict caries is not recommended.

The stimulation of salivary flow to inhibit enamel demineralization should be considered with the use of chewing sugarless (sorbitol) gum within 5 minutes after eating and continuing for at least 15 minutes.

A vigilant approach in monitoring optimal fluoride levels in the water supply is required, as is the formulation of specific guidelines to prevent any fluoride overfeed.

The effect of fluoride in prevention now seems to be more a surface phenomenon, with remineralization as its primary mechanism.

G. Fräns Currier, D.D.S., M.S.D., M.Ed.

Risk Assessment

Modern Management of Dental Caries: The Cutting Edge Is Not the Dental Bur
Anderson MH, Bales DJ, Omnell K-A (Univ of Washington, Seattle)
J Am Dent Assoc 124(6):37–44, 1993   105-94-6–1

Introduction.—New materials and techniques have led to great advances in what dentistry can accomplish. Changes have also occurred in the management of the 2 primary diseases of the mouth: caries and periodontal diseases. In a subtle shift, dentistry is moving from the traditional surgical model of care to a more modern medical model. The conventional treatment of caries and methods of modern management were reviewed.

The Conventional Model.—The view that dental caries is a bacterially mediated disease was codified in 1890. Treatment has followed the assumption that plaque is odontopathic. Dentists have surgically excised the diseased tooth structure and filled the area with a restorative material, but they have not addressed the underlying infection. With the causative organisms of dental caries identified, the treatment plan can now include an attack on the infection.

Specific Plaque Hypothesis.—This hypothesis states that plaque per se is not odontopathic. Instead, a finite and identifiable number of organisms within the plaque of some patients result in caries. Caries is diagnosed, the patient is treated for the infection, and the dentist regularly recalls the patient to ensure that the infection has not been reacquired. Two of the primary organisms involved in human caries are mutans streptococci and lactobacilli species. Studies have shown that dental ca-

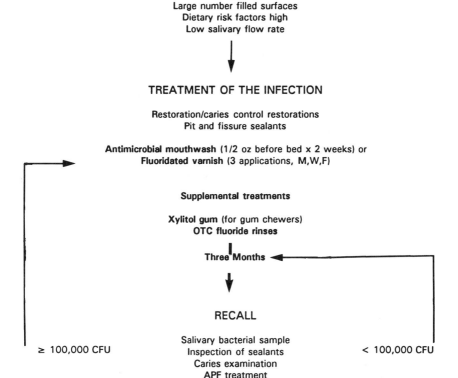

HIGH CARIES RISK
(one or more factors)

Two carious lesions
Large number filled surfaces
Dietary risk factors high
Low salivary flow rate

TREATMENT OF THE INFECTION

Restoration/caries control restorations
Pit and fissure sealants

Antimicrobial mouthwash (1/2 oz before bed x 2 weeks) or
Fluoridated varnish (3 applications, M,W,F)

Supplemental treatments

Xylitol gum (for gum chewers)
OTC fluoride rinses

Three Months

RECALL

≥ 100,000 CFU   Salivary bacterial sample   < 100,000 CFU
Inspection of sealants
Caries examination
APF treatment

Fig 6–1.—Managing patients with caries. (Courtesy of Anderson MH, Bales DJ, Omnell K-A: *J Am Dent Assoc* 124(6):37–44, 1993.)

ries is the clinical symptom of a bacterial infection, mediated primarily by mutans streptococci. Lactobacilli appear to be secondary caries organisms. The treatment of dental caries is based on this knowledge (Fig 6–1).

Treatment of Caries.—The first step is to restore the existing carious lesions with frank cavitation. Simultaneously, a fluoride-releasing pit and fissure sealant is applied. Sealants are also used in questionable and early carious pit and fissure sites. Antimicrobials are then applied intensively, on a short-term basis. Chlorhexidine (CHX) is highly effective against mutans streptococci infections. The patient uses a half-ounce, 30-second CHX rinse just before bedtime. Adjunctive therapies include salivary substitutes for people with xerostomia, xylitol gum, and over-the-counter fluoride rinses. As a final step, the patient is recalled to determine whether infection has recurred. Several simple media culture tests can diagnose the presence and severity of mutans streptococci infection.

▶ A newer orientation is toward caries as a disease (infection) rather than as a symptom (lesion), with a medical model rather than a surgical model of care. This new model addresses the lesion as a clinical manifestation of the infection and the cause of the disease process from a finite and identifiable number of organisms within the plaque of some patients. The 2 primary organisms in human caries are mutans streptococci and lactobacilli species. The median age of mutans streptococci transmission to a child is 24 months (between 19 and 28 months of age); they are not found in predentulous newborns. Dental caries is the clinical symptom of a bacterial infection that is transmitted by salivary exchange within the family unit. Lactobacilli are secondary caries organisms that generally do not predict the carious process.

As stated by the authors, the rational steps in infection control include:

1. Restoration of existing carious lesions with frank cavitation (not white spots or incipient radiographic lesions without cavitations).

2. Fluoride-releasing pit and fissure sealants, especially primary second molars, and all questionable pit and fissure sites on permanent teeth.

3. Short-term antimicrobials such as CHX (the positive charge of this strongly cationic drug causes it to adhere to almost everything, because almost all oral surfaces are negatively charged). This 14-day period is followed by fluoride rinses. Because CHX is poorly absorbed in the gastrointestinal tract, the lethal dose for 50% of a human population (LD_{50}) is 2,000 mg/kg body weight. For a 110-pound child, this translates to 83 liter bottles of a .12% solution in a short time to have a 50/50 chance of dying.

In addition to these 3 areas, options for infection control include dietary restriction of large amounts of frequent sugars; maintenance of good salivary flow for buffering and remineralization; xylitol gum for patients who chew gum (xylitol is a 5-carbon sugar alcohol that is not a fermentable substrate for mutans streptococci); and fluoride rinses and dentifrices (fluoride is a powerful bactericidal agent for mutans streptococci, a remineralization facilitator, and a former of acid-resistant carbonate apatite crystals).

Recalls should consist of levels of mutans streptococci and a clinical examination, including the status of sealant for any repair. An infection of 3,000 CFU/mL of mutans streptococci in saliva can colonize a susceptible pit or fissure (sealant importance here). A level of 43,000 CFU/mL is needed for establishing a smooth surface infection. There are in-office tests for mutans streptococci infections. They have rather low sensitivity for caries (true positive) but relatively high specificity (true negative); they are poor in predicting who will get carious lesions but are good in predicting low caries levels when a patient has low mutans streptococci counts. The retreatment value is more than 100,000 CFU/mL of mutans streptococci.

The caries treatment described is directed toward the causative organisms. New schema can evolve, but the underlying model will remain the same.—G.F. Currier, D.D.S., M.S.D., M.Ed.

Need for Change in Standards of Caries Diagnosis: Perspective Based on the Structure and Behavior of the Caries Lesion
Hume WR (Univ of California, San Francisco)
J Dent Educ 57:439–443, 1993   105-94-6–2

Objective.—With advances in our understanding of the nature of dental caries should come changes in the rational forms of management. Changes in the understanding of this disease are summarized, and standards for diagnosis that will be most useful in clinical management are proposed.

Nature of Caries.—Caries may be defined as progressive loss of the mineral composition of the enamel, then the dentin. It is in various respects a microbial and a dietary disease. The balance between demineralization and remineralization is affected by a number of factors, including salivary composition and flow and fluoride concentration at the plaque-hydroxyapatite interface. Caries is most often associated with organisms that produce a gel matrix of extracellular glucans, the development of which relies on sucrose. Once glucan is established, a large bacterial population may develop simply through adhesion. A substrate for bacterial metabolism is provided by frequent ingestion of simple carbohydrates. Once pH decreases at the interface between the tooth surface and gel plaque, the main buffering mechanism is dissolution of the apatite phase, with fluorapatite dissolving at a slightly lower pH than hydroxyapatite.

Diagnosis and Therapy.—A diagnosis-based treatment approach begins with the concept of a range of risk and activity states for dental caries. The early enamel lesions and all cementum and dentinal lesions are reversible to some degree; arrested caries is a commonly observed clinical phenomenon. Thus, nonsurgical healing should be considered a care option. A different therapeutic option is indicated for the various risk and disease states, ranging from behavioral reinforcement and monitoring for a patient at low risk to surgical removal of infected tissue for those with active and rapid disease. Present diagnostic tools, many of them subjective, include radiographic density, color, and hardness. Some short-term index of mineral loss or gain would be a useful tool, as would a simple test of demineralization/remineralization balance.

Conclusion.—Caries is a dynamic disease process with definable risk factors. The approach to prevention and cure can be enhanced by the concept of demineralization/remineralization balance. With increased understanding of the nature of the disease come new challenges in diagnosis and management.

▶ When pH (power of hydrogen) falls at the interface between the tooth surface and a gel plaque of moderate thickness, the principal buffering mechanism is dissolution of the apatite (mineral) phase. Hydroxyapatite dissolves at pH 5.5, and fluorapatite dissolves at a slightly lower pH. The balance between demineralization and remineralization depends primarily on the time balance between acid and neutral conditions within the plaque. Microbial composition of plaque, plaque thickness, and frequency of eating and drinking are the determinants of this time balance.

The 3 most common sites for the initiation of enamel caries are pits and fissures, the area beneath the contact, and the junction of the enamel and gingiva. Caries diagnosis and therapy should include risk assessment and a range of possible activity states (early reversible and arrested caries as reversed demineralization need greater consideration).—G.F. Currier, D.D.S., M.S.D., M.Ed.

Diagnostic Standards

Validity of Probing for Fissure Caries Diagnosis
Penning C, van Amerongen JP, Seef RE, ten Cate JM (Academic Centre for Dentistry, Amsterdam)
Caries Res 26:445–449, 1992   105-94-6–3

Purpose.—Discolored fissures are routinely investigated with an explorer and a mirror, even though there is increasing evidence that this method has important drawbacks and is not as reliable for diagnosing fissure caries as previously thought. The sensitivity and specificity of probing for stickiness in the diagnosis of fissure caries was investigated in an in vitro study.

TABLE 1.—Comparison of Sticking and Nonsticking Sites on Probing to Presence of Caries Lesions in the Dentine (Scores 2–4) on X-Ray Films

Probings	n	Caries lesions (scored on X-rays)	
		caries	sound
Sticking	41	36 (true positive)	5 (false positive)
Non-sticking	1,009	112 (false negative)	987 (true negative)
Total	1,140	148	992

(Courtesy of Penning C, van Amerongen JP, Seef RE, et al: *Caries Res* 26:445–449, 1992.)

TABLE 2.—Comparison of Sticking and Nonsticking Sites on Probing to the Presence of Caries Lesions in Enamel and Dentine (Scores 1–4) on X-Ray Films

Probings	n	Caries lesions (scored on X-rays)	
		caries	sound
Sticking	41	38 (true positive)	3 (false positive)
Non-sticking	1,009	181 (false negative)	918 (true negative)
Total	1,140	219	921

(Courtesy of Penning C, van Amerongen JP, Seef RE, et al: *Caries Res* 26:445–449, 1992.)

Methods.—Fifty upper and 50 lower molars with discolored fissures but no visible carious lesions were mounted, probed in every fissure, and marked for sticky spots. Color slides were made of the occlusal surfaces. The crowns were then embedded in epoxy resin and sectioned in a facial-lingual direction. The sections were radiographed and scored for caries by placing a measuring grid over each radiograph. The results were compared with the color slides.

Results.—Only 24% of the actual caries lesions were discovered by probing for stickiness (Table 1). The results obtained when the enamel lesions were also included in the calculations are shown in Table 2.

Conclusion.—The sensitivity of the explorer probing method is much lower than has been presumed and further confirms that this method is unreliable for the diagnosis of fissure caries.

▶ "Sticking" of an explorer in a sound fissure seldom occurs (a negative predictive value of 90% per fissure, not per tooth). However, with the average number of probings per tooth being more than 11, each tooth analyzed is likely to contain one undiagnosed lesion.

The sensitivity of the explorer probing method (36/148, or 24.3%, in Table 1 and 38/219, or 17.4%, in Table 2) is much lower than presumed. The specificity was 99.5% (987/992 in Table 1 and 918/921 in Table 2). The positive predictive value was 88% in Table 1 (36/41) and 93% in Table 2 (38/41), and the negative predictive value was 90% (987/1,099) in Table 1 and 84% (918/1,099) in Table 2. (Readers should note an error in Tables 1 and 2: The nonsticking number equals 1,099 *not* 1,009.)

The days of the explorer in diagnosis of fissure caries are numbered.—G.F. Currier, D.D.S., M.S.D., M.Ed.

Need for Change in Standards of Caries Diagnosis: Epidemiology and Health Services Research Perspective
Bader JD, Shugars DA (Univ of North Carolina, Chapel Hill)
J Dent Educ 57:415–421, 1993   105-94-6-4

Introduction.—The methods and criteria of caries diagnosis currently used in North America are in need of reevaluation. Development of new

test result	true condition		total
	carious	sound	
carious	400	25	425
sound	100	475	575
total	500	500	1000

Caries Prevalence = 0.50
Sensitivity = 0.80 (400/(400 + 100))
Specificity = 0.95 (475/(475 + 25))
Positive Predictive Value = 0.941 (400/(400 + 25))
Negative Predictive Value = 0.826 (475/(475 + 100))

test result	true condition		total
	carious	sound	
carious	80	45	125
sound	20	855	875
total	100	900	1000

Caries Prevalence = 0.10
Sensitivity = 0.80 (80/(80 + 20))
Specificity = 0.95 (855/(855 + 45))
Positive Predictive Value = 0.640 (80/(80 + 45))
Negative Predictive Value = 0.977 (855/(855 + 20))

Fig 6–2.—Test performance at high (**top**) and moderate (**bottom**) caries prevalance. (Courtesy of Bader JD, Shugars DA: *J Dent Educ* 57:415-421, 1993.)

methods depends on an accurate understanding of how caries are actually diagnosed and restored. A review of 5 outcomes of current methods and criteria for caries diagnosis may be useful in the development of new approaches.

Agreement on Treatment Decisions.—Dentists often disagree on restorative treatment decisions. A recent study of the nature, extent, and reasons for those disagreements found disagreement for treatment of almost one third of the teeth. The presence of a restoration was associated with a lesser extent of agreement, whether or not caries was clinically present.

Restorative Decision-Making.—In a model of dentists' restorative decision-making processes, no distinct step of diagnosis was found. Rather, in most cases, no treatment decision is made because there is no condition requiring treatment or a condition is present that requires routine treatment. Thus, treatment becomes a repetition of a learned behavior.

Influence of Tactile Information.—In a study to determine the extent to which treatment decisions are influenced by tactile examination, the absence of tactile information tended to inhibit the identification of caries and to promote the condemnation of existing restorations.

Effect of Caries Prevalence on Treatment Validity.—Although diagnostic tests are traditionally evaluated in terms of sensitivity and specificity, the individual dentist must determine whether a particular finding is correct for a given patient. A high positive predictive value becomes more important as the prevalence of caries declines (Fig 6–2). Thus, a test that is acceptable when caries is prevalent may have an unacceptably high false positive rate when caries is less prevalent.

Validity of Caries Incidence Determinations.—More and more, knowledge of caries incidence is derived from practitioners' treatment decisions, rather than from epidemiologic observations. In a study of 27 patients, caries-related treatment recommendations accounted for an average of 4 of 8 newly filled surfaces, about half of the total detectable increment. Treatment recommendations accounted for about two thirds of the increment for teeth with previous restorations, compared with two thirds for teeth without previous restorations.

Conclusion.—An appropriate treatment decision is the ultimate goal of the caries diagnostic process. This outcome depends on interactions among practitioner behaviors, caries detection methods and associated criteria, and changes in the nature of the disease. Considerable effort will be required to meet the obvious need for improvement.

▶ Substantial variations exist among dentists regarding treatment decisions, including criteria for intervention, identification of carious conditions, and diligence in the search for lesions. The restorative decision-making process might necessitate new criteria, diagnostic techniques, and revised criteria for intervention. New roles of visual and tactile assessment are warranted. A test with acceptable performance when caries is prevalent may be unacceptable in terms of its false positive rate when the prevalence of caries is lower. With the lower rate of caries and the decreasing validity of older tests, risk determination of caries based on decayed or filled surface scores may not reflect the true caries experience.—G.F. Currier, D.D.S., M.S.D., M.Ed.

Current Methods and Criteria for Caries Diagnosis in North America
Chan DCN (Univ of Texas Health Science Ctr, San Antonio)
J Dent Educ 57:422–427, 1993   105-94-6-5

Background.—In recent years, European researchers have paid more attention to caries research than North American researchers have. Although the North American procedure relies on finding actual, frequently small cavities, the European system is based on a longer, detailed visual examination. Both systems detect caries by 4 basic techniques: visual examination, tactile examination, radiographic diagnosis and transillumination. Current North American methods and criteria of caries diagnosis were reviewed.

Diagnostic Criteria.—In this era of fluoridated water and increased patient awareness, traditional methods of caries diagnosis may no longer be sufficiently specific or sensitive. Occlusal caries may account for a greater percentage of the caries seen. In North American dental schools, the diagnosis and treatment of caries are often addressed by several departments. The main difference between the North American and European methods of caries detection may be the use of sharp explorers (Table 1). The Europeans believe this method is misleading at best and potentially damaging at worst. It remains useful in the detection of secondary caries in restorations. Binocular magnification loupes and elective temporary tooth separations are potentially useful techniques.

TABLE 1.—The Teaching of the Use of an Explorer in Occlusal Caries Diagnosis

1924	Black	"Passing the explorer into pits...noting whether or not there is any softening, and whether the instrument catches or enters at any point."
1956	Simon	"Recognize change in the continuity of enamel or marginal and submarginal changes around a previously placed restoration. This can be accomplished with a mirror and explorer."
1982	Gilmore	"Susceptible site can be entered using a small sharp explorer or if the enamel is rough, decalcified, or opens to the dentin."
1985	Marzouk	"Sharp explorer...pressing this tip into pits and fissures with forces parallel to the blade will cause it to penetrate the enamel and/or dentinal caries cone, making a definitive diagnosis of decay."
1985	Sturdevant	"Defects are best detected when an explorer placed into a pit or fissure provides tug-back or resistance to removal."

(Courtesy of Chan DCN: *J Dent Educ* 57:422–427, 1993.)

TABLE 2.—Guidelines for Prescribing Dental Radiographs Adapted From HHS
Publication FDA 88-8273, 1987

Patient Category	Child		Adolescent	
	Primary Dentition	Transitional Dentition	Permanent Dentition	Dentulous
New Patient				
All new patients to assess dental diseases and growth and development	Posterior BW exam if proximal surfaces of primary teeth cannot be visualized or probed	Individualized radiographic exam consisting of periapical/ occlusal views and posterior BWs or panoramic exam & posterior BW	Individualized radiographic exam consisting of posterior BWs & elected periapicals. A full mouth intraoral radiographic exam is appropriate when the patients presents with evidence of generalized dental disease or a history of extensive dental treatment	
Recall Patient				
Clinical caries or high-risk factors for caries	Posterior BW exam at 6-month intervals or until no carious lesions are present		Posterior BW exam at 6- to 12-month intervals or until no carious lesions are evident	Posterior BW exam at 12- to 18-month intervals
No clinical caries and no high-risk factors for caries	Posterior BW exam at 12- to 24-months' intervals if proximal surface of primary teeth cannot be visualized or probed.	Posterior BW exam at 12- to 24-month intervals	Posterior BW at 18- to 36-month intervals	Posterior BW at 24- to 36-month intervals

(Courtesy of Chan DCN: *J Dent Educ* 57:422–427, 1993.)

Diagnostic Requirements.—Various stages or grades of caries may be established by visual or radiographic examination, yet most trials use one grade only. Dental schools should emphasize prevention as well as diagnosis and restoration. Prevention requires early diagnosis, and present criteria of diagnosing caries only when cavitation is present do not meet current clinical needs.

Diagnostic Methods.—Radiographic examination is an often essential aspect of caries diagnosis. With the changing pattern and incidence of caries, even the 1987 guidelines of the U.S. Department of Health and Human Services may be excessive (Table 2). Caries risk assessment can permit distinction of patients at high vs. low risk for caries, thus directing the appropriate diagnostic tests and radiographic examination. Although not yet clinically available, dye uptake by enamel lesions would be helpful in diagnosing early caries. In terms of restorations, it seems likely that many carious lesions are being overtreated and retreated.

Conclusion.—The clinician should be careful to choose the best explorer for each application and recognize the different requirements of caries diagnosis. Operative dentistry should treat caries as an infectious disease and adopt standards of diagnosis, recording, and management of initial caries. Educational programs should emphasize initial caries, root caries, and recurrent caries.

▶ Caries is a disease of multifactorial etiology and pathogenesis. The differences in progression of the disease in primary and permanent teeth, in addition to the risk assessment of the patient, necessitate general radiographic guidelines. The radiographic examination should be individualized for each patient, based on the needs from the history and the clinical examination. There is no such word as routine when one is discussing ionizing radiation.—G.F. Currier, D.D.S., M.S.D., M.Ed.

Dilemmas in Caries Diagnosis: Applications to Current Practice and Need for Research
Dodds MWJ (Univ of Texas Health Science Ctr, San Antonio)
J Dent Educ 57:433–438, 1993   105-94-6–6

Objective.—Recent decades have seen significant changes in the nature of dental caries. Along with worldwide reductions in prevalence have come decreases in the predictive values of diagnostic tests. New technologies for caries diagnosis have been developed, but they are unlikely to be incorporated into routine practice in the foreseeable future. An approach to caries diagnosis that will recognize the problems inherent in the diagnostic system is needed.

Sensitivity vs. Specificity.—There are 2 approaches to diagnosing the level of caries activity, one limited to the tooth or tooth surface and the other applied to the patient as a whole. With every treatment decision there is the possibility of a false positive or false negative outcome. Visual diagnosis appears to have a sensitivity of about 60% and a specificity of about 85%, so more lesions may be missed than overdiagnosed. In risk assessment, a false positive result is less harmful than a false negative result.

Classification.—Classification of caries lesions according to tooth site, although helping to define the different diagnostic problems at various sites, does not determine the dynamics of the lesion. The different diagnostic methods are of varying value in the various sites (table). The dentist should use the best available scientific methods for diagnosis while keeping the treatment and outcome possibilities in mind, rather than combining the decision-making processes of diagnosis and treatment. In questionable cases, having more treatment options may ease diagnosis.

Recommendations.—Raising awareness of the need to improve diagnosis will be a major first step in improving caries diagnosis. Educators should know about the new methods of diagnosis and new restorative materials and methods. High-risk patients should be identified by a systematic approach to caries risk, including caries history, diet, fluoride use, microbiological testing, and evaluation of salivary flow rates and

Relative Utility of the Available Diagnostic Systems in Diagnosis of Early (Noncavitated) Lesions

Method	Tooth Site				
	Occlusal	Approximal	Smooth Surface	Root Caries	Recurrent Caries
Visual	+	+*	+	+	-
Tactile	-#	-#	-	+	-
Radiographic	+	+	-	+ (approximal)	+
FOTT[a]	+/-	+	-	-	-
ERM[b]	+	-	-	-	-

[a]Fiber optic transillumination.
[b]Electric resistance measurements.
Note: + indicates that the method is useful; - indicates that the method is not useful; +/- indicates equivocal findings; * after tooth separation; # indicates potential for fracture of intact surface enamel into subsurface demineralized areas.
(Courtesy of Dodds MWJ: *J Dent Educ* 57:433-438, 1993.)

buffer capacity. Assessment of lesion status and activity, sometimes available only by longitudinal evaluation, may also be useful. Additional research is needed in key areas, such as the natural progression of the lesion, data on specific risk groups, and better ways to differentiate progressive from static or remineralizing lesions.

▶ The sensitivity of a given test is defined by the probability of that test giving a positive finding when the disease is present; specificity is the probability of a negative finding when the disease is absent. With 60% sensitivity and 85% specificity, more lesions are potentially missed than are overdiagnosed. A false positive result from a risk assessment test would be less harmful than a false negative finding, because a caries-active patient might be missed and he or she might have disease develop without preventive intervention.—G.F. Currier, D.D.S., M.S.D., M.Ed.

Salivary Flow

Salivary Clearance From Different Regions of the Mouth in Children
Watanabe S (Higashi Nippon Gakuen Univ, Hokkaido, Japan)
Caries Res 26:423–427, 1992   105-94-6-7

Background.—Nursing bottle caries in very young children is a well-known condition that causes rampant decay on the buccal surface of the upper anterior primary teeth. Although microorganisms, tooth structure, and diet as etiologic factors have been studied, there has been little information about the salivary flow rate in children. The rates of salivary clearance in children were investigated.

Methods.—Potassium chloride in an agarose matrix was placed in small acrylic chambers that were attached to the teeth with dental floss. The diffusion chambers were removed from the mouth at selected time intervals and the saliva flow rates were determined by using atomic absorption spectrophotometry to measure the extracted potassium chloride. Seven different sites in the mouth were selected for measurements. Three of the sites were tested while the salivary flow rate was stimulated by having the child suck on sour lemon drops with the diffusion chambers in place. Clearance half-time was defined as the time it took for the initial potassium concentration to decrease by half.

Patients.—The study was done with parental permission in 12 children who had complete primary dentitions. Six children had spaces between their anterior teeth, and 6 children did not. All the children were age 5 years at the time of the study.

Results.—The rate of clearance of substances from agarose gels into saliva varied markedly at different sites. When the salivary flow was unstimulated, the lower anterior lingual (LALi) region had the lowest clearance halftime and the upper anterior buccal (UAB) region had the highest halftime (Table 1). When the salivary flow was stimulated, the clearance halftimes for both the lower anterior buccal (LAB) and the

TABLE 1.—Halftimes (Mean ± Standard Deviation) and Salivary Flow Rates When Salivary Flow Was Unstimulated

Location	LALi	UPLi	LPLi	UPB	LAB	LPB	UAB
Spacing arch (n = 6)							
Halftime, min	5.9 ± 2.8 ‡	9.6 ± 4.8*	9.4 ± 5.4*	14.2 ± 8.8	11.5 ± 6.4	16.1 ± 7.4	24.6 ± 11.4
Flow rate, ml/min	0.4 ± 0.3	0.4 ± 0.2	0.5 ± 0.2	0.4 ± 0.2	0.6 ± 0.3	0.5 ± 0.3	0.6 ± 0.4
No-spacing arch (n = 6)							
Halftime, min	5.3 ± 2.1 ‡	9.1 ± 4.4 †	10.1 ± 5.3*	13.8 ± 6.8	13.8 ± 7.0	17.4 ± 8.1	25.9 ± 9.4
Flow rate, ml/min	0.5 ± 0.3	0.4 ± 0.2	0.5 ± 0.3	0.7 ± 0.4	0.5 ± 0.3	0.4 ± 0.2	0.6 ± 0.4

Abbreviations: UPLi, upper posterior lingual; LPLi, lower posterior lingual; UPB, upper posterior buccal; LPB, lower posterior buccal.
Notes: Halftime in large volume at 37°C = 3.9 minutes. Statistical analyses were done between UAB site and other sites in each group.
* $P < .05$.
† $P < .01$.
‡ $P < .001$.
(Courtesy of Watanabe S: *Caries Res* 26:423–427, 1992.)

TABLE 2.—Halftimes (Mean ± Standard Deviation) and Salivary Flow
Rates When Salivary Flow Was Stimulated

	Location		
	LALi	LAB	UAB
Spacing arch (n = 6)			
Halftime, min	4.0 ± 0.3 †	4.5 ± 0.8 †	11.3 ± 4.5
Flow rate, ml/min	3.4 ± 1.5	4.1 ± 2.1	3.9 ± 1.8
No-spacing arch (n = 6)			
Halftime, min	4.0 ± 0.2 †	9.4 ± 2.8*	15.4 ± 4.2
Flow rate, ml/min	3.7 ± 1.2	3.9 ± 1.7	4.8 ± 1.7

Notes: Halftime in large volume at 37°C = 3.9 minutes. Statistical analyses were done
between UAB site and other sites in each group.
* $P < .05$.
† $P < .01$.
(Courtesy of Watanabe S: *Caries Res* 26:423–427, 1992.)

UAB regions in the 6 children without spaces between their anterior
teeth were significantly higher than those in the 6 children with spaces
(Table 2).

Conclusion.—The UAB region, the site most prone to nursing bottle
caries, has the longest saliva clearance halftime.

▶ One of the reasons that the mandibular teeth usually do not get caries is
the high salivary clearance rate in that region, whereas the maxillary anterior
facial region is worse in terms of salivary clearance. Clearance of stimulated
saliva is poor with nonspaced anterior segments compared with spaced segments. Therefore, the greatest risk for nursing bottle caries is with nonspaced anterior segments, because they have the lowest rate of salivary
clearance. Sleeping children are considered to have even less salivary flow,
which would worsen the problem. However, 5-year-old children have almost
the same mean salivary film thickness as adults.—G.F. Currier, D.D.S., M.S.D.,
M.Ed.

**Intra- and Inter-Individual Variation in Salivary Flow Rate, Buffer Ef-
fect, Lactobacilli, and Mutans Streptococci Among 11- to 12-Year-Old
Schoolchildren**
Tukia-Kulmala H, Tenovuo J (Public Health Care, Salo, Finland; Univ of Turku,
Finland)
Acta Odontol Scand 51:31–37, 1993   105-94-6–8

Objective.—Within-individual and between-individual variations in salivary flow rate, buffer effect, and bacterial counts were analyzed in 128

Clinical Caries Data, Salivary Flow Rate, and Mutans Streptococci of Study Population at Baseline of 9-Month Follow-Up

	Boys ($n = 68$)		Girls ($n = 56$)		
	Mean	SD	Mean	SD	Significance*
DMFS	0.63	1.43	0.70	1.74	NS
DS$_{inc}$†	0.16	0.41	0.37	0.87	NS
Flow rate (ml/min)	1.64	0.57	1.48	0.53	NS
Mutans streptococci‡	5.34	5.64	5.59	5.94	NS

Abbreviation: NS, not significant.
* Student's t test.
† New decayed surfaces (caries increment) during 1-year follow-up.
‡ Log colony-forming units per milliliter; mutans streptococci quantitated with mitis-salivarius-bacitracin agar plates.
(Courtesy of Tukia-Kulmala H, Tenovuo J: *Acta Odontol Scand* 51:31–37, 1993.)

children aged 11 years who were followed up for 9 months. The 68 boys and 60 girls were living in an area where there was less than .3–1 ppm of fluoride in the drinking water. Levels of both streptococci and lactobacilli were estimated. The chairside method (Strip mutans test) was compared with the conventional agar plate method of quantifying mutans streptococci.

Findings.—There were no significant initial differences in decayed, missing, or filled-teeth surfaces (DMFS) indices or salivary variables, ex-

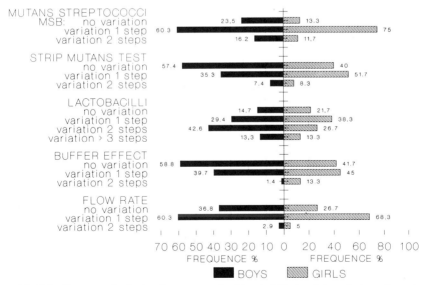

Fig 6–3.—Frequency distribution (in percentages) of intraindividual variations during a 9-month follow-up (6 samples) in salivary mutans streptococci, lactobacilli, buffer effect, and stimulated flow rate of 128 children. (Courtesy of Tukia-Kulmala H, Tenovuo J: *Acta Odontol Scand* 51:31–37, 1993.)

cept for a higher buffer effect in boys (table). The 2 methods for quantifying salivary mutans streptococci correlated to a highly significant degree. Correlations between mutans streptococci and lactobacilli were statistically significant in children with and without earlier caries. Baseline bacterial counts correlated significantly with caries indices, baseline DMFS, and the 1-year caries increment. Intraindividual variations in salivary factors are shown in Figure 6–3. The buffer effect was the most stable variable and lactobacilli the least stable during the 9-month follow-up.

Discussion.—Salivary flow rates in young teenagers continue to increase with age, possibly explaining part of the intrasubject variation observed. The within-subject variation in buffer effect is much greater in girls than in boys. Single-point measurements of salivary variables should not be used to diagnose or predict caries in children whose dentition is developing.

▶ Boys and girls, approximately 11 years of age, demonstrated large intraindividual and interindividual variation in salivary flow rate (65% to 75% had intraindividual variation) and buffer effect (girls lower than boys at 40% vs. 60% with the effect from female sex steroids). The buffer effect was clearly the most stable of the 4 variables; the least stable variable was the lactobacilli during the 9-month follow-up for both boys and girls. A single measure of salivary variables is not good enough to diagnose or predict caries in the developing dentition.—G.F. Currier, D.D.S., M.S.D., M.Ed.

Effect of Time and Duration of Sorbitol Gum Chewing on Plaque Acidogenicity
Park KK, Schemehorn BR, Stookey GK (Indiana Univ, Indianapolis)
Pediatr Dent 15:197–202, 1993   105-94-6-9

Introduction.—Studies have shown that chewing sugarless gum increases the rate of salivary flow, pH, and the buffering capacity of saliva. Results may vary, however, according to the time interval between food ingestion and use of the gum and the duration of gum chewing. How to obtain the maximum reduction of the acidogenic challenge through chewing sorbitol gum was determined.

Methods.—Four starch-containing snacks known to produce a significant plaque pH response were used in the study: pretzels, potato chips, corn chips, and granola bars. The 5 participants (mean age, 37.8 years) were fitted with an indwelling plaque pH telemetry system that continuously monitored the plaque pH responses for 2 hours. After a baseline session in which the foods were ingested according to a randomized block design, the test was repeated with the use of a sorbitol-containing gum. Gum was chewed for 10 minutes beginning after a 15-minute wait in the first test and for 15 minutes after a 5-minute wait in the second test.

TABLE 1.—Area of Plaque pH Curve (pH/Time) Under 5.5

Test Snack	Baseline (No Gum)	Gum Chewing		Chewing Impact (% Reduction)	
		Test 1	Test 2	Test 1	Test 2
Pretzels	6995 ± 1735*	2559 ± 881	197 ± 165 †	64.7 ‡	96.1
Potato chips	9822 ± 1039	1583 ± 836	539 ± 537 ‡	84.3	91.5
Granola bar	10447 ± 1844	3710 ± 2209	292 ± 292	64.5	98.1
Corn chips	12069 ± 1220	7395 ± 3171	4142 ± 1665	34.1	60.5

Test 1: 5-minute baseline pH; 2-minute snack ingestion; 15-minute wait; 20-minute gum chewing; 88-minute monitor.
Test 2: 5-minute baseline pH; 2-minute snack ingestion; 5-minute wait; 15-minute gum chewing; 93-minute monitor.
* Mean ± SEM ($n = 5$).
† Underlined values do not differ significantly.
‡ Percent decrease in area resulting from gum chewing; values are significantly different.
(Courtesy of Park KK, Schemehorn BR, Stookey GK: *Pediatr Dent* 15:197–202, 1993.)

TABLE 2.—The Effect of Gum Chewing on Minimum Plaque pH

Test Snack	No Gum		Gum Chewing Regimen			
			Test 1		Test 2	
Pretzels	4.53 ±	0.10*	4.89 ±	0.11†	5.64 ±	0.26
Potato chips	4.43	0.05	4.90	0.17	5.59	0.28
Granola bars	4.48	0.25	4.90	0.22	5.83	0.16
Corn chips	4.01 ±	0.07	4.48 ±	0.22	4.83 ±	0.25

Test 1: 5-minute baseline pH; 2-minute snack ingestion; 15-minute wait; 10-minute gum chewing; and 88-minute monitor.
Test 2: 5-minute baseline pH; 2-minute snack ingestion; 5-minute wait; 15-minute gum chewing; and 93-minute monitor.
* Mean ± SEM ($n = 5$).
† Underlined values do not differ significantly.
(Courtesy of Park KK, Schemehorn BR, Stookey GK: *Pediatr Dent* 15:197–202, 1993.)

Results.—The acidogenic challenge induced by snack foods was significantly reduced by the salivary stimulation caused by chewing sorbitol gum (Table 1). The gum was more effective when chewing was initiated after 5 minutes than after 15 minutes, and when chewing continued for 15 rather than 10 minutes. In the shorter gum chewing session, only the potato chip group had a significantly higher minimum plaque pH relative to the no-gum session (Table 2). Analysis of the maximum plaque pH decrease from baseline resting plaque pH showed that the first test regimen significantly reduced plaque pH with only 2 of the snack foods; the second test regimen, with the longer period of gum chewing, provided a significant reduction in plaque pH from all 4 snack foods (Table 3).

TABLE 3.—The Effect of Sorbitol Gum Chewing on Maximum Plaque pH Drop
(Baseline Resting pH − Minimum pH Attained)

Test Snack	Baseline (–No Gum)		Gum Chewing Regimen			
			Test 1		Test 2	
Pretzels	2.41 ±	0.08*	2.05 ±	0.08	1.29 ±	0.24
Potato chips	2.47	0.07	2.01	0.15	1.31	0.31†
Granola bars	2.50	0.25	2.08	0.22	1.14	0.17
Corn chips	2.94 ±	0.08	2.47 ±	0.22	2.12 ±	0.30

Test 1: 5-minute baseline pH; 2-minute snack ingestion; 15-minute wait; 10-minute gum chewing; and 88-minute monitor.
Test 2: 5-minute baseline pH; 2-minute snack ingestion; 5-minute wait; 15-minute gum chewing; and 93-minute monitor.
* Mean ± SEM ($n = 5$).
† Underlined values do not differ significantly.
(Courtesy of Park KK, Schemehorn BR, Stookey GK: *Pediatr Dent* 15:197–202, 1993.)

Conclusion.—Chewing sugarless gum after meals and snacks stimulates salivary flow, thereby inhibiting enamel demineralization. If toothbrushing is not possible and chewing gum is recommended, the patient should be advised to use a sugarless gum within 5 minutes after eating and to continue chewing for at least 15 minutes.

▶ Chewing sorbitol gum after eating starch-containing snacks seems to be better than just okay. If one likes to chew gum, one should use the sugarless variety within 5 minutes after eating food, with the idea that sooner is better than later, and one should continue chewing for at least 15 minutes to receive the maximum benefit. Chewing sugarless gum is an adjunct to prevention of caries, but it is not a substitute for tooth brushing. The decrease in plaque acidity is the result of a combination of increased salivary flow and increased buffering capacity attributed to the salivary bicarbonates.—G.F. Currier, D.D.S., M.S.D., M.Ed.

Infectivity

Initial Acquisition of Mutans Streptococci by Infants: Evidence for a Discrete Window of Infectivity
Caufield PW, Cutter GR, Dasanayake AP (Univ of Alabama, Birmingham)
J Dent Res 72:37–45, 1993   105-94-6-10

Introduction.—Because dental caries in animals was ascribed to a transmissible cause, a group of phenotypically similar bacteria, the mutans streptococci, has been implicated as the chief bacterial factor re-

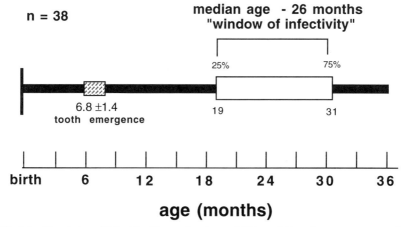

Fig 6–4.—The window of infectivity. The median time to initial acquisition of mutans streptococci for 38 infants is depicted as a function of infant age in months. The average age and standard deviation at emergence of the first primary tooth are also shown for these 38 infants. (Courtesy of Caufield PW, Cutter GR, Dasanayake AP: *J Dent Res* 72:37–45, 1993.)

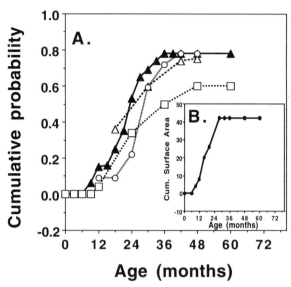

Fig 6–5.—The cumulative probability of mutans streptococci acquisition as a function of child's age in months from the present study (*filled triangle*), and from 3 other longitudinal studies by Carlsson et al. (1975) (*square*), Kohler et al. (1988) (*open triangle*) and Masuda et al. (1979) (*circle*). **B,** the cumulative surface area of the primary dentition as a function of infant age in months. The value for surface area was derived for each tooth type relative to the surface area of the primary incisor, which was assigned a value of 1. Compared with the surface area of an incisor, first molars were assigned a value of 3, second molars were assigned a value of 4, and canines were assigned a value of 1.5. The cumulative surface area at a given period is based on the teeth emerging multiplied by their assigned surface area. Age of emergence represented the average infant age for emergence of each of the primary teeth (Lunt and Law, 1974). (Courtesy of Caufield PW, Cutter GR, Dasanayake AP: *J Dent Res* 72:37-45, 1993.)

sponsible for caries in humans. Mutans streptococci require a hard, non-desquamating surface to colonize, and infants do not harbor them until sometime after the teeth emerge. The mother's salivary level of mutans streptococci may or may not influence the extent of colonization and later caries activity in a child.

Objective.—The levels of oral bacteria were monitored for up to 5 years in 46 mother-child pairs to determine when mutans streptococci are acquired.

Findings.—Thirty-eight of the 46 infants acquired mutans streptococci at a median age of 26 months (Fig 6-4), and three fourths of these infants had acquired mutans streptococci by age 31 months. Although noncolonized children were more often black, gender and the mother's dental history were not significant factors. In infants with mutans streptococci, 58% of subsequent saliva samples and 85% of plaque samples were positive. Mothers of noncolonized children consistently had lower levels of mutans streptococci and lactobacilli in saliva than did mothers of colonized children. The 2 groups of children had had similar numbers of illness episodes necessitating antibiotics.

Discussion.—Children acquire mutans streptococci during a defined time in early life. Acquisition is related to age (Figure 6–5). Several of the children in this study who were not colonized were cared for by persons other than their mothers. The mother's salivary level may be a factor in the acquisition of mutans streptococci by her child.

▶ Dental caries is an infectious, transmissible disease (1). This longitudinal study from birth to between 3 and 6 years of age demonstrated a "window of infectivity" past the median age of 26 months, which is about the time that all 20 primary teeth have erupted. This could be an initial window period, with a second window between 6 and 12 years of age with permanent tooth eruption. However, further evidence is needed to demonstrate this. The principal source of mutans streptococci is the mother, not other individuals.—G.F. Currier, D.D.S., M.S.D., M.Ed.

Reference

1. Keyes PH: *Arch Oral Biol* 1:304, 1960.

Fluoride

Feeding Patterns, Water Sources and Fluoride Exposures of Infants and 1-Year-Olds

Levy SM, Maurice TJ, Jakobsen JR (Univ of Iowa, Iowa City)
J Am Dent Assoc 124(4):65–69, 1993   105-94-6–11

Introduction.—The wide use of fluoride in various forms probably is the chief reason for the decline in caries in children in developed countries, but at the same time there is concern over an increasing prevalence of dental fluorosis. Relatively few studies have dealt with fluoride exposures of young children and the relation between various sources of fluoride and the occurrence of fluorosis.

Study Plan.—Exposure to fluoride was investigated from birth to age 18 months. A group of 107 women who were pregnant or had infants younger than age 6 months participated in the study. Questionnaires dealing with their children's fluoride exposure were completed at 3-month intervals.

Findings.—About 37% of the children received dietary fluoride supplements, more than half of them on a daily basis. Brushing at least once a day increased to 69% at age 18 months. For about 50% of the children aged 12–18 months less than .1 mg of fluoride was used per brushing, but for as many as 16% about .5 mg was used.

Conclusion.—There was considerable variation in young infants with respect to feeding habits, water sources, and the use of dietary fluoride supplements and fluoridated toothpaste. The use of fluoride dentifrices in small amounts is recommended to minimize the risk of fluorosis.

High-concentration dentifrices should be avoided in young children. Dietary fluoride supplements should be used conservatively and only after all sources of water fluoride have been taken into account.

▶ This is an important period to study, because fluoride supplements given up to the age of 2 years are only .25 mg, even though the peak period of potential aesthetic fluorosis is 22 to 28 months. The recommended total intake of fluoride based on caloric needs is around .5 mg from 12 to 18 months. In this study, breast-fed infants aged 3 months were one third of the sample, but at 12 months they were not part of the sample. Mothers were the primary oral hygiene caregivers from 9 to 18 months (65%). Daily toothbrushing increased from 45% to 70% from 12 to 18 months.

This study demonstrated wide variations in feeding habits, water sources, dietary fluoride supplements, and fluoridated toothpastes from birth to 18 months. Even though small amounts of fluoride toothpastes are recommended, no standard method of dispensing such a dentifrice to infants is currently available. Dietary fluoride supplements should be conservatively applied after considering all sources of water fluoride, such as tap, bottled, or filtered, found at home and at child care.—G.F. Currier, D.D.S., M.S.D., M.Ed.

Fluoride Overfeeds in Public Water Supplies
Flanders RA, Marques L (Illinois Dept of Public Health; Illinois Environmental Protection Agency)
Ill Dent J 62:165–169, 1993   105-94-6-12

Two Incidents.—A fluoride overfeed took place in the community water system of Hooper Bay, Alaska, in 1992. About 90 individuals became ill, mainly with nausea, vomiting, and abdominal pain. There was 1 death. Most of those who became ill lived in a part of town that obtained water from a well. Water samples from the well contained as much as 150 ppm of fluoride. When the well was turned off, the water in the holding tank contained 61 ppm. In 1988, a water sample from a subdivision in Illinois was found to contain 1,289 ppm of fluoride. There was no illness, and an investigation showed that this value was not representative of water in the system at the subdivision, but rather had been collected at an outlet close to the fluoride injection port where a slug of fluoride solution was in the line.

Overview.—Most deaths from fluoride toxicity have occurred when fluoride compounds were accidentally substituted for household cooking ingredients or have resulted from industrial accidents. Two deaths have been reported from fluoride used in dental prophylaxis. One death associated with community drinking water occurred after a renal dialysis procedure. Acute fluoride toxicity produces chiefly gastrointestinal problems. A number of overfeeds in school water fluoridation systems have produced illness in school children. Because of the many factors influencing absorption of fluoride, it is quite difficult to specify the exact level of fluoride in drinking water that will have adverse effects on health.

Recommendation.—The continuing safety of fluoridation programs depends on maintaining optimal fluoride levels, and this in turn depends on monitoring and on the formulation of specific guidelines to prevent fluoride overfeeds.

▶ The 1992 Alaskan case was the first reported death resulting from fluoride toxicity caused by drinking water from a community water system. More than 9,000 water systems in 8,081 communities that provide fluoridated drinking water to more than 130 million individuals in the United States. Daily monitoring of fluoride levels is essential. Most of the overfeeds have occurred in small water supplies (fewer than 2,000 individuals). In the Hooper Bay incident, the holding tank had 61 ppm of fluoride.

Three factors contribute most often to overfeeds: (1) operator error resulting from inadequate knowledge; (2) defective design of equipment; (3) equipment failure.

The 2 fatal cases of fluoride toxicity related to dental prophylaxis occurred in 3-year-old children. One went into cardiorespiratory arrest after apparently swallowing several ounces of a 4% stannous fluoride solution after prophylaxis, and the other swallowed 200 1-mg sodium fluoride tablets. The child reportedly vomited and seemed to recover but later died of cardiorespiratory arrest.

The probable toxic dose (PTD) of oral fluoride is 5 mg/kg of body weight. In a child younger than 7 years of age, a dose of 4 mg/kg could be fatal. In children aged 7 to 18 years, 15 mg/kg could be fatal. In an adult, 32 mg/kg could be fatal.

Symptoms of acute fluoride toxicity resulting from any source include sudden onset of nausea and vomiting, with burning, cramplike abdominal pains and diarrhea. Other signs and symptoms may include salivation, tearing, oral or nasal mucous discharge, headache, and generalized weakness.—G.F. Currier, D.D.S., M.S.D., M.Ed.

Appropriate Use of Fluorides in the 1990s
Clark DC (Univ of British Columbia, Vancouver)
J Can Dent Assoc 59:272–279, 1993   105-94-6–13

Objective.—A workshop was conducted in 1992 to review and revise the existing recommendations for the use of fluorides in Canada. One reason for the meeting was the recognition that the levels of fluoride in dental materials may no longer be appropriate, because most Canadians today are exposed to fluoride from more than 1 source.

Caries Prevention.—Previously, fluorides were thought to prevent caries mainly by increasing tooth resistance to acid demineralization when incorporated into the outer enamel surface. Inhibition of bacterial en-

TABLE 1.—Prevalence of Dental Fluorosis Scores Reported From Nonfluoridated Areas

Study Group	Exam Year	Age	Fluoride Intake Period	Percent Distribution of Scores			
				None	Very mild/mild	Mod/severe	Total*
Segreto et al.	1980	7-18	1962-79	74.6	25.4		25.4
Driscoll et al.	1980	8-16	1964-78	94.1	5.9	0.0	5.9
Leverett	1981	7-17	1964-80	95.6			4.4
Ismail et al.	1987 Public	11-17	1970-82	68.9			31.1
	Private	11-17		69.9			30.1

zymes also was implicated. Recent studies have suggested that remineralization is the chief mechanism involved in preventing caries. Another has suggested that the most critical time for fluoride exposure is from tooth emergence to the establishment of interproximal contact and full occlusion.

Fluorosis.—Dental fluorosis may have increased in recent years in Canada. Prevalence rates probably range from 20% to 45% in non-

Study	Year	Age	Period				
Hargreaves et al.	1987	6-13	1974-87	85			15
Pendrys et al.	1988	11-14	1974-83	74.8			25.2
Woolfolk et al.	1987	9-13	1974-84	77.7	21.4		21.4
Szpunar & Burt	1986	6-12	1974-86	87.8	12.2	0.0	15.0
Ismail et al.	1991	10-12	1979-87	41.5			41.5
Clark et al	1991	6-14	1977-91	45.0	53.0	1.0	55.0

* Percent of tooth surfaces affected.
(Courtesy of Clark DC: *J Can Dent Assoc* 59:272-279, 1993.)

fluoridated areas (Table 1) and from 35% to 60% in fluoridated communities (Table 2). The chief sources of ingested fluoride are fluoridated water, drinks, and juices and dentifrices. Children younger than age 6 years take in significant fluoride from dentifrices (Table 3).

Forms of Fluoridation.—It is now recommended that chewable fluoride supplements be used in targeted individuals and groups of children aged 3 years and older in areas where the water fluoride level is less than

TABLE 2.—Prevalence of Dental Fluorosis Reported From Optimally Fluoridated Areas

Study Group	Exam Year	Age	Fluoride Intake Period	Percent Distribution of Scores			
				None	Very mild/mild	Mod/severe	Total*
Segreto et al.	1984	7-18	1962-78	39.6	60.1	0.3	60.4
Driscoll et al.	1980	8-16	1964-78	84.5	15.5	0.0	15.5
Leverett	1981	7-17	1964-80	73.1			26.9
Heifetz et al.*	1980	8-10	1970-78	81.1	8.7	0.1	18.8
	1980	13-15	1965-73	88.6	11.4	0.0	11.4
		8-10	1975-83	72.0	28.0	0.1	28.1
		13-15	1970-78	70.7	29.3	0.0	29.3
Szpunar & Burt	1986	6-12	1974-84	51.0	49.0	0.0	48.4
Williams & Zwemer	1988	12-14	1974-82	19.1	66.9	14.0	80.9
Ismail et al.	1991	10-12	1979-87	31.8			69.2
Clark et al.	1991	6-14	1977-91	35.0	63.0	2.0	65.0

* Percent of surfaces affected.
(Courtesy of Clark DC: J Can Dent Assoc 59:272–279, 1993.)

.3 ppm (Table 4). Patient compliance is an important factor in the overall efficacy of fluoride supplements. Ending the use of supplements probably would reduce dental fluorosis at the cost of a small increase in caries in a small segment of school-age children. The use of a fluoride dentifrice by young children should by supervised by adults. Only a pea-

TABLE 3.—Dentrifice Usage and Ingestion by Young Children (per Toothbrushing)

Age of Child	Dentifrice Used (g)*	Dentifrice Ingested (%)	Fluoride Intake (mg)
2	0.62	65	0.33
3	0.50	36	0.18
4	0.45	49	0.22
3-6	1.38	28	0.39
6-7	0.44	27	0.12
7	0.50	34	0.16

(Courtesy of Clark DC: *J Can Dent Assoc* 59:272-279, 1993.)

sized amount of toothpaste should be used. Professionally applied topical fluorides are useful on a selective basis, although there are problems in defining a high risk of caries.

▶ Posteruptive remineralization is the current fluoride-tooth preventive model. The cumulative effect on the overall growing population from water fluoridation and fluoride toothpastes has focused attention on the more limited use of fluoride supplements and professionally applied topical fluorides. Ingestion of toothpaste and an excess quantity of paste given to children younger than 6 years of age remain a large problem.—G.F. Currier, D.D.S., M.S.D., M.Ed.

TABLE 4.—Revised Fluoride Supplement Regimen

Age of Child	Fluoride in Water Supply < 0.3 ppm F
3,4, & 5	0.25 mg* F/day
6 + years	1.0 mg F/day

* If there is no regular use of fluoridated toothpaste, then .5 mg is recommended.
(Courtesy of Clark DC: *J Can Dent Assoc* 59:272-279, 1993.)

7 Endodontics and Pulp Biology

Introduction

In the 1993 YEAR BOOK OF DENTISTRY, I discussed the fact that end-odontic practice is very dependent on techniques and devices. When new developments arrive on the endodontic scene, they are often heavily promoted long before adequate scientific investigation is complete. We must, as dental professionals, critically review the scientific literature relative to such developments before embracing them.

I believe every practitioner has the right to ask whether a new development will lead to better care or facilitate the delivery of care. If a new development does not do one or both of these, then we must question whether there is any reason to adopt this development in our practices. Indeed, we have seen that, time and again, when new developments with no scientific basis were introduced, they actually led to less effective or efficient dental care.

This year I have selected 12 articles for inclusion in this chapter; they provide scientific insights important to the delivery of effective and efficient endodontic therapy, address important new areas in the field of endodontics, and contribute significantly to the scientific basis of clinical endodontics. The articles address endodontic anesthesia, the use of sonics and ultrasonics in canal preparation, endodontic irrigation effectiveness, endodontic leakage from the coronal aspect, and endodontic aids to facilitate treatment.

In the 1993 YEAR BOOK, I stated that although the articles reviewed did shed considerable scientific light on the topics addressed, no individual article provided complete definitive answers, nor were all the facets of a particular clinical question addressed. This comment is also apropos for the articles included in the 1994 YEAR BOOK. Because of this, in addition to the short comments that follow each abstract, I have provided more extensive comments overviewing a topic area, e.g., endodontic anesthesia, where appropriate. This is designed to provide a more comprehensive look at the topic while highlighting unanswered questions and discussing their clinical relevance.

Kenneth L. Zakariasen, D.D.S., M.S., Ph.D.

Endodontic Anesthesia

Endodontic Anesthesia in Mandibular Molars: A Clinical Study

Cohen HP, Cha BY, Spångberg LSW (New Haven, Conn; Univ of Connecticut, Farmington)
J Endodont 19:370–372, 1993   105-94-7-1

Objective.—The anesthetic effectiveness of 3% mepirocaine was compared with that of 2% lidocaine containing 1:100,000 epinephrine in 61 patients with mandibular molar teeth affected by irreversible pulpitis.

Methods.—Twenty-seven patients received an inferior alveolar nerve block with 2% lidocaine with epinephrine, and 34 others received 3% mepivacaine with no vasoconstrictor. Pulp anesthesia was estimated using dichlorodifluormethane (DDM). Patients whose response to DDM was positive received a periodontal ligament injection of lidocaine with epinephrine. All of the teeth were responsive to cold.

Results.—More than a third of the patients given lidocaine remained sensitive to the DDM cold test after 5 minutes. Two DDM-insensitive teeth required intrapulpal injection to achieve surgical anesthesia. The success rate of lidocaine was 55%, and the rate for mepivacaine was the same. Of 23 teeth that remained sensitive to the DDM cold test after inferior alveolar nerve block, 73% were insensitive after the initial periodontal ligament injection. Six teeth required a second injection, and 1 of these required intrapulpal anesthesia. The DDM cold test was 92% effective overall in confirming pulpal anesthesia.

Implications.—When the standard inferior alveolar nerve block fails to provide adequate pulpal anesthesia, periodontal ligament injection is quite effective. Apparent lip anesthesia does not ensure adequate pulpal anesthesia. All vital teeth should be tested before treatment begins. Dichlorodifluormethane is a simple and very reliable indicator of pulpal anesthesia.

▶ This study is noteworthy for several reasons. It evaluated patients who exhibited irreversible pulpitis, and the research methods included obtaining access to the pulp. In clinical practice, vital teeth being opened for endodontic reasons usually exhibit irreversible pulpitis that may affect the responses to anesthesia; therefore, the anesthesia must be profound enough to allow access to the pulp with no or minimal discomfort to the patient. This study included these factors in its design, and it thus maintained very good clinical relevancy.

In addition, it found that cold, at least in the form of DDM, was a reliable method for determining pulp anesthesia, whereas lip anesthesia was not a reliable indicator. In clinical practice, one could very quickly and easily test an anesthetized tooth with DDM to assess pulpal anesthesia before beginning endodontic therapy. Many practitioners begin endodontic therapy only to find that their anesthesia is less than profound, making it necessary to reanesthetize the area of treatment. Testing with DDM before initiating treatment would eliminate this problem in most cases.

It is interesting to note that the inferior alveolar nerve block (IANB) alone resulted in only slightly more than half of the patients exhibiting pulpal anesthesia. However, in most cases where the IANB was not successful, the periodontal ligament (PDL) injection resulted in pulpal anesthesia. In those few patients who experienced some discomfort on entering the pulp chamber, an intrapulpal injection was used to attain pulpal anesthesia. Thus, in the case of mandibular molar teeth, the practitioner has in his or her armamentarium the IANB, the PDL, and the intrapulpal injection with which to attain profound pulpal anesthesia.—K.L. Zakariasen, D.D.S., M.S., Ph.D.

An Evaluation of 4% Prilocaine and 3% Mepivacaine Compared With 2% Lidocaine (1:100,000 Epinephrine) for Inferior Alveolar Nerve Block

McLean C, Reader A, Beck M, Meyers WJ (York, Pa; Ohio State Univ, Columbus)

J Endodont 19:146–150, 1993   105-94-7-2

Background.—An inferior alveolar nerve block (IANB) does not always provide total pulpal anesthesia. Both 3% mepivacaine and 4% prilocaine are commonly used for dental anesthesia. Most studies evaluating these preparations have not used standard stimuli to quantify anesthesia.

Objective and Methods.—The degree of anesthesia achieved with 3% mepivacaine and 4% prilocaine was compared with that obtained using 2% lidocaine with 1:100,000 epinephrine when used for IANB. Thirty adults aged 24–43 years participated in the study. Each subject received each of the preparations at 1-week intervals. A 1.8 mL volume was used in all instances. The first molar, first premolar, lateral incisor, and contralateral canine were pulp tested in a blind manner over 50 minutes. A successful result was defined as a lack of subject response to the maximum output (80 reading) within 16 minutes.

Results.—All subjects achieved lip and tongue numbness, and at least 90% gained mental and lingual mucosal anesthesia. The rate of buccal nerve anesthesia was 73%. Excluding failures, pulpal anesthesia began after 8–17 minutes with all anesthetics. The time course of pulp anesthesia was similar for the various preparations in most comparisons. Anesthetic failures were least frequent in premolar teeth and most frequent in the lateral incisors. Success rates were comparable with all the anesthetics, as were the rates of slow-onset and noncontinuous anesthesia and anesthesia of short duration.

Implications.—Numbness of the lip and mucosa may not necessarily indicate pulp anesthesia. The preparations tested in this study were equally effective in blocking the inferior alveolar nerve. Once pulpal anesthesia was achieved, its duration was generally adequate.

▶ This study varies substantially from the previous study (Abstract 105-94-7-1) in that patients with normal pulpal tissues were used and no access was made into the pulp. However, the results for successful mandibular molar pulpal anesthesia were very similar, i.e., 43% to 63% of molars. In the previous study, 55% of molars exhibited pulpal anesthesia after the IANB. Comparing the results of this study with those of the first study would seem to indicate that inflammation of the pulp does not in fact make pulpal anesthesia less effective. This was also the opinion of the authors of the first study. It appears that, whether the pulp is inflamed, the incidence of anesthetic success with the IANB is far less than we would desire. This points out the need for adjunctive anesthetic methods as discussed in the first study, i.e., periodontal ligament and intrapulpal injections.

This study found no differences between the various anesthetics that were used. The first study tested 2 of these anesthetics and likewise found no significant differences. Prilocaine, mepivacaine, and lidocaine are 3 of the most frequently used local anesthetics in dentistry. Many practitioners would claim that there are distinct differences in anesthetic effectiveness among these various anesthetics. This highlights the importance of testing anecdotal reports using well-designed clinical trials.—K.L. Zakariasen, D.D.S., M.S., Ph.D.

Electron Microscopic Changes in Human Pulps After Intraligamental Injection
Torabinejad M, Peters DL, Peckham N, Rentchler LR, Richardson J (Loma Linda Univ, Calif; Corona, Calif)
Oral Surg Oral Med Oral Pathol 76:219–224, 1993   105-94-7-3

Introduction.—Intraligamental injections are commonly used for supplemental local anesthesia in patients undergoing dental procedures. The advantages of intraligamental injection have made the technique popular for teeth with normal and diseased pulps. This is the first electron microscopic study to investigate changes in human pulps after intraligamental injection.

Methods.—Specimens were obtained from 96 human mandibular and maxillary premolar teeth extracted for orthodontic reasons. Only teeth without prior decay, restoration, or peridontal involvement were used. Teeth that did not respond to an electric pulp tester were not included. Forty-two teeth were randomly anesthetized with intraligamental injections of 2% lidocaine, 1:100,000 epinephrine through a 30-gauge short needle (experimental group). The contralateral premolars were anesthetized by either nerve or field blocks of the same anesthetic solutions (control group). Six teeth were extracted for each time interval of 0 to 15 minutes, 1 hour, 6 hours, 24 hours, 72 hours, 1 week, and 4 weeks. Twelve premolars (group C) were anesthetized with the control technique, extracted, and their pulps placed in physiologic saline solution for periods ranging from 15 minutes to 6 hours. These pulp specimens were used to study the effects of ischemia on odontoblasts.

Results.—Fifteen-minute and 1-hour samples from both experimental and control groups showed no cellular changes. Odontoblasts in both groups showed mitochondrial swelling, some chromatin clumping, and irregular nuclear membranes in the 6-hour and 72-hour specimens. No significant cellular changes were observed in the 1-week and 4-week samples. After 1 hour of ischemia, however, group C samples showed distinct chromatin clumping in the nuclei of odontoblasts. Wrinkling of the nuclear membrane and cytoplasmic mitochondrial swelling were also apparent.

Conclusion.—No permanent odontoblastic changes were found in these young human premolars.

▶ It was pointed out in the first 2 abstracts on dental anesthesia (Abstracts 105-94-7–1 and 105-94-7–2) that injection of the periodontal ligament (PDL) is frequently necessary to achieve satisfactory pulpal anesthesia. Most studies in the literature report that damage to the periodontal ligament from the PDL injection is minimal and transient. However, it is known that PDL injection of local anesthetics with epinephrine can cause marked reduction in pulpal blood flow, thus raising questions as to how this may affect pulpal tissues. When the PDL injection is being used for pulpal anesthesia during endodontic therapy, the pulp is removed and pulpal effects caused by ischemia would not be of concern. However, the PDL injection is also used for restorative procedures where the pulp is vital and normal, and we wish it to remain that way. Light microscopic examination of pulps anesthetized by PDL injection have not shown pathologic changes.

This study uses electron microscopic examination to look for changes in human pulps after the PDL injection. Although a previous electron microscopic study showed that odontoblasts are the cells most sensitive to ischemia, this study found that the PDL injection appears to cause no long-term pathologic effects on the pulps of young human premolars. However, these teeth had not experienced decay, restoration or periodontal involvement. As the authors of this paper point out, further study is needed on the possible effects of the PDL injection on vital pulps of mature teeth, both with and without permanent restorations. Until that is done, definitive answers will not be known regarding the potential effects on vital human pulps after the PDL injection.—K.L. Zakariasen, D.D.S., M.S., Ph.D.

▶ *Additional Comment:* The first 2 studies in this group compared local anesthetics without vasoconstrictors with a local anesthetic containing a vasoconstrictor. Although neither study shows differences in the anesthetic effects, as practitioners we must be concerned with both the local and systemic effects of vasoconstrictors. For example, in a medically compromised patient, vasoconstrictors may be contraindicated. If the inferior alveolar nerve block is administered and is not successful, the dentist is then faced with using the periodontal (PDL) injection. However, it has been reported that the PDL injection does not work well without the vasoconstrictor, i.e., the success rate for anesthesia is low and, even when successful, the duration of anesthesia is very short. If the dentist were to use local anesthetic with vasoconstrictor for the PDL injection, the reality is that an intraosseous injection is actually being used, which can lead to a vascular introduction of epinephrine and systemic effects. Each practitioner must thoroughly understand the systemic conditions of each patient and what potential complications could arise. For medically compromised patients, it is often very helpful to seek a medical consultation to arrive at the safest method for handling the patient in question.—K.L. Zakariasen, D.D.S., M.S., Ph.D.

Sonics and Ultrasonics

Today's Sonics: Using the Combined Hand/Sonic Endodontic Technique

Zakariasen KL, Zakariasen KA, McMinn MM (Dalhousie Univ, Halifax, NS)
J Am Dent Assoc 123(10):67–78, 1992   105-94-7-4

Introduction.—A technique has been developed that uses sonics to effectively and safely prepare most root canals. Apical preparations should be done with hand instrumentation, but sonic instrumentation may be used to achieve a smooth, tapered root canal by reducing dentin.

Instrumentation.—The Rispisonic and Canal Shaper instruments of the Sonic Air system can efficiently flare even small, curved root canals without ledging when properly used. These instruments have small rounded barbs that constitute their cutting edge. The completed preparation has an apical canal diameter that is much smaller than the coronal diameter.

Technique.—For this combined technique, hand instruments always are used for initial canal penetration, the apical preparation, and final smoothing or finishing of the tapered canal preparation. Most practitioners prefer the K-type file, but the Hedstrom file makes it easier to flare or taper the canal, particularly when used in a circumferential filing action. The access opening is placed so as to gain unrestricted straight-line access to the root canals. The canal is penetrated to within about 3 mm of the apex and then gently filed to smooth and slightly enlarge the canal. Sonic preflaring follows, using a continuous circumferential technique and copious irrigation. The working length generally is .5–1 mm short of the radiographic apex. Finally, the canal is penetrated to full working length by using a precurved no. 10 K-type or Hedstrom file. The last step is to blend the apical preparation with the preflared canal space and provide a more marked flare.

Discussion.—This approach effectively combines hand instrumentation for some aspects of the preparative procedure with sonics for the bulk of the canal flaring and enlargement. Both hand and sonic techniques require a light hand and care to avoid ledging when making curvatures.

▶ This article presents a very simple and straightforward technique for the application of sonics to the preparation of root canals before obturation. It is important to note that the technique uses hand instrumentation as the preferred method for initial canal penetration, apical preparation, and finishing of the prepared canal. Sonics, on the other hand, is used for the majority of the canal flaring, i.e., tapered enlargement, even in small curved canals.

It should be noted that all root canal instrumentation is very technique-sensitive. However, with the use of sonics, an overly aggressive, "heavy-handed" technique will almost certainly result in ledges being formed. When using sonics, it is important that the practitioner pull back immediately if it feels like the instrument tip is "bottoming out" in a curvature. When the instrument is "bottoming out", the tip is actually hitting the outside of the curvature and a ledge can quickly form.—K.L. Zakariasen, D.D.S., M.S., Ph.D.

An In Vivo Evaluation of the Efficacy of Ultrasound After Step-Back Preparation in Mandibular Molars
Archer R, Reader A, Nist R, Beck M, Meyers WJ (Naval Hosp, Portsmouth, Va; Ohio State Univ, Columbus)
J Endodont 18:549–552, 1992   105-94-7–5

Objective.—A histologic study was undertaken to compare the effectiveness of a step-back technique with that of a combined step-back and ultrasound method when debriding the mesial root canals of vital mandibular molars in vivo. Thirty-seven healthy adults participated in the study.

Methods.—The 17 mesial roots in group 1 were prepared by a step-back technique using intermittent irrigation with 5.25% sodium hypochlorite. Each canal was enlarged about 3 file sizes more than the first file that bound at the working length. The 17 mesial roots in group 2 were treated similarly, followed by 3 minutes of ultrasonic instrumentation using a no. 15 Endosonic file in an Enac unit set at 3.5. Additional sodium hypochlorite was used during ultrasonic preparation. Eight noninstrumented molars served as histologic controls.

Results.—The canal and isthmus were significantly cleaner at all apical levels when the ultrasonic technique was used.

Conclusion.—If the goal of treatment is complete debridement, adding ultrasound treatment to the step-back preparation should improve the outcome.

▶ This study demonstrates that the addition of ultrasonic cleaning of the root canal after hand step-back preparation can lead to significantly cleaner canals. Similar results have been found by other investigators for both ultrasonics and sonics. In this particular study, the ultrasonic preparation added an additional 3 minutes of canal preparation beyond the normal step-back filing used in both the control and experimental groups. It would have been interesting if the canals in the experimental groups had been flared by ultrasonic preparation instead of by step-back filing with the ultrasonic preparation as an add-on step. In the practice situation, it would be much more desirable to use the ultrasonic system for canal flaring in place of the step-back filing so that both canal enlargement and cleansing were being accomplished by the ultrasonics. Otherwise, ultrasonic preparation is simply an added step that will make the instrumentation time longer.

The increased cleanliness in the canals demonstrated in this study is not surprising given that sonic and ultrasonic devices are extremely effective in carrying irrigants to the tip of the instrument. The irrigant then flows back out through the canal orifice, ensuring that there is constant flow of irrigant through the root canal system during sonic and ultrasonic instrumentation. This certainly does not occur during hand instrumentation using syringe irrigation of the canals.—K.L. Zakariasen, D.D.S., M.S., Ph.D.

▶ *Additional Comment:* It has been my observation both from clinical practice and research investigations that sonic and ultrasonic devices generally irrigate extremely well down to the tip of the instrument. Thus, if the sonic or ultrasonic file is placed into the apical region, these devices will irrigate very effectively most of the canal space. However, it is also my experience that there are considerable differences between the various sonic and ultrasonic devices regarding their ability to cut dentin and thus effectively flare the root canal during instrumentation. If you are considering the use of sonics or ultrasonics in your practice, it is a wise idea to try the various devices on simulated plastic canals or extracted teeth to determine which device and files works best for you. Doing so will avoid the purchase of an instrumentation system that does not measure up to your expectations for both canal enlargement and irrigation and therefore sits on a shelf in the back room. We have all had too many experiences with materials and devices that do not live up to their claims.—K.L. Zakariasen, D.D.S., M.S., Ph.D.

Endodontic Irrigation

Efficacy of Several Concentrations of Sodium Hypochlorite for Root Canal Irrigation

Baumgartner JC, Cuenin PR (United States Army Inst of Dental Research, Washington, DC)

J Endodont 18:605–612, 1992   105-94-7-6

Objective.—Sodium hypochlorite (NaOCl) has several properties that provide effective chemomechanical débridement of the root canal system. Several concentrations of NaOCl, delivered with a needle or an ultrasonic device in the middle third of the root canal, were evaluated.

Methods.—Matched pairs of single canal bicuspids, extracted for orthodontic purposes, were used to compare the effects of NaOCl when used in concentrations of .5%, 1%, 2.5%, and 5.25%. Both instrumented and noninstrumented surfaces of root canal walls were examined by scanning electron microscopy.

Results.—All concentrations of NaOCl, delivered by either method, were effective in flushing out loose debris from the root canals. All instrumented surfaces exhibited a smear layer with some exposed dentinal tubules. All preparations except .5% NaOCl totally removed pulp remnants and predentin from the uninstrumented canal surfaces. The weak preparation removed most of this material, but left some fibrils on the surface of the mineralized dentin and adjacent calcospherites.

Conclusion.—Sodium hypochlorite can physically remove superficial debris from the root canal surfaces and can at the same time chemically remove organic pulp debris and predentin from noninstrumented areas of the root canal.

▶ This study found that 1%, 2.5%, and 5.25% NaOCl solutions were equally effective in cleansing canals whether they were delivered by endodontic irrigation needle or an ultrasonic device. However, it must be noted that large, single-canal bicuspid teeth were used for this study, and that the middle thirds of the root canals were studied. As the authors point out, it is probable that different results would have been obtained in the apical third of small curved canals. It is in this region that it is difficult to irrigate with an endodontic syringe, and it is also in such areas where sonics and ultrasonics are particularly effective in carrying the irrigation solution apically. Thus, although the results of this study verify the effectiveness of NaOCl as an endodontic irrigating solution, it should not be assumed that the beneficial effects of this irrigant will be obtained where syringe tips cannot enter. Sonics and ultrasonics clearly have an advantage in such areas.—K.L. Zakariasen, D.D.S., M.S., Ph.D.

Antibacterial Effects of Various Endodontic Irrigants on Selected Anaerobic Bacteria

Ohara P, Torabinejad M, Kettering JD (Loma Linda Univ, Calif)
Endodont Dent Traumatol 9:95–100, 1993   105-94-7-7

Objective.—Several irrigant solutions have been used to treat root canal infections. Most past studies were focused on irrigant effects against facultative or aerobic organisms; in the present study, selected anaerobic bacteria that often are found in infected root canals were examined.

Methods.—The irrigants tested included 5.25% sodium hypochlorite, 3% hydrogen peroxide, 17% ethylenediamine tetraacetic acid (EDTA), .2% chlorhexidine, saturated calcium hydroxide solution, and .9% saline. The organisms (*Peptococcus, Propionibacterium acnes, Veillonella par-*

vula, Lactobacillus, Bacteroides gingivalis, and *Fusobacterium*) were mixed separately with dilutions of each of the irrigants in tubes of fluid thioglycollate broth, and growth was assessed after varying times.

Results.—Chlorhexidine was the most consistently effective antibacterial agent tested. It prevented bacterial growth at all dilutions and all time intervals. Hydrogen peroxide was relatively effective, but lower concentrations required longer exposure times. The EDTA preparation prevented growth at many dilutions, but exposure for longer than 1 hour generally was required. Calcium hydroxide and saline solutions were totally ineffective.

Conclusion.—Chlorhexidine was the most effective antibacterial irrigant in this study, and it may prove useful in endodontic treatment.

▶ This in vitro study of anaerobic bacteria showed that chlorhexidine was the most effective irrigant for antibacterial effects, even in very small concentrations. Sodium hypochlorite was also shown to be very effective in a .5% solution. Although these results are promising, the authors point out that further studies are necessary before chlorhexidine is adopted for use in endodontic therapy. In vitro studies such as this are important, but they are only the first step in assessing chlorhexidine's value for clinical application. At the present time, sodium hypochlorite is still the most widely used endodontic irrigant because of its antibacterial properties *and* its ability to dissolve organic tissues and removed debris.—K.L. Zakariasen, D.D.S., M.S., Ph.D.

Coronal Leakage

Coronal Dye Penetration of the Apical Filling Materials After Post Space Preparation
Ravanshad S, Torabinejad M (Shiraz Univ, Iran; Loma Linda Univ, Calif)
Oral Surg Oral Med Oral Pathol 74:644–647, 1992   105-94-7–8

Introduction.—Most past studies have emphasized leakage in an apical-coronal direction after post space preparation. The integrity of the coronal seal is equally important, because exposure of the coronal seg-

Means and Standard Deviations of Coronal Leakage in Various Groups

Experimental group	Mean leakage (mm)	Standard deviation (mm)
Lateral	1.94	1.022
Vertical	2.15	0.599
Thermafil	3.53	0.944

(Courtesy of Ravanshad S, Torabinejad M: *Oral Surg Oral Med Oral Pathol* 74:644–647, 1992.)

ment of a filled root canal to the oral flora can lead to total recontamination in a brief time.

Methods.—Forty canals of palatal and distal mandibular molar roots were cleaned and shaped using a step-back technique. Thirty of them then were obturated using a lateral, vertical, or Thermafil technique. A thin layer of Roth's root canal sealer was applied to the surfaces of root canals in experimental teeth. Five root canals were obturated without a root canal sealer, and 5 others were obturated and had their coronal halves sealed with sticky wax. The apical 5–6 mm of filling material were exposed to India ink for 48 hours to estimate the degree of leakage.

Results.—Coronal dye leakage was most marked in the apical plugs of the Thermafil group (table). Canals filled by lateral condensation had about the same amount of coronal leakage as those filled by vertical condensation. Ink penetrated the entire root canals in positive control specimens, whereas no dye penetration occurred in the negative control specimens.

Conclusion.—The lateral and vertical condensation techniques produce a better seal, with less coronal leakage, than does the Thermafil method.

▶ It is now thought that coronal leakage is at least as important as apical leakage in regard to endodontic success or failure. Coronal leakage can very easily lead to recontamination of the root canal system and provide a pathway for pathogens to the periapical tissues. This study demonstrates that different obturation techniques can lead to differing amounts of coronal leakage. It should be noted that in this study, the coronal gutta-percha was only exposed to the India ink for a 48-hour period, and yet in the most extensive leakage group, an average of 3.5 mm of leakage had occurred. These teeth only had 5–6 mm of gutta-percha remaining in the apical portion of the canal. It would seem highly probable that given a long-term exposure to coronal fluids, the leakage figures would be much greater than those observed in this study.

The data on coronal microleakage that have appeared in the endodontic literature during the past few years indicate that we must consider coronal leakage very seriously as a potential cause of endodontic failure. Most recall radiographs to determine endodontic success or failure are taken at either 6 months or 1 year. It is quite possible that coronal microleakage clinically may take longer than this to occur, and that cases we initially classify as being successful may, in fact, become failures at some later date because of coronal leakage.—K.L. Zakariasen, D.D.S., M.S., Ph.D.

An Evaluation of Three Materials As Barriers to Coronal Microleakage in Endodontically Treated Teeth

Beckham BM, Anderson RW, Morris CF (Med College of Georgia, Augusta)
J Endodont 19:388–391, 1993   105-94-7-9

Background.—Often only the apical seal is considered when performing endodontic obturation, but the coronal seal may be just as important to the ultimate outcome. Coronal leakage may be a concern in endodontically treated teeth with clinically intact restorations.

Objective.—The efficacy of 3 materials as barriers against coronal microleakage was examined in 70 extracted single-rooted anterior teeth having single canals and intact crowns.

Methods.—The materials evaluated included Barrier Dentin Sealant, GC Glass Ionomer Lining Cement, and TERM. The root canals were accessed, cleaned, shaped, and then obturated with gutta-percha and sealer. Specimens were either stored in a humidor or immersed in artificial saliva for 1 week before being exposed to methylene blue dye.

Results.—Each group had some teeth that exhibited coronal microleakage. Leakage was most marked for glass ionomer-treated specimens stored in artificial saliva and least marked for those treated with Barrier Dentin Sealant and not exposed to saliva. There is relatively great microleakage associated with the use of glass ionomer cement and exposure to saliva.

Recommendation.—The efficacy of Barrier Dentin Sealant, the ease with which it is placed, and its compatibility with amalgam and composite restorations commend its use. A thin layer of the material is used, so that retention of the final restoration is not compromised.

▶ The authors of this study recognize the potential importance of coronal microleakage in the success or failure of endodontic therapy. Under the conditions of this study, glass ionomer cement was unacceptable as a coronal leakage barrier. Although Barrier Dentin Sealant and TERM both showed very good results, the authors note that Barrier Dentin Sealant has advantages clinically; it can be easily placed in a thin layer, and it is compatible with both amalgam and composite restorations. Thus, from both the leakage perspective and the perspective of ease of clinical use and materials compatibility, this material may have significant potential.

This study used very short exposure times to the methylene blue dye solution. In my opinion, this may lead to serious underestimation of the coronal microleakage that can occur. I believe that to be more clinically relevant, such studies should use much longer exposure times to the dyes.—K.L. Zakariasen, D.D.S., M.S., Ph.D.

Clinical Aids

Using Cyanoacrylate to Facilitate Rubber Dam Isolation of Teeth

Roahen JO, Lento CA (Naval Dental School, Bethesda, Md)
J Endodont 18:517–519, 1992   105-94-7–10

Introduction.—Rubber dam isolation is a critical aspect of nonoperative endodontic treatment, but microbiological leakage reportedly occurs in more than half of the procedures. Cyanoacrylate might provide an efficient means of rapidly isolating structurally compromised teeth.

Technique.—After removing any soft caries and drying the tooth, a hole is punched in the rubber dam and the dam is stretched over the remaining tooth structure or surrounding tissue. Isobutyl cyanoacrylate is flowed liberally about the area as the dam is held tightly against the gingival tissue. Either an endodontic plugger or a disposable micropipette may be used. The material air dries in 1-2 minutes. The rubber dam frame then is applied and the procedure is begun. A leak-proof seal will endure for about 60–90 minutes.

Clinical Use.—This method may be used without a rubber dam clamp, such as when there are retained roots that provide alveolar bone height for an overdenture. Cyanoacrylate also may be used in place of a rubber dam clamp in hemophiliac patients and postradiation patients, or when part of the tooth may break away during treatment.

Precautions.—Skin and glove contact must be avoided while the adhesive dries, and patients and staff should wear eye protection. The patient should be asked about a past allergic reaction to adhesive. The pungent fumes can be lessened by high-speed evacuation while drying the adhesive.

▶ This article describes a very interesting and simple way of isolating broken-down teeth with the rubber dam. The obvious advantages are that little tooth preparation is necessary and no restorative material build-up needs to be placed. However, if this technique does not provide sufficient rubber dam retention in a particular case, a bonded composite core can be placed that will allow the placement of a rubber dam clamp for retention of the rubber dam. This bonded composite core technique likewise requires very little preparation of the tooth except for caries removal, but it does require more time to place than does the cyanoacrylate.—K.L. Zakariasen, D.D.S., M.S., Ph.D.

Endodontic Case Selection: To Treat or To Refer

Rosenberg RJ, Goodis HE (Univ of California, San Francisco)
J Am Dent Assoc 123(12):57–63, 1992   105-94-7–11

The Problem.—The conscientious dentist often must decide whether to treat a patient or to make a referral to an endodontic specialist. Most often the decision has been based on a brief assessment and a radiograph. The clinician, in effect, made a personal assessment of how difficult treatment would be.

A Case Selection System.—The University of California at San Francisco (UCSF) Endodontic Case Selection System is a means by which the clinician can evaluate each patient to determine the degree of therapeutic difficulty. A number of factors related to the patient and to the tooth are rated as uncomplicated, moderately complicated, or complicated. If all ratings are uncomplicated, the general dentist usually will do the procedure if experienced with it. Moderate complications or perhaps a single complicating rating may indicate the need for referral to a specialist.

Considerations.—The patient's health and medical history must be taken into account as well as his ability to withstand local anesthesia and any physical limitations that may make treatment more difficult. An accurate diagnosis is basic to any endodontic treatment. A periapical and possibly a bite-wing radiograph must be evaluated. A number of anatomical features must be considered, including the pulp chamber, root curvature, canal calcification, and apex development. The degree of carious tooth destruction is an important factor, as is the type of restoration that exists. If the periodontal status is uncertain, the patient should see a periodontist. All perforating resorptions should be referred for evaluation and treatment. Retreatment is more difficult than initial treatment.

▶ The decision to treat or to refer an endodontic case to a specialist should be made on the basis of an appropriate set of criteria. The UCSF Endodontic Case Selection System brings together all of the pertinent criteria that are necessary for making such a decision. This system appears quick and easy to use, but at the same time it delineates for the practitioner all of the criteria that should be considered. The use of this system will ensure that all appropriate criteria are being considered in a systemic way.—K.L. Zakariasen, D.D.S., M.S., Ph.D.

Accuracy of an Electronic Apex Locator: A Clinical Evaluation in Maxillary Molars
Hembrough JH, Weine FS, Pisano JV, Eskoz N (Loyola Univ, Maywood, Ill)
J Endodont 19:242–246, 1993   105-94-7-12

Introduction.—An accurate estimate of root canal length is critical to the success of endodontic treatment. Maxillary molar teeth have proved to be the major source of problems when calculating endodontic working length.

Objective.—The accuracy of an electronic apex locator was determined, by comparison with radiographic and direct anatomical measurements of tooth length, in 26 maxillary molars from 14 men, aged 47–75 years. The Sono-Explorer Mark III was used to determine root canal length to the apical foramen.

Results.—Radiography provided acceptably accurate estimates of root canal length in 88.5% of the cases, but the electronic method was accurate in only 73.1%. The inaccurate electronic estimates were invariably too long. The distobuccal canal was accurately estimated in only 69.2% of the instances using the electronic method, and the palatal canal was accurately estimated in 76.9%. In 3 instances, the Sono-Explorer failed to indicate the site of the apical foramen.

Conclusion.—Accurate radiographs still are necessary for successful endodontic treatment. An electronic device may prove useful in certain types of cases, but it does not determine root canal length as accurately as the radiograph.

▶ Although the predominant method for determining root length during endodontic therapy has been the radiographic method, electronic apex locators have also been available to practitioners for this purpose. Some practitioners have adopted them for use as an adjunct to the radiographic method, and others have gone so far as to replace the radiographic method with the electronic apex locator method. This in vivo research study comparing radiographic and electronic lengths to direct anatomical measurements indicates that the electronic method is not as reliable as the radiographic method, and that when an error occurs, it is consistently long in determining the length. The radiographic method gave the best results, in spite of the maxillary molar area presenting the most complications for radiographic root length determination. However, there are certainly situations in which the radiographic method is very difficult to use because of factors such as anatomical complexities. In such situations, the electronic apex locator may be a very valuable adjunct to the radiographic method. The results of this study and of several others in the literature do not support the replacement of the radiographic method with the electronic apex locator method.—K.L. Zakariasen, D.D.S., M.S., Ph.D.

8 Lasers in Dentistry

Introduction

The inclusion of a chapter on the use of lasers in dentistry in the 1994 YEAR BOOK OF DENTISTRY is very pertinent given the tremendous interest the dental profession has shown toward the potential applications of this technology to clinical dentistry. An impressive body of scientific literature is developing relative to laser applications in dentistry, and few dental meetings can now be found that do not have at least one presentation on lasers. A review of the literature suggests that lasers will ultimately have a multitude of applications in clinical dentistry. Soft tissue surgery, hard tissue surgery to remove decay and shape cavity preparations, laser etching of tooth structure, laser inhibition of the caries process, endodontic procedures, and laser diagnosis of incipient decay are some of the areas that show much promise today. Research into these and other areas will certainly lead to other applications for lasers in dentistry that we have not even contemplated at present.

However, as with most new developments in dentistry, some proponents of this new technology have heavily promoted it for clinical applications far before scientific investigation is complete. This has the potential for serious consequences, given that laser energy, when used improperly, can cause serious damage to biological tissues. It is extremely important to know how laser light interacts with tissues and that these interactions are highly dependent on the laser wavelength being used.

The six articles selected for this chapter cover a wide variety of laser topics. The first article addresses laser tissue interactions and will help to clarify the role of lasers as described in the subsequent articles. These articles cover the potential use of lasers for cutting dental hard tissues, for curing composite resins, for inhibiting the formation of carious lesions, and, in endodontics, for sealing off dental tubules and killing microorganisms. These articles should provide valuable perspectives on these fascinating new developments in dentistry. As someone who has been involved in researching the applications of lasers in dentistry for the past 10 years, I am confident that lasers will play a very large role in the provision of dental care. However, it is incumbent on the profession to only implement new applications when they are properly validated by very good dental science.

Kenneth L. Zakariasen, D.D.S., M.S., Ph.D.

Laser/Tissue Interaction: What Happens to Laser Light When It Strikes Tissue?

Dederich DN (Univ of Alberta, Edmonton)
J Am Dent Assoc 124(2):57–61, 1993   105-94-8-1

The Fate of Laser Light.—Laser light that strikes a tissue surface may be reflected outward, scattered, absorbed after a characteristic amount of scattering, or transmitted beyond a given tissue boundary. It is absorption that is responsible for the thermal effects of laser energy within the tissue.

Factors in Absorption.—The wavelength of laser light is the primary determinant of its absorption, and it therefore determines the type of reaction that takes place between the laser energy and the tissue. The extent of this interaction depends on the amount of energy delivered and the properties of the tissue. Pigmented tissue, for instance, absorbes more Nd:YAG laser energy than do nonpigmented tissues, making it necessary to consider the risk to periradicular tissues if this laser is used within a root canal or to remove caries. The Nd:YAG laser eventually will warm dentin to the point of charring, at which point tissue darkening abruptly increases the absorption of light. Both the continuous-wave and the pulsed Nd:YAG lasers have unreliable effects on dentin. Energy from the CO_2 laser is so well absorbed by tissues that virtually none penetrates beyond .1 mm.

▶ An understanding of laser/tissue interactions and the importance of the laser wavelength is critical when considering the use of lasers in dental practice. Without this understanding, inappropriate lasers or inappropriate exposure parameters can easily be selected that may lead to serious tissue damage. With appropriate attention to these factors, lasers have enormous potential in the practice of dentistry.—K.L. Zakariasen, D.D.S., M.S., Ph.D.

The Effect of Lasers on Dental Hard Tissues

Wigdor H, Abt E, Ashrafi S, Walsh JT Jr (Ravenswood Hosp, Chicago; Univ of Illinois, Chicago)
J Am Dent Assoc 124(2):65–70, 1993   105-94-8-2

Background.—The dental community is actively seeking a method to remove diseased and healthy dental hard tissues without the negative effects associated with dental handpieces. Lasers are currently being considered as possible replacements. A study was undertaken to evaluate the effects of the erbium:YAG (Er:YAG) Nd:YAG, and CO_2 lasers on dentin and pulpal tissues.

Methods.—In vitro studies were first conducted using 4 freshly extracted, enamel-free, human anterior teeth. Teeth were treated with 1 of 4 modalities, including a size-4 round carbide bur on a slow-speed den-

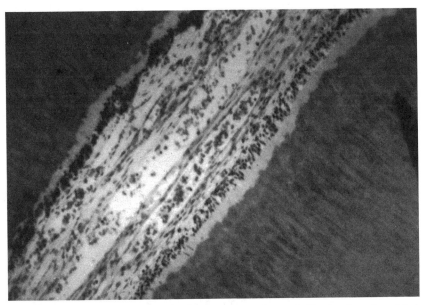

Fig 8–1.—Photomicrograph of dental pulp in an untreated control. Hematoxylin-eosin; original magnification, ×400. (Courtesy of Wigdor H, Abt E, Ashrafi S, et al: *J Am Dent Assoc* 124(2):65–70, 1993.)

tal handpiece at about 10,000 rpm; a CO_2 laser set to emit .1-second-long pulses of 10.6-μm radiation at 5 Hz; an Nd:YAG laser adjusted to 12.5 W continuous wave, 1.06-μm radiation through a 2-mm quartz fiber; or an Er:YAG laser set to 250 microsecond-long pulses of 2.94-μm radiation at 3 Hz, with an energy pulse of 500 mJ. Scanning electron microscopy (SEM) was used to examine teeth after dehydration, drying, and mounting. In vivo dentin and pulpal studies were next undertaken using the incisors, canines, and premolars of 2 male canines. Experimental teeth were treated using the in vitro protocol to make 1-mm deep cuts into the dentin. Four teeth were included in each experimental group. Two teeth were left untouched and served as controls. One animal died 6–12 hours after treatment, and the teeth were not available. The other animal was euthanized 4 days after treatment, and the teeth were harvested and processed for light microscopy.

Results.—When compared with untreated control dentin, the Er:YAP laser caused the least effect of the lasers studied in vitro. In the in vivo studies, there was marked evidence of a thermal effect on dentin, caused by both the CO_2 and Nd:YAG lasers, whereas no evidence of the effect was noted with the Er:YAG laser or the slow-speed rotary instrument. The histologic changes were most dramatic when the Nd:YAG laser was used. A total disruption of the normal architecture, including destruction of the odontoblastic cell layer, was observed (Fig 8–1). The CO_2 laser–treated teeth revealed several responses close to the laser surface, including loss of the odontoblastic cell layer, absence of the predentin layer, and congestion of the blood vessels with extravasation. A normal architecture of the odontoblastic cell layer and the predentinal layer was maintained when the Er:YAG laser was used, with vascularity and cellularity of the connective tissue comparable to that of untreated controls. No difference between slow-speed treated teeth and control specimens were observed.

Conclusion.—No laser can currently match the same degree, efficiency, and speed of cut achieved when using dental handpieces. However, the Er:YAG laser produced effects similar to dental handpiece preparations at both the light and SEM levels of analyses.

▶ The studies reported in this paper are not definitive studies but, rather, should be considered as pilot studies that attempt to compare several laser systems as they might be used clinically. The authors recognize this and point out the need for extensive research in the application of lasers to dentistry. However, this report is valuable because it demonstrates the importance of laser/tissue interactions. The authors use 3 different laser systems to produce cutting of dentin that was similar to that achieved with a traditional bur. The effects on the dentin and pulp varied among the laser systems. This is not unexpected, because different wavelengths absorb differently in the tooth structure. When less of the energy is absorbed at the cutting site and is instead transmitted through the tooth structure, more energy will be available for absorption at deeper sites, e.g., the dental pulp. When this energy is absorbed, heat will be produced and damage can potentially occur.

Although lasers appear to have great potential in dentistry, these authors are very realistic in stating that "to date, no laser can cut to the same degree, efficiency and speed of the existing dental handpieces." Perhaps, someday!—K.L. Zakariasen, D.D.S., M.S., Ph.D.

Influence of Argon Laser Curing on Resin Bond Strength
Hinoura K, Miyazaki M, Onose H (Nihon Univ, Tokyo)
Am J Dent 6:69–71, 1993   105-94-8-3

Background.—Light-cured resin composites are commonly cured with halogen lamps. However, light output decreases with time and distance to the resin surface when halogen lamps are used. Thus, the efficacy of the light source should be considered an important factor for polymerization. It has been suggested that the argon laser may be a valuable polymerization method, because its light intensity remains stable over time. The bond strengths of resins were compared to tooth structure cured with an argon laser or a standard halogen light.

Methods.—Wet no. 240 grit SiC paper was first used to grind the labial surfaces of bovine incisors. After removal of the roots, the teeth

TABLE 1.—Enamel and Dentin Bond Strengths With Argon Ion Laser and Activator Light

	Adherend surface	Argon ion laser MPa (SD)	Activator light MPa (SD)	Significant differences*
Scotchbond 2/ Silux	enamel	14.05 (1.03)	14.18 (1.14)	No
	dentin	13.33 (1.32)	12.97 (1.82)	No
Clearfil Photo Bond/Photo Clearfil A	enamel	16.27 (2.09)	15.39 (1.72)	No
	dentin	8.33 (1.11)	7.63 (1.39)	No

* Significant differences in the same plane ($P < .05$).
(Courtesy of Hinoura K, Miyazaki M, Onose H: *Am J Dent* 6:69-71, 1993.)

were mounted in cold-curing acrylic resin to expose the flattened area. A 4-mm diameter area of enamel and dentin surface was next exposed using wet no. 600 grit SiC paper, and a 4×2-mm mold was placed on the tooth surface. Scotchbond 2/Silux and Clearfil Photobond/Photo Clearfil A were placed in the molds and cured with either a quick light or an argon laser. Exposure times were 10, 20, and 30 seconds, at distances of .0, .5, 1, and 1.5 mm from the resin surface. The quick light intensity was

TABLE 2.—Effect of Distance From Light Tip to Resin Paste on Dentin Bond Strength

	Distance	Argon ion laser MPa (SD)	Activator light MPa (SD)	Significant Differences*
Scotchbond 2/Silux	0 cm	13.33 (1.32)	12.97 (1.82)	No
	0.5 cm	13.29 (1.25)	12.91 (2.16)	No
	1.0 cm	13.03 (1.92)	10.54 (1.92)	No
	1.5 cm	12.82 (1.82)	5.36 (1.47)	Yes
Clearfil Photo Bond/Photo	0 cm	8.33 (1.11)	7.63 (1.39)	No
Clearfil A	0.5 cm	8.27 (1.06)	7.36 (1.31)	No
	1.0 cm	8.05 (1.31)	5.17 (1.30)	Yes
	1.5 cm	7.88 (0.99)	3.63 (0.94)	Yes

* Significant differences in the same plane ($P < .05$). Values connected by vertical lines are not significantly different ($P > .05$). Irradiation times: Scotchbond 2: 20 seconds; Silux, 30 seconds; Clearfil Photo Bond: 10 seconds; Phto Clearfil A: 30 seconds.
(Courtesy of Hinoura K, Miyazaki M, Onose H: Am J Dent 6:69-71, 1993.)

measured as 510 mW/cm² at 470 ± 15 nm. Before curing with the agron laser, light intensity was also adjusted to 510 mW/cm². After 24 hours of storage in water, shear bond tests using a crosshead speed of 1. mm/min were undertaken.

Results.—When the same exposure times at distances of .0 and .5 from the resin surface were used, no significant differences in bond strength were observed between the methods (Table 1). However, at distances greater than .5 mm, a significant decrease in halogen lamp bond strength was noted for both resins. Laser-cured bond strength did not decrease, despite increases in distance (Table 2).

Conclusion.—In instances where the light source cannot be brought into proximity to the resin surface, use of the argon laser may prove to be clinically advantageous. However, lasers are more expensive than the conventional halogen lamp. Further studies to determine the benefits of laser for curing light-cured resin composites are suggested.

▶ This study points out that lasers may have significant value in obtaining maximum resin bond strengths when the curing light cannot be brought into the immediate proximity of the surface of resin. As the authors point out, that factor alone can hardly justify the cost of a laser in a dental practice. However, the literature indicates that some lasers can cause etching of enamel and an increase in caries resistance of enamel, cutting of tooth structure, soft tissue surgery, caries diagnosis, and a number of other functions. At some point in time, the curing of resins with the laser may be practical if the same laser can be used for other functions. Then, the increased frequency of use could justify the cost of the laser.—K.L. Zakariasen, D.D.S., M.S., Ph.D.

Caries-Like Lesion Initiation and Progression in Sound Enamel Following Argon Laser Irradiation: An In Vitro Study

Hicks MJ, Flaitz CM, Westerman GH, Berg JH, Blankenau RL, Powell GL (Baylor College of Medicine, Houston; Univ of Texas Health Science Ctr, Houston; Creighton Univ, Omaha, Neb; et al)
J Dent Child 60:201–206, 1993   105-94-8-4

Background.—There has recently been renewed interest in the role of lasers in preventing and treating enamel and dentinal caries. The effect of argon laser irradiation on the development of carieslike lesions and progression in human enamel was investigated in an in vitro study.

Methods.—Twenty caries-free human molars were used. One buccal window and 1 lingual window in each specimen were exposed to argon laser irradiation at 250 mW for 10 seconds. The remaining buccal and lingual windows were protected from irradiation and served as controls. Longitudinal sections were prepared for assessment after a 6-week exposure period.

Results.—Argon laser irradiation significantly reduced the body of the lesion depths after lesion initiation and progression periods (table). Exposure of sound enamel surfaces to irradiation increased the ability of lased enamel to resist a constant in vitro cariogenic challenge.

Conclusion.—The precise mechanism of caries resistance after argon laser irradiation is unknown. Most likely, a change occurs in the pore

Argon Laser Irradiation Effect on Caries Initiation and Progression

	Control lesions (mean depth ± sd)	Lased lesions (mean depth ± sd)
Lesion initiation period		
Surface zone (n = 40)	33 ± 7um	31 ± 8um
Body of lesion* (n = 40)	117 ± 24um	69 ± 18um
Lesion progression period I		
Surface zone (n = 40)	34 ± 8um	33 ± 10um
Body of lesion† (n = 40)	158 ± 29um	103 ± 22um
Lesion progression period II		
Surface zone (n = 40)	29 ± 9um	36 ± 11um
Body of lesion‡ (n = 40)	221 ± 32um	135 ± 21um

* Lesion initiation period: $P < .05$ for body of lesion depth between lased and control groups.
† Lesion progression period I: $P < .05$ for body of lesion depth between lased and control groups.
‡ Lesion progression period II: $P < .05$ for body of lesion depth between lased and control groups.
(Courtesy of Hicks MJ, Flaitz CM, Westerman GH, et al: *J Dent Child* 60:201–206, 1993.)

structure of lased enamel with entrapment and reprecipitation of mineral phases released during demineralization.

▶ The caries process and various preventive methods to reduce caries are widely studied in in vitro studies such as this, using artificial caries systems. These authors as well as many other independent researchers have found that laser energy applied in small amounts to human enamel can impart caries resistance to the tooth structure. A number of authors have studied the CO_2 laser and found very similar results. Laser energy at relatively low levels does appear to have significant potential as a preventive tool. Although considerably more research is necessary in this area, such research is moving ahead quite rapidly among a number of independent research groups.—K.L. Zakariasen, D.D.S., M.S., Ph.D.

Sealing of Human Dentinal Tubules by XeCl 308-nm Excimer Laser
Stabholz A, Neev J, Liaw L-HL, Stabholz A, Khayat A, Torabinejad M (Hebrew Univ-Hadassah, Jerusalem; Univ of California, Irvine; Shiraz Univ, Iran; et al)
J Endodont 19:267–271, 1993   105-94-8-5

Background.—Exposed dentinal tubules can result in root hypersensitivity. Different techniques and materials have been tried to occlude such tubules. The effects of XeCl excimer laser on exposed dentinal tubules on extracted human teeth were investigated.

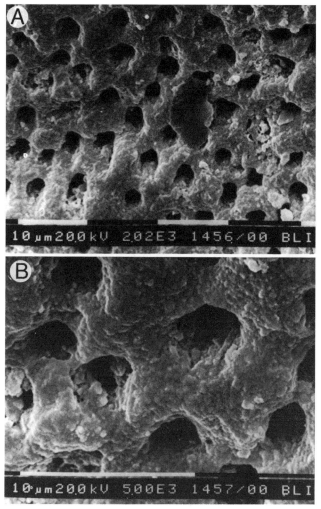

Fig 8–2.—**A,** photomicrograph of a nonlased dentin surface showing exposed dentinal tubules almost without smear layer (original magnification, ×2,000). **B,** photomicrograph of a nonlased dentin surface showing exposed dentinal tubules almost without smear layer (original magnification, ×5,000). (Courtesy of Stabholz A, Neev J, Liaw L-HL, et al: *J Endodont* 19:267–271, 1993.)

Methods.—Fifteen slices, 3-mm thick, were cut at the cementoenamel junction from 15 extracted teeth using an electric saw. A diamond bur was used to remove the cementum layer and expose the dentinal tubules. Slices were then scored by a permanent marker into 4 quadrants of equal size. Three quadrants were lased for 4 seconds with an XeCl excimer laser. Fluences ranged from .5 to 7 J/cm², and the pulse repetition was 25 Hz. The last quadrant on each specimen was not lased and

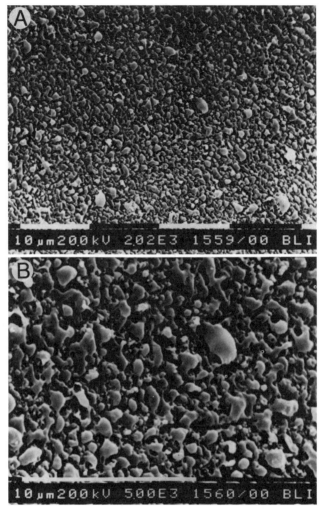

Fig 8–3.—Photomicrographs of lased area with fluence of .5 J/cm². **A,** the surface is composed of finer grain of melted material spread uniformly throughout the surface (original magnification, ×2,000). **B,** ×5,000 (original) magnification of the same area. Original location of tubules openings cannot be observed. (Courtesy of Stabholz A, Neev J, Liaw L-HL, et al: *J Endodont* 19:267-271, 1993.)

served as a control. The specimens were examined by scanning electron microscopy.

Findings.—Many exposed dentinal tubules were observed on the un-lased surfaces. However, all surfaces lased at fluences of up to 1 J/cm² showed melted dentin that closed the tubules. Molten material rupture and dentinal tubule exposure occurred at fluences of 4 J/cm² and greater (Figs 8-2, 8-3, and 8-4).

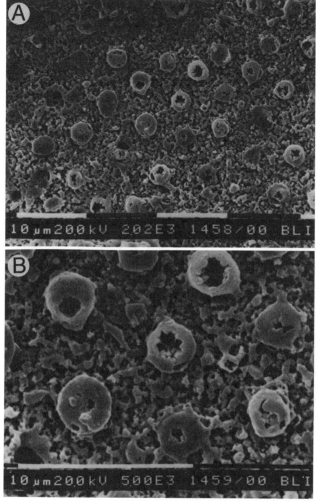

Fig 8–4.—Photomicrographs of lased area with fluence of 7 J/cm². **A,** the beads are dominant and numerous on the surface. **B,** almost all of the beads appear to be ruptured, exposing the dentinal tubules (original magnification, ×5,000). (Courtesy of Stabholz A, Neev J, Liaw L-HL, et al: *J Endodont* 19:267–271, 1993.)

Conclusion.—The use of a 308-nm excimer laser at fluences of .7 and 1 J/cm² can modify dentin surfaces and occlude dentinal tubule openings. This may be accepted as a treatment modality in the future, because the melting and resolidification of the dentin and tubule closure may be permanent.

▶ Root hypersensitivity is a significant problem in dental practice. This in vitro study suggests that the 308-nm XeCl excimer laser may have significant potential for occluding open dentinal tubules. The authors recognize that thermal damage to surrounding tissues can occur with lasers, but they suggest that this could be avoided by using very short pulse durations so that heat accumulation does not occur. However, this study does not directly address this question, and research is necessary to verify that unwanted tissue damage is not occurring. In addition, research is necessary to determine whether tubule closure is permanent. This is only conjecture at this time. Should this technique ultimately be found to be effective and safe, it would provide yet another useful dental application of lasers.—K.L. Zakariasen, D.D.S., M.S., Ph.D.

Effects of the XeCl Excimer Laser on *Streptococcus mutans*
Stabholz A, Kettering J, Neev J, Torabinejad M (Hebrew Univ-Hadassah, Jerusalem; Loma Linda Univ, Calif; Beckman Laser Inst, Irvine, Calif)
J Endodont 19:232–235, 1993   105-94-8-6

Background.—The main etiologic factor in the development of pulpal and periapical lesions is thought to be bacterial contamination of the root canal system. Laser irradiation has the potential to eliminate bacteria in various infected regions of the body and may be used in endodontic therapy. The effects of an XeCl excimer laser on the growth of mutans streptococci in liquid media and agar plates were studied.

Methods.—Ninety-six wells of mutans streptococci bacterial suspensions were studied. Three experimental groups of 24 wells each were lased for 2, 4, and 8 seconds, respectively. The remaining 24 wells served as controls. Blood agar plates were also inoculated with mutans strepto-

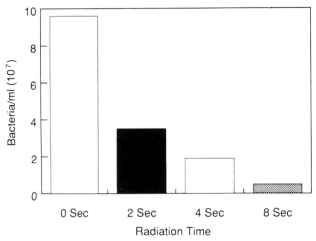

Fig 8–5.—Antibactericidal effects of the XeCl excimer laser for radiation times of 0, 2, 4, and 8 seconds. (Courtesy of Stabholz A, Kettering J, Neev J, et al: *J Endodont* 19:232–235, 1993.)

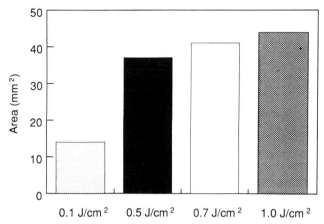

Fig 8–6.—The mean size of the zones of inhibition produced by the different fluences. (Courtesy of Stabholz A, Kettering J, Neev J, et al: *J Endodont* 19:232-235, 1993.)

cocci and lased with different fluences, and bacterial inhibition zones were measured.

Findings.—The length of radiation time and the bactericidal effects of laser treatment were directly correlated. Irradiation for 4 and 8 seconds had a significantly greater bactericidal effect than did no treatment or 2-second exposure. In blood agar plates, higher fluences produced larger zones of inhibition than the lowest fluence. Laser application to the surface of the agar plates resulted in an indentation with a surrounding halo. These indentations and the inhibition zones were more marked with increasing fluences (Figs 8-5 and 8-6).

Conclusion.—The XeCl 308-nm excimer laser apparently kills mutans streptococci. The effect of this laser on other bacteria common in infected root canals should be investigated.

▶ This study found that, like the CO_2 laser, the XeCl excimer laser can kill oral microbes. Such lasers have been suggested for use in sterilizing root canals, which is very difficult to do by current endodontic therapeutic means. However, microbes will only be killed if they are directly irradiated by the laser beam. Given that the root canal is very irregular and contains such complex spaces as fins and spaces between canals in molars, it is doubtful that the laser light can be delivered to all areas. As this technology progresses, it should be possible to design fiberoptic tips shaped to disperse the laser light, leaving the tip in all directions to cover the maximal amount of canal surface as the fiberoptic tip is withdrawn from the canal. The combination of traditional chemomechanical methods for preparing canals with laser irradiation may lead to significantly reduced numbers of organisms left in canals as compared with traditional chemomechanical preparation alone.—K.L. Zakariasen, D.D.S., M.S., Ph.D.

9 Periodontics

Introduction

The pattern of new information influencing our approach to the care of a patient with one of the periodontal diseases begins with the ever-increasing body of evidence that these diseases are a complex of distinct infectious diseases whose expression can be modified by a variety of factors that, by themselves, are not primary etiologic agents. As students, we were required to memorize classification systems for various oral diseases. In some cases, the distinctions seemed of great importance only to academicians. Our understanding of the periodontal diseases has reached a point where both general practitioner and specialist need a framework within which to conceptualize the periodontal diseases. The recently proposed classification by Dr. Richard R. Ranney (1) is a clear and logical synthesis of current information and, at the same time, provides a basis for developing plans of treatment that recognize both the primary etiology as well as those factors modifying the expression of the disease. Familiarity with the Ranney classification will facilitate an appreciation for how information contained in the papers selected for this section of the YEAR BOOK can be applied to everyday practice.

The intense interest in identifying diagnostic tools that are capable of reliably detecting active disease is a reflection of the current understanding that periodontal disease activity is site-specific, that is, can be limited to a specific surface of a specific tooth at any given point in time. Much of this research seeks to bring molecular biology into the clinical environment. New diagnostic tools that are appearing on the market have significant commercial value. The practitioner must be well informed as to the limitations of such diagnostic tools, lest they be depended on to provide information they are not capable of generating.

The recognition that periodontal diseases are simply inflammatory diseases of bacterial origin has led to a search for the most appropriate use of antimicrobial agents delivered both locally and systemically. Just as with new diagnostic capabilities, the practitioner must be knowledgeable about the relationship between the bacterial spectrum of the antibiotic chosen and the specificity of the primary putative pathogens involved in the disease.

Finally, the literature in periodontology continues to add significant assessments of the outcomes of therapy that not only provide guidance in matching a specific therapeutic approach to a specific clinical situation, but also allow a better estimation of the results that can reasonably be anticipated, as well as provide projections of the risk for future disease.

Those articles selected for review in the 1994 YEAR BOOK OF DENTISTRY provide a substantial, but necessarily limited, survey of these areas. For the reader who wishes more information in a concise format, the Periodontics sections in the 1991 through 1993 volumes of the YEAR BOOK together provide a comprehensive review of these subjects so important to the successful management of the patient with a periodontal disease.

James E. Kennedy, D.D.S., M.S.

Reference

1. Ranney RR: *Periodontology 2000* 2:13, 1993.

Etiology and Pathogenesis

Periodontal Disease in the Life Stages of Women
Folkers SA, Weine FS, Weissman DP (Loyola Univ, Maywood, Ill)
Compend Contin Educ Dent 13:852–865, 1992   105-94-9-1

Introduction.—The occurrence of periodontal disease in women is, to a significant degree, a function of the stage of life and the endocrine status.

Periodontal Disease Throughout Life.—Periodontal disease is infrequent before puberty, but gingival changes are more prominent in puberty when cycling begins. Juvenile periodontitis begins at about this time. Many affected patients have deficient neutrophilic chemotaxis and, therefore, are less able to defend against periodontal pathogens. Rapidly progressive periodontitis is more frequent in young adult women than in young adult men. Adult periodontitis is a slowly progressive disorder that ususally does not become clinically significant until the middle 30s. No sex predilection is established.

Pregnancy.—Gingivitis is described in widely varying proportions of pregnant women. Hormonal changes may not be the sole cause of gingivitis, but they may increase tissue responses to local irritants. Tooth mobility often increases even in the absence of gingivitis. The proportion of *Bacteroides intermedius* within the microbial flora has been reported to increase during pregnancy. The so-called "pregnancy tumor" is a gingival lesion resembling pyogenic granuloma. Although it often recurs if removed during pregnancy, it frequently regresses spontaneously after delivery. Similar but less marked gingival changes may be seen in women using oral contraceptives.

Postmenopause.—Osteoporosis is prevalent in postmenopausal women and may result in dental osteopenia that predominantly affects the mandible.

▶ The national emphasis on women's health is not without good reason. The periodontal diseases are but one more example of the difference in women's susceptibility to what is essentially the same disease that occurs in men, but where the expression of the disease can be significantly modified.—J.E. Kennedy, D.D.S., M.S.

Changes of Facial Gingival Dimensions in Children: A 2-Year Longitudinal Study
Andlin-Sobocki A (Univ of Umeå, Sweden)
J Clin Periodontol 20:212–218, 1993   105-94-9–2

Objective.—A wide zone of keratinized and attached gingiva appears to be preferable to a narrow one or no zone at all. Although some studies suggest that the width of the attached gingiva increases with aging, others have found no such increase. This may be because of variations in the criteria used for the selection of children in these studies. Taking previously neglected factors into account, facial gingival surfaces of maxillary and mandibular anterior teeth were monitored to evaluate age-related changes in the width of the keratinized and attached gingiva.

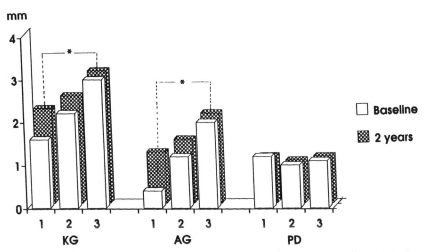

Fig 9–1.—*Abbreviations:* KG, keratinized gingiva; AG, attached gingiva; PD, probing depth. The mean width of KG, AG, and mean PD at baseline, and differences between baseline and 2-year examinations for mandibular anterior permanent teeth with various baseline amounts of attached gingiva; group 1: ≤ .5 mm (6 children); group 2: > .5 but < 1.5 mm (19 children); group 3: ≥ 1.5 mm (38 children). Asterisk significant difference, P < 0.05, for changes 0 to 2 years between indicated groups. (Courtesy of Andlin-Sobocki A: J Clin Periodontol 20:212–218, 1993.)

Methods.—The study sample comprised 96 6- to 12-year-old children, who underwent 2 examinations within an interval of 2 years. At each examination, dental plaque, gingival inflammation, probing depths, and width of the keratinized and attached gingiva were measured. Facial/lingual tooth position was studied by means of study models; the analysis included well-aligned teeth only.

Results.—During the 2 years, the widths of the facial keratinized and attached gingiva increased significantly (Fig 9–1). This was so for the different dental regions studied as well as for the deciduous and permanent teeth. Variable patterns of change were noted during the transition from the deciduous to the permanent dentition. Areas in which the width of the attached gingiva was smallest showed the greatest increases in gingival width, whereas those with the greatest baseline width showed the smallest increases.

Conclusion.—These findings call into question the need for gingival grafting for children with minimal widths of attached gingiva. In well-aligned teeth at least, a period of monitoring before surgical intervention seems appropriate. Longitudinal observations in adults seem to further validate such an approach.

Dimensional Alterations of the Gingiva Related to Changes of Facial/ Lingual Tooth Position in Permanent Anterior Teeth of Children: A 2-Year Longitudinal Study
Andlin-Sobocki A, Bodin L (Univ of Umeå, Sweden; Med Ctr Hosp, Örebro, Sweden)
J Clin Periodontol 20:219–224, 1993   105-94-9–3

Purpose.—Teeth in lingual position appear to have a wider facial zone of gingiva and those in facial position appear to have a narrower facial zone of gingiva in proper arch position. There are contradictory results as to the association between widths of keratinized and attached gingiva and alterations in tooth position. This question was studied using data from a previous study of the dimensional changes of keratinized and attached gingiva in children.

Methods.—Data on maxillary and mandibular anterior permanent teeth in 38 7- to 12-year-old children were used. The children were examined twice in 2 years, including measurements of dental plaque, gingival inflammation, probing depth, and width of keratinized and attached gingiva. Crown height and tooth position were assessed in study casts from both examinations.

Results.—Teeth that changed position in either the facial or lingual direction showed significant changes in the widths of their keratinized and attached gingiva (table). Gingival width changes were at least somewhat related to alterations in clinical crown height. Teeth that moved lingually were associated with increasing gingival width and decreased

Means and Standard Deviations (mm) for Width of Keratinized Gingiva, Width of Attached Gingiva, and Probing Depth for the Various Malposition Groups and Well-Aligned Control Groups at Baseline and the Change Between Baseline and 2-year Examinations

Group	Number of subjects	Keratinized gingiva		Attached gingiva		Probing depth	
		baseline mean SD	change mean SD	baseline mean SD	change mean SD	baseline mean SD	change mean SD
Malposition groups							
A-L	9	4.0±1.5	2.1±1.4**	2.4±1.6	2.3±1.4***	1.6±0.4	−0.2±0.6
L-A	9	4.2±0.6	−0.7±0.7**	2.4±0.8	−0.2±1.2	2.1±0.8	−0.5±0.6*
A-F	9	3.3±1.3	−0.5±0.6*	2.2±1.2	−0.4±0.6*	1.2±0.4	−0.1±0.4
F-A	8	2.6±1.4	1.1±0.8***	1.5±1.1	1.0±0.6**	1.1±0.2	0.2±0.3
L-L	7	4.5±0.9	0.6±1.2	3.2±0.8	0.8±1.0	1.3±0.5	−0.1±0.4
F-F	9	2.5±0.8	0.0±0.5	1.3±0.6	0.0±0.6	1.1±0.2	0.1±0.1
Control groups							
C-A-L	9	3.3±0.8	0.3±0.4	2.0±0.8	0.3±0.3*	1.3±0.2	0.1±0.2
C-L-A	9	3.2±1.1	0.3±0.2**	2.0±0.9	0.2±0.2*	1.3±0.2	0.1±0.1**
C-A-F	9	3.8±0.8	0.2±0.5	2.6±0.7	0.1±0.3	1.2±0.2	0.2±0.1***
C-F-A	8	3.4±0.9	0.3±0.6	2.2±0.8	0.2±0.5	1.2±0.1	0.1±0.1*
C-L-L	7	3.4±0.7	0.2±0.4	2.2±0.6	0.1±0.5	1.2±0.2	0.1±0.4
C-F-F	9	3.2±0.6	0.4±0.6*	2.0±0.7	0.4±0.6*	1.2±0.1	0.0±0.1

*P < .05.
**P < .01.
***P < .001.

(Courtesy of Andlin-Sobocki A, Bodin L: *J Clin Periodontol* 20:219–224, 1993.)

clinical crown height. Those that moved facially were associated with decreasing gingival widths and, in some cases, recession of the facial gingiva.

Conclusion.—Changes in the amount of keratinized and attached gingiva after spontaneous tooth movements were documented. Associations with clinical crown height may also be observed. Gingival examination would be a useful aspect of monitoring of the development of the permanent dentition.

▶ Every dentist has had the experience of answering the questions of an anxious parent concerned that their child has or is developing a problem with the labial gingiva of an anterior tooth. Abstracts 105-94-9-2 and 105-94-9-3 provide a comprehensive basis on which to answer such questions. The dimensions of keratinized and attached gingiva will change over time, and for teeth that are well aligned, the increase will be greatest where the initial amount is minimal. Although this is good information, the critical elements of the evaluation are the tooth position at the time the patient is examined and the analysis that allows a prediction of how tooth position might change over time. Unnecessary surgery to increase the zone of attached gingiva must be avoided. Conversely, anticipating the possibility of recession allows a preventive surgical procedure, e.g., a free gingival graft, to be done and the stripping of the labial gingiva to be minimized, if not totally avoided.—J.E. Kennedy, D.D.S., M.S.

Periodontal Disease Experience in Adult Long-Duration Insulin-Dependent Diabetics

Thorstensson H, Hugoson A (Inst for Postgraduate Dental Education, Jönköping, Sweden)
J Clin Periodontol 20:352–358, 1993   105-94-9-4

Purpose.—Several studies have reported an increased incidence of periodontal disease among persons with diabetes, but the association is still inconclusive. In a randomized, cross-sectional study, periodontal disease experience among patients with long-duration insulin-dependent diabetes was compared with that among nondiabetic controls.

Patients.—The study population consisted of 83 patients aged 40–69 years with insulin-dependent diabetes and 99 sex-matched nondiabetic controls. Only diabetic patients with a disease duration of more than 7 years were included in the analysis. The mean disease duration was 25.6 years for diabetic patients aged 40–49 years, 20.5 years for those aged 50–59 years, and 18.6 years for those aged 60–69 years. All study participants were given clinical and radiographic examinations, which included recording the number of remaining teeth, plaque status, gingival health, probing pocket depth, and alveolar bone level.

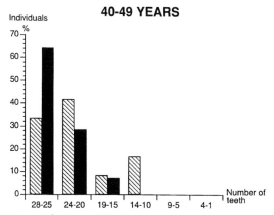

Fig 9–2.—Distribution of the subjects (%) in the age group 40–49 years by number of teeth. Diabetic patients (*hatched bars*); nondiabetic controls (*filled bars*). (Courtesy of Thorstensson H, Hugoson A: *Clin Periodontol* 20:352–358, 1993.)

Results.—Thirty-four diabetic patients and 13 nondiabetic controls were edentulous. The difference was statistically significant. Diabetic patients aged 40–49 years had fewer remaining teeth (Fig 9–2), more periodontal pockets with a probing depth of 6 mm or greater (Fig 9–3), and more extensive alveolar bone loss (Fig 9–4) than nondiabetic controls in the same age group. Severe periodontal disease was significantly more common among diabetic patients than among nondiabetic controls, with the difference most pronounced for the 40- to 49-year-old age group.

Conclusion.—Younger patients with diabetes have more periodontal destruction than nondiabetic persons of the same age, suggesting that

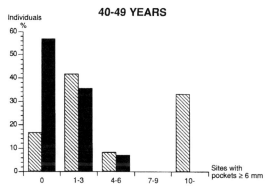

Fig 9–3.—Distribution of the subjects (%) in the age group 40–49 years by number of sites with periodontal pockets ≥ 6 mm. Diabetic patients (*hatched bars*); nondiabetic controls (*filled bars*). (Courtesy of Thorstensson H, Hugoson A: *J Clin Periodontol* 20:352–358, 1993.)

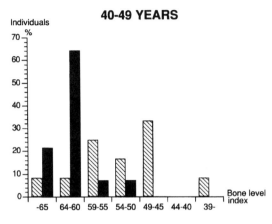

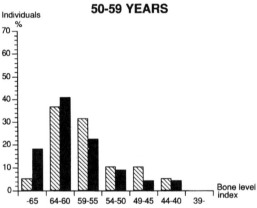

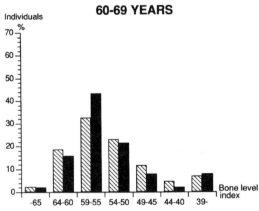

Fig 9-4.—Distribution of the subjects (%) according to bone level index. Diabetic patients (*hatched bars*); nondiabetic controls (*filled bars*). (Courtesy of Thorstensson H, Hugoson A: *J Clin Periodontol* 20:352–358, 1993.)

early disease onset is a much greater risk factor for periodontal loss than mere disease duration.

▶ This study gives strong evidence that age at onset is a very critical factor in the relationship between type 1 diabetes and the severity of adult-onset periodontitis. For patients whose diabetes began in the fourth decade of life, it would be advisable for the practitioner to consider a more intense approach to maintenance and detailed documentation of the status of the periodontium to include measurements of *both* pocket depth and attachment levels. Reassessments as frequent as 6-month intervals would be in order. Treatment of an active site of periodontitis should be monitored to ensure that the desired outcome has been achieved.—J.E. Kennedy, D.D.S., M.S.

Transmission of *Porphyromonas gingivalis* Between Spouses
van Steenbergen TJM, Petit MDA, Scholte LHM, van der Velden U, de Graaff J (Academic Centre for Dentistry, Amsterdam)
J Clin Periodontol 20:340–345, 1993   105-94-9–5

Objective.—*Porphyromonas gingivalis* is specifically associated with severe periodontitis in adults. It is not known whether this organism is part of the normal oral flora, perhaps present in undetectable levels, or is transmitted between persons. The possible transmission of *P. gingivalis* between spouses was studied.

Patients and Results.—The spouses of 18 patients with severe periodontitis from whom *P. gingivalis* had been isolated were examined for the presence of *P. gingivalis*. *Porphyromonas gingivalis* was isolated from 10 of 18 spouses studied. Eight patients and their colonized spouses underwent further clinical and microbiologic studies. Seven

---

Colonization Level of *Porphyromonas gingivalis* (Percent of Total Cultivable Flora) in the Oral Cavity of 8 Patients with Severe Periodontitis and Their Spouses

Couple no.	Periodontitis patient					Spouse				
	pocket	tóngue	buccal mucosa	tonsils	saliva	pocket	tongue	buccal mucosa	tonsils	saliva
1	12	–	–	–	0.4	13	–	0.1	2.0	0.2
2	51	–	6.0	0.7	2.0	20	–	0.4	–	–
3	24	–	0.01	–	0.03	38	0.01	0.8	–	6.0
4	36	–	3.0	0.03	–	3.1	0.4	0.6	1.2	0.3
5	38	0.06	7.3	2.7	0.8	61	0.03	0.1	0.7	0.08
6	31	–	0.8	1.5	2.9	60	1.9	0.3	3.5	0.3
7	32	0.01	2.8	–	1.5	–	0.2	0.9	14.6	2.8
8	5	–	0.3	1.7	0.9	0.2	–	–	0.4	0.2

Note: –, Not detected.
(Courtesy of van Steenbergen TJM, Petit MDA, Scholte LHM, et al: *J Clin Periodontol* 20:340–345, 1993.)

spouses had high percentages of *P. gingivalis* in their periodontal pockets (table). This species was also often isolated from saliva, the tongue, the buccal mucosa, and the tonsillar area of both patients and spouses. The DNA patterns of *P. gingivalis* isolates from husband and wife were clearly distinct from each other in 2 couples but indistinguishable from each other in 6.

Conclusion.—*Porphyromonas gingivalis* can be transmitted between spouses. Whether transmission is a risk factor for the development of periodontal destruction remains to be determined.

▶ *Porphyromonas gingivalis* is one of the organisms frequently isolated from active sites of adult-onset periodontitis. Therefore, the use of this single indicator organism, though having inherent limitations, is not inappropriate. This study seeks to provide information regarding one of the hallmark characteristics of an infectious disease, the transmission to a susceptible host. Although acknowledging that the results do not allow the conclusion that the clinician should modify his or her approach to treatment, it does give some reason to suggest that the spouse of the patient with active periodontal disease be evaluated. This whole question of transmission needs further research and should be followed by all practitioners managing patients with adult-onset periodontitis.—J.E. Kennnedy, D.D.S., M.S.

Diagnostics

Granulocyte Elastase in Gingival Crevicular Fluid: A Possible Discriminator Between Gingivitis and Periodontitis

Gustafsson A, Åsman B, Bergström K, Söder P-Ö (Huddinge Hosp, Sweden)
J Clin Periodontol 19:535–540, 1992   105-94-9-6

Background.—In periodontitis, the periodontal ligament is lost behind a defending barrier of granulocytes. Collagen destruction may result from granulocyte enzymes. Elastase is a serine protease stored in granulocyte granules that is able to degrade various functionally and structurally important molecules, including collagen and proteoglycans.

Objective.—Both the granulocyte elastase activity and the immunoreactive (antigenic) granulocyte elastase were studied in gingival crevicular fluid (GCF) samples from 16 patients with periodontitis and 10 with gingivitis. The periodontitis patients had at least 5 pockets more than 5 mm deep and an attachment loss exceeding 4 mm.

Results.—Elastase activity in the GCF increased with the degree of periodontal disease (Fig 9–5). Both elastase activity per site and activity per microliter correlated with probing depth and with attachment loss, but no such correlations were evident for antigenic elastase. Patients with periodontitis had significantly higher values of elastase activity than did those with a diagnosis of gingivitis (Fig 9–6).

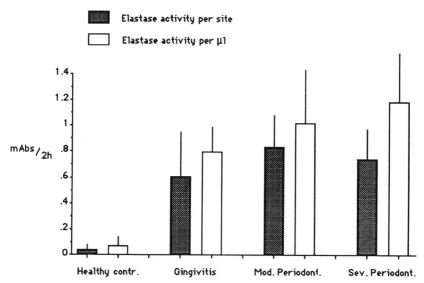

Fig 9–5.—Granulocyte elastase activity per site and per microliter in GCF. The mean and standard deviation of 6 sites in each of 4 patients with different periodontal status: 1 healthy control, 1 with gingivitis, 1 with moderate periodontitis, and 1 with severe periodontitis. (Courtesy of Gustafsson A, Åsman B, Bergström K, et al: *J Clin Periodontol* 19:535–540, 1992.)

Conclusion.—Increased granulocyte elastase activity in GCF may be independent of inflammation, and therefore it may be a useful indicator of patients at risk for periodontitis.

▶ The search for an indicator that would alert the practitioner that a patient or, more appropriately, a specific area of the periodontium is at risk for an acute exacerbation of periodontal infection and rapid loss of attachment has increasingly focused attention on the contents of the GCF. Elastase is among the most promising of the various compounds evaluated thus far. The relationship of flow rates (1) to elastase activity must be taken into account when evaluating the results of this and similar studies.—J.E. Kennedy, D.D.S., M.S.

Reference

1. Darany D, et al: *J Periodontol* 63:743, 1992.

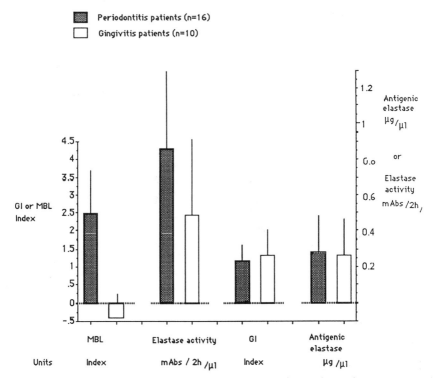

■ Periodontitis patients (n=16)

□ Gingivitis patients (n=10)

Fig 9–6.—Mean marginal bone loss (MBL) as well as site-specific granulocyte elastase activity per microliter, clinical inflammation (GI), and antigenic elastase per microliter in patients with periodontitis and in patients with gingivitis. *Bars* indicate +1 standard deviation. (Courtesy of Gustafsson A, Åsman B, Bergström K, et al: *J Clin Periodontol* 19:535–540, 1992.)

Five Parameters of Gingival Crevicular Fluid From Eight Surfaces in Periodontal Health and Disease

Smith QT, Au GS, Freese PL, Osborn JB, Stoltenberg JL (Univ of Minnesota, Minneapolis)
J Periodont Res 27:466–475, 1992   105-94-9-7

Introduction.—Many studies have sought to establish specific relationships between periodontal disease and gingival crevicular fluid (GCF) parameters. Additional data are required, however, for a fuller understanding of the relationship of GCF composition to periodontal health status. The volume and amounts of the GCF constituents myeloperoxidase (MPO), lactoferrin (LF), aryl sulfatase (AS), and lactate dehydrogenase (LDH) were measured in samples collected from the mesial and distal proximal surfaces of the premolars and first and second molars of 3 subject groups.

Methods.—The 3 groups represented 3 levels of periodontal health. There were 19 subjects in the healthy group, 18 in disease group 1, and

15 in disease group 2. Those in disease group 1 had moderate gingival inflammation, shallow probing depth (PD), and only minimal attachment loss (ATL). The subjects in disease group 2 had moderate gingival inflammation, but intermediate to deep PD and moderate to severe ATL. At most sites, ATL was 0–1 mm in the healthy group, 1–2 mm in the disease 1 group, and 4–9 mm in the disease 2 group. Gingival crevicular fluid was collected from the proximal stites that were clinically measured. Supragingival plaque was removed from all sites that were to be sampled.

Results.—Analyses revealed that GCF volumes and amounts of the 4 GCF constituents varied with periodontal health status. In each of the 3 experimental categories, the volume of GCF differed among the 8 surfaces and 4 teeth and between premolars and molars. The greater amount of GCF collected from posterior locations was not related to gingival index and PD. Differences with sampling location in amounts of GCF constituents were restricted to MPO and LF. Most differences were associated with more severe periodontal disease. At all surfaces, the quantity of MPO was the only measure that differed between the 2 disease groups at all surfaces.

Conclusion.—Because of its ability to differentiate between level of severity in periodontal disease, MPO appears to have the greatest potential as a marker for advanced periodontal disease.

▶ This study has the advantage of assessing multiple potential molecular indicators of periodontal disease activity in the same patient, at the same site, and at the same time. Although promising, it must be remembered that the results are drawn from sites of existing disease, so no conclusions can be drawn regarding the ability of these indicators to also predict subsequent breakdown. Practitioners must become sophisticated consumers of the various diagnostic kits that are becoming commercially available, lest they overestimate their potential value in reliably monitoring a patient's periondontal status.—J.E. Kennedy, D.D.S., M.S.

Peripheral Inflammatory Root Resorption: A Review of the Literature With Case Reports
Gold SI, Hasselgren G (Columbia Univ, New York)
J Clin Periodontol 19:523–534, 1992   105-94-9-8

Introduction.—External inflammatory resorption of root surfaces is triggered by the destruction of cementoblasts and cementoid and maintained by necrotic, and probably also infected, pulp tissue. Another type of external resorption involves a communication with the periodontal pocket, and there is no involvement of the pulp. The latter form of resorption has been given many names, including subosseous and cervical resorption, but it is better referred to as peripheral inflammatory root resorption (PIRR).

Clinical Aspects.—Most root surface resorptions appear to be self-limiting and reversible. Lesions of PIRR usually are asymptomatic and most often are found on routine clinical or radiographic examination. Lesions that begin marginally may be associated with granulation tissue. Radiographs are positive after lesions have reached a certain size. Knife-edged borders are characteristic.

Mechanisms.—Both ostoclasts and osteocytes are involved in the resorption of hard tissues. It may be that highly vascularized tissue adjacent to an unprotected root surface is necessary for root resorption to take place. Multinucleated giant cells have been described in some studies. Newly formed, uncalcified tissue on cemental surfaces is resistant to resorption, and a resorption inhibitor has been demonstrated in hyaline cartilage. It has been proposed that cementum may inhibit resorption on the root surface. Ongoing resorption requires an inflammatory component that may arise from infection in the root canal, orthodontic force or, in the case of PIRR, marginal periodontal inflammation. Animal studies have shown that various cellular elements and enzyme systems participate in resorptive processes.

Conclusion.—Destruction of the surface covering of mineralized tissue creates an environment that favors resorption. Vascular connective tissue is an important element of the resorptive process, as is the presence of an inflammatory stimulus in the form of bacterial infection or both bacterial and traumatic factors.

▶ This study is a good reminder that not all gingival inflammation is what it seems to be, and that clinical findings together with radiographs must be reviewed. The author's description of the environment that favors the resorptive process serves as a guide to therapy in that correction of the environment, to the extent possible, is a major goal.—J.E. Kennedy, D.D.S., M.S.

Personal Oral Hygiene

Comparison Between Mechanical Cleaning and an Antimicrobial Rinse for the Treatment and Prevention of Interdental Gingivitis

Caton JG, Blieden TM, Lowenguth RA, Frantz BJ, Wagener CJ, Doblin JM, Stein SH, Proskin HM (Eastman Dental Ctr, Rochester, NY)
J Clin Periodontol 20:172–178, 1993   105-94-9–9

Background.—Although antimicrobial mouthrinses have been shown to reduce supragingival plaque and gingival inflammation, previous studies have not assessed the midinterproximal area. Mechanical therapies can eliminate plaque and reduce inflammation in the interdental area, but it is unknown whether antimicrobial mouthrinses can reduce inflammation in the interdental area. It is possible that mouthrinses may be unable to penetrate the interdental region at therapeutic concentrations.

Methods.—Ninety-two men with a total of 8 interproximal bleeding sites were studied to compare the efficacy of .12% chlorhexidine gluco-

TABLE 1.—Mean Percentages of Bleeding Sites at Baseline and 3 Months for the 2-Exam and 4-Exam Half-Mouth Scores

Regimen	Two-exam ½ mouth		Four-exam ½ mouth	
	Baseline	3 months	Baseline	3 months
control	51.56	44.57	47.50	40.46
mouthrinse	61.37	52.17	54.65	47.08
mechanical	60.49	7.82	56.09	5.70

(Courtesy of Caton JG, Blieden TM, Lowenguth RA, et al: *J Clin Periodontol* 20:172–178, 1993.)

nate plus toothbrushing, mechanical interdental cleaning plus toothbrushing, and toothbrushing alone in the reduction and prevention of interdental gingival inflammation. The presence of inflammation was assessed at baseline and then every 3 months by the Eastman interdental bleeding index. The results were expressed in terms of the percentage of available sites that bled at examination.

Results.—With mechanical cleaning, bleeding sites decreased from 57% at baseline to 13% at 1 month, to 6% at 3 months (Table 1). The full benefit of mechanical interdental cleaning was noted after 2 months. No important reduction in bleeding was noted in either the antimicrobial or control group. The proportion of bleeding was always greater in posterior than in anterior sites, but there were no differences on analysis of maxillary vs. mandibular or buccal vs. lingual sites. In the mechanical cleaning group, sites that bled at baseline were likely to stop bleeding, and those that did not bleed at baseline were unlikely to start bleeding (Table 2).

Conclusion.—The efficacy of mechanical interdental plaque removal plus toothbrushing in the reduction or prevention of interdental inflammation is demonstrated. Toothbrushing alone or with an antimicrobial

TABLE 2.—Percentage of Sites That Did Not Bleed at Baseline but Subsequently Bled, for Each Treatment Regimen by Time at Which Bleeding Began

Time at which bleeding began	% of sites Treatment regimen		
	Control	Mouthrinse	Mechanical
month 1	28.5	30.4	7.2
month 2	10.9	14.8	4.3
month 3	7.5	9.8	0.8
% which began to bleed during study	46.9	55.0	12.3
% not bleeding at baseline	100	100	100

(Courtesy of Caton JG, Blieden TM, Lowenguth RA, et al: *J Clin Periodontol* 20:172–178, 1993.)

rinse cannot achieve the same results. Mechanical interdental cleaning is important in the prevention of interdental inflammation.

▶ This study would indicate that there is no substitute, chemical or otherwise, for the mechanical removal of plaque from interdental surfaces and gives reason to reassess the use of chlorhexidine alone or in combination with brushing alone as an adequate plaque control regimen. The use of the Eastman Interdental Bleeding Index may account in part for the difference in these findings compared with others in studies that used the more universally accepted Löe gingival index.—J.E. Kennedy, D.D.S., M.S.

Nonsurgical Therapy

Effect of Subgingival Irrigation With Chlorhexidine During Ultrasonic Scaling

Chapple ILC, Walmsley AD, Saxby MS, Moscrop H (Dental School, Birmingham, England)
J Periodontol 63:812–816, 1992   105-94-9-10

Introduction.—Inflammatory periodontal disease may be treated by combining the antimicrobial action of a chemical agent such as chlorhexidine with mechanical plaque removal. A new ultrasonic saline instrument allows irrigating solution to be delivered via a specially designed insert to the scaling tip.

Objective.—The new ultrasonic scaler was compared with a conventional ultrasonic scaler, with and without chlorhexidine, in 17 patients with moderately advanced adult periodontitis. Each patient had 1 quadrant treated with the traditional ultrasonic scaler and water, the traditional scaler with .2% chlorhexidine, the new scaler with water, and the new scaler with chlorhexidine.

TABLE 1.—Plaque Index Expressed as Percentage Decrease at Post-Oral Hygiene Stage and at 1, 3, and 6 Months Post Treatment in All 4 Groups ± Standard Error of Mean

Treatment Regimen	Post-Oral Hygiene	1 Month	3 Months	6 Months
CM-CHX	− 3.9 ± 6.4	− 9.90 ± 5.3	− 19.4 ± 4.6	− 32.5 ± 3.2
US-CHX	− 9.9 ± 3.1	− 12.9 ± 3.6	− 19.6 ± 4.5	− 26.6 ± 4.4
CM-water	− 3.1 ± 4.4	− 7.50 ± 4.6	− 4.00 ± 7.0	− 17.2 ± 3.4
US-water	− 5.0 ± 4.9	− 7.30 ± 4.0	− 11.5 ± 4.4	− 23.0 ± 4.7

Abbreviations: CM, sealer with insert; US, traditional sealer; CHX, chlorhexidine.
(Courtesy of Chapple ILC, Walmsley AD, Saxby MS, et al: *J Periodontol* 63:812–816, 1992.)

TABLE 2.—Mean Tolerance Levels for 4 Treatment Regimens

	US-Water	US-CHX	CM-Water	CM-CHX
Mean discomfort value	3.7	2.5	3.0	2.0
Standard error of mean	0.8	0.6	0.8	0.6

Abbreviations: US, traditional scaler; CHX, chlorhexidine. CM, sealer with insert.
Note: Expressed in centimeters along 10-cm visual analogue scale.
(Courtesy of Chapple ILC, Walmsley AD, Saxby MS, et al: *J Periodontol* 63:812–816, 1992.)

Results.—Oral hygiene reduced plaque and bleeding indices in the 14 evaluable patients, and a significant gain in attachment also was observed. There were no significant differences between the 4 treatment methods at 1, 3, or 6 months (Table 1). Chlorhexidine increased tolerance in three fourths of the cases, compared with the use of a water irrigant. The scaler with the insert was tolerated better than the conventional ultrasonic device in 70% of cases, although there were no significant group differences (Table 2).

► The ability to combine ultrasonic scaling with the delivery of an antimicrobial has definite advantages. A practitioner considering the purchase of new equipment should certainly consider such capability in deciding what to buy.—J.E. Kennedy, D.D.S., M.S.

Clinical Effects of Simultaneous Ultrasonic Scaling and Subgingival Irrigation With Chlorhexidine: Mediating Influence of Periodontal Probing Depth
Reynolds MA, Lavigne CK, Minah GE, Suzuki JB (Univ of Maryland, Baltimore; Vermont Dept of Health, Burlington)
J Clin Periodontol 19:595–600, 1992   105-94-9-11

Objective.—The efficacy of a single treatment combining ultrasonic scaling with subgingival chlorhexidine (CHX) irrigation was examined in 60 patients with adult periodontitis, using clinical probing depth as a criterion.

Study Design.—Thirty-two women and 28 men, aged 28–58 years, participated in the study. All were in good general health and had early or moderate adult periodontitis. None had received professional periodontal therapy in the past 6 months. The patients were assigned to receive subgingival irrigation under cavitation with either water or .12% CHX, delivered through the tip of an ultrasonically activated scaler.

Results.—Plaque and gingival indices were significantly reduced at 2 weeks in both treatment groups (Fig 9–7). There was no further reduction in scores at 4 weeks. Clinical probing depths also were significantly

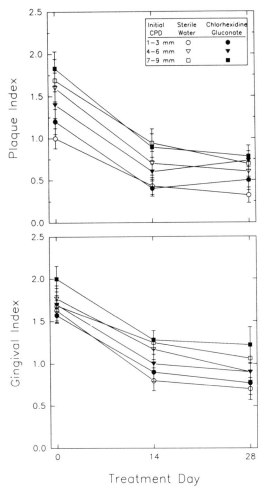

Fig 9-7.—Effects of subgingival irrigation with water and CHX on a Plaque Index and Gingival Index (mean ± SEM) among sites with initial clinical probing depths (CPD) of 1-3 mm, 4-6 mm, and 7-9 mm. Scores on the plaque index and gingival index were significantly (P < .05) reduced among all sites within both groups at 14 and 28 days post treatment. (Courtesy of Reynolds MA, Lavigne CK, Minah GE, et al: *J Clin Periodontol* 19:595-600, 1992.)

reduced at 2 weeks in both groups (Fig 9-8), with a modest trend toward further improvement at 4 weeks. Probing depths were reduced more in patients having irrigation with CHX than in those irrigated with water. Counts of motile organisms and spirochetes were quite variable in both treatment groups and did not change significantly over time.

Conclusion.—Subgingival irrigation with CHX during ultrasonic scaling can be expected to reduce clinical probing depths more than irrigation with water in patients with adult periodontitis.

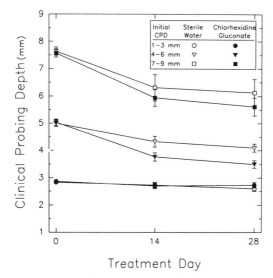

Fig 9–8.—Comparative, temporal effects of subgingival irrigation with water and CHX on clinical probing depth (CPD; mean ± SEM) among sites initially probing 1-3 mm, 4-6 mm, and 7-9 mm. Significant reductions in CPD were observed among all sites within both treatment groups at 14 and 28 days post treatment. The relative reduction was significantly greater among sites 4-6 mm within the CHX group than in the control (sterile water) group. (Courtesy of Reynolds MA, Lavigne CK, Minah GE, et al: *J Clin Periodontol* 19:595-600, 1992.)

▶ It is becoming increasingly apparent that subgingival instrumentation for the purpose of removing calculus and other root accretions is not all that needs to be accomplished. The introduction of ultrasonic instruments that allow an antimicrobial to be delivered at the same time has a clear advantage in deeper pockets. Depending on the number of patients in a practice that have the characteristics of the group that benefited most in this study, investment in an instrument that has an antimicrobial delivery capability would seem worthy of serious consideration.—J.E. Kennedy, D.D.S., M.S.

The Effect of a Number of Commercial Mouthrinses Compared With Toothpaste on Plaque Regrowth

Binney A, Addy M, Newcombe RG (Univ of Wales, Cardiff)
J Periodontol 63:839–842, 1992   105-94-9-12

Background.—Plaque formation is a progressive process, and tooth-cleaning is intended to regularly remove enough plaque so as to leave no more than is consistent with health. Effective mechanical cleaning requires a degree of dexterity that often is lacking. For this reason, a number of chemical plaque control agents have been incorporated in toothpastes or mouthwashes, but except for chlorhexidine, their efficacy has been limited.

Means and Standard Deviations for Plaque Index and Area by Treatment

Mouthwash	Plaque Index	Plaque Area
Bocasan	1.94 (0.31)	1.45 (0.68)
Colgate*	2.30 (0.23)	2.26 (1.06)
Corsodyl	1.60 (0.31)	0.86 (0.41)
Saline	2.28 (0.33)	2.26 (0.98)
Reach	2.22 (0.32)	2.17 (1.22)
Plax	2.19 (0.22)	2.09 (0.82)

Summary Statistics

	Bocasan	Colgate*	Corsodyl	Saline	Reach	Plax
Bocasan		$P<0.01$		$P<0.01$	$P<0.01$	$P<0.01$
Colgate*				ns	ns	ns
Corsodyl	$P<0.01$	$P<0.01$		$P<0.01$	$P<0.01$	$P<0.01$
Saline		ns†			ns	ns
Reach		ns	ns			ns
Plax		ns	ns	ns		

* Toothpaste.
† Not significant.
(Courtesy of Binney A, Addy M, Newcombe RG: J Periodontol 63:839–842, 1992.)

Objective.—A single-blind, crossover study was carried out to compare 6 mouthrinses for their ability to inhibit the regrowth of plaque.

Study Design.—Eight men and 10 women, aged 20–29 years, were assigned to rinse with cetylpyridium chloride (Reach), sodium benzoate solution (Plax) before brushing, a peroxyborate preparation (Bocasan), a slurry of toothpaste (Colgate), chlorhexidine gluconate (Corsodyl), or saline. Plaque was scored after 4 days, and washout periods of at least 3 days were allowed between regimens.

Results.—Compliance with treatment was rated as good. Plaque regrowth was significantly reduced by chlorhexidine compared with peroxyborate, whereas peroxyborate was significantly more effective than the other rinses (table). There were no significant differences in efficacy between the other treatments.

Conclusion.—Both chlorhexidine and peroxyborate effectively countered the reformation of dental plaque in this study, and a detergent prebrushing rinse and a cetylpyridinium chloride rinse were not especially effective.

▶ This well-designed study allows the comparison of a large number of compounds, all of which are purported to have a beneficial effect on plaque reduction or control gingivitis, or both. The results provide the basis for advising patients or responding to their questions regarding the efficacy of various over-the-counter products.—J.E. Kennedy, D.D.S., M.S.

Antibiotics in Periodontal Therapy: An Update

Rams TE, Slots J (Univ of Pennsylvania, Philadelphia; Univ of Southern California, Los Angeles)
Compend Contin Educ Dent 13:1130–1146, 1992   105-94-9-13

Etiology.—There is increasing evidence that human periodontitis represents specific microbial infections. If this is the case, anti-infective measures may be formulated that focus on suppressing or eliminating periodontal pathogens in the subgingival flora and other oral sites. The range of potential pathogens associated with progressive periodontitis is wider than previously thought. Juvenile periodontitis is closely associated with *Actinobacillus actinomycetemcomitans,* but adult periodontitis generally features a combination of anaerobic and facultative bacteria that may include gram-negative and gram-positive species. In addition, less common organisms (e.g., enteric rods, pseudomonads, enterococci, and yeasts) may colonize periodontal pockets.

Antibiotics.—Clinical studies of various antimicrobial regimens are summarized in Table 1. Systemic tetracyclines are marginally effective in adult patients. Metronidazole has proved useful after periodontal debridement. Clindamycin also is a useful adjunct to debridement. Combination regimens may prove useful in refractory or difficult-to-treat periodontal cases. Local antibiotic therapy can deliver much higher subgingival doses than are achieved with systemic regimens, but adjunctive local treatment has produced little or no benefit beyond that resulting from conventional mechanical débridement alone (Table 2).

Recommendations.—A conservative, highly selective approach to periodontal antibiotic therapy is suggested, rather than routinely administering antibiotics to all patients with periodontal disease. Treatment should focus on periodically reducing the supragingival and subgingival microbiota and calculus. Appropriate antimicrobial treatment may be decisive in patients with actively progressing periodontitis or infectious failure of a dental implant. Healing is best when mechanical débridement precedes antibiotic therapy. Microbiological assessment is indicated 1–2 months after local chemomechanical therapy is completed. Systemic antimicrobial therapy is useful in cases of recalcitrant periodontal infection involving A. acetinomycetemcomitans, black-pigmented anaerobic rods, *Peptostreptococcus micros,* enteric rods/pseudomonads, and perhaps other species (e.g., *Staphylococcus aureus* and *Enterococcus faecalis*).

▶ The extensive search of the literature and the terse statements of pertinent outcomes serve as an excellent reference for choosing an antibiotic to fit a particular clinical problem. Accessing the entire article or, even better, several of the reference papers (see the information on Mosby's Document Express following the Table of Contents) will benefit any practitioner who uses antibiotics as an adjunct in the management of periodontal infections.—J.E. Kennedy, D.D.S., M.S.

TABLE 1.—Clinical Studies of Systemically Administered Antibiotics in Periodontitis Therapy

Study Single Antibiotic Regimens	No. of Patients	Antibiotic and Dose	Concurrent Treatment	Control	Length of Follow-up	Outcome
Tetracyclines Miller et al (1989)	15 AP	MINO 100 mg bid for 21 d	Sc, MWF	-	3 mo	Aa eliminated from 2 patients with MINO alone, and 8 patients with MINO+Sc and MINO+MWF. Clinical improvements directly related to elimination of Aa.
de Graaff et al (1989)	12 LJP 21 RPP	MINO or DOXY (dosages not reported)	Sc	-	10 mo	MINO and DOXY failed to eliminate Aa and arrest disease activity in 82% of patients.
Muller et al (1990)	8 LJP 13 RPP 4 AP	MINO 100 mg bid for 7 d alone or 21 d with Sc	Sc	-	1 mo	MINO alone eliminated Aa from only 18% of positive sites, and initially low Aa-infected sites demonstrated increases in Aa from 2.7% to 15.7% of flora.
Asikainen et al (1990)	16 LJP	DOXY 200 mg LD, then 100 mg daily for 13 d	Sc	P	2 mo	No clinical or microbial adjunctive benefits of DOXY+Sc vs P+Sc. DB study
Saxén et al (1990)	14 LJP	DOXY 200 mg LD, then 100 mg daily for 13 d	Sc	P	20 mo	DOXY reduced Aa better than P. DB study
McCulloch et al (1990) Kulkarni et al (1991)	55 R AP	DOXY 100 mg daily for 21 d	Sc	P	7 mo	43% reduction in disease activity risk with DOXY vs P. However, 45% of DOXY group developed abscesses within 7 mo. DOXY reduced Pg, Pi, Fusobacterium spp, and spirochetes, but not Aa. DB study
Novak et al (1991)	4 LJP	TET 250 mg qid for 42 d	none	-	12 to 48 mo	TET without Sc reduced PD, AL, and BL up to 4 years

Study						
Westergaard & Fiehn (1991) Fiehn & Westergaard (1991)	8 R AP	DOXY 100 mg daily for 21 d	MWF	-	24 mo	DOXY+MWF temporarily suppressed periodontal pathogens, but improved clinical parameters and arrested AL in 7/8 patients. One patient experienced further AL at 6 sites.
Freeman et al (1992)	30 AP	MINO 100 mg either once daily or bid for 8 d	-	-	15 d	No clinical or microbial differences between regimens. Fewer side effects with lower doses.
Metronidazole Jenkins et al (1989)	10 AP	MET 200 mg tid for 5 d	Sc	-	3 mo	No adjunctive benefit of MET on moderate pockets.
Soder et al (1990)	98 AP	MET 400 mg tid for 7 d	Sc	P	6 mo	MET better reduced number of patients with ≥ 5 mm PD than P. DB study.
Eisenberg et al (1991)	10 AP	MET 200 mg tid for 7 d	Sc	P	3 wks	MET + Sc better reduced PD and motile organisms.
Loesche et al (1991)	39 AP	MET 250 mg tid for 7 d	Sc	P	27 to 44 mo	MET + Sc better reduced surgical needs and spirochetes compared to P + Sc. DB study.
Loesche et al (1992)	33 AP	MET 250 mg tid for 7 d after completion of Sc	Sc	P	1 to 1.5 mo	MET after Sc better reduced surgical needs, PD, AL, *Bi* and motile organisms as compared to P after SC. DB study.
Loesche et al (1992)	74 AP	MET 500 mg bid or DOXY 100 mg daily for 14 d	Sc	P	?	MET or DOXY after Sc reduced initially estimated surgical needs by 75%, and better than P after Sc. DB study.
Paquette et al (1992)	14 AP	MET 250 mg tid for 7 d or after completion of Sc	Sc	Sc	6 mo	MET + Sc better reduced rate of AL over 6 mo as compared to P + SC
Saxén & Asikainen (1992)	27 LJP	MET 200 mg tid for 10 d or TET 250 mg qid for 12 d	Sc	Sc	18 mo	Best clinical results with MET + Sc. *Aa* eliminated in 100% of MET group but in only 44% of TET group and 67% of Sc-only group

(continued)

Table 1 (*continued*)

Penicillins Magnusson et al (1989)	10 R AP	AUG 250 mg tid for 14 d	Sc	-	12 mo	AUG reduced AL, PD, and disease active sties from 14% initially to 7% at 9 mo. One subject had 10% active-sites with additional AL at 9 and 12 mo.
Abu Fanas et al (1990)	8 RPP	AUG 250 mg tid or TET 250 mg qid for 14 d	Sc	-	4 mo	AUG and TET equally improved clinical and microbial parameters
Magnusson et al (1992)	21 R AP	AUG or CLIN (dosages not reported)	Sc	P	24 mo	AUG or CLIN better reduced disease activity rate and improved clinical parameters as compared to P. However, further AL tended to occur at 12 to 15 mo postantibiotic.
Clindamycin Gordon et al (1990) Walker & Gordon (1990)	24 R AP	CLIN 150 mg qid for 7 d	Sc	-	24 mo	CLIN improved clinical parameters, reduced annual disease activity rate from 8% to 0.5% active sites/patient and increased time between active episodes from 5 mo to 17 mo. *Pg, Pi, and P micros* reduced or absent at 12 mo.
Quinolones Slots et al (1990)	3 R AP	CIP 500 mg bid for 10 d	Sc	-	12 mo	CIP eliminated superinfecting enteric rods from subgingival flora and improved clinical parameters.
Serial Drug Regimens Matisko & Bissada (1992)	11 R AP	DOXY 200 mg LD, then 100 mg daily for 4 d, followed by AUG 500 mg tid for 5 d	Sc	DOXY for 9 d	6 mo	DOXY + AUG sustained reductions in PD and AL better than DOXY alone.

Reference	Patients	Drug regimen	Sc		Duration	Results
Aitken et al (1992)	23 R AP	DOXY 200 mg LD, then 100 mg daily for 21 d, followed by (if disease active) MET 250 mg tid for 10 d	Sc	P before MET	7 mo	DOXY + MET group exhibited less disease recurrence than P+MET group (9% vs 42% patients) and showed better reductions in AL and periodontal pathogens.
Combination Drug Regimens Rams et al (1990)	5 R AP	MET + AUG 250 mg tid of each for 7 d	Sc	-	12 mo	MET + AUG eliminated *Aa* in all patients and improved clinical parameters.
Goené et al (1990)	4 R AP	MET 250 mg plus AMOX 375 mg each tid for 7 d	Sc	-	2 to 9 mo	MET + AMOX eliminated *Aa* in all patients and improved clinical parameters.
van Winkelhoff et al (1992)	28 LJP 50 AP 40 R AP	MET 250 mg + AMOX 375 mg each tid for 7 d	Sc	-	3 to 9 mo	MET + AMOX improved clinical status, and eliminated *Aa* in 97% and *Pg* in 82% of patients. However, additional AL occurred in 6 patients despite antibiotic regimen.
Pavicic et al (1992)	40 AP	MET 250 mg plus AMOX 375 mg each tid for 7 d	Sc	-	14 to 36 mo	MET + AMOX eliminated *Aa*, *Pg*, and further AL in 39/40 patients.
Rams et al (1992)	17 R AP	MET + CIP 500 mg each bid for 8 d	Sc	-	18 mo	MET + CIP improved clinical parameters and reduced periodontal pathogens, resulting in a predominately streptococcal subgingival flora and no postantibiotic AL at any site.

Abbreviations: AP, adult periodontitis; RAP, adult periodontitis with unknown disease activity rate; RAP, adult periodontitis with recent disease activity or refractory to prior treatment; LJP, localized juvenile periodontitis; RPP, rapidly progressive periodontitis; MNO, minocycline; DOXY, doxycycline; TET, tetracycline HCl; MET, metronidazole; AUG, Augmentin®; AMOX, amoxicillin; CLIN, clindamycin; CIP, ciprofloxcin; bid, 2×/day; tid, 3×/day; qid, 4×/day; LD, loading dose; Sc, subgingival débridement; MWF, modified Widman flap surgery; - - - -, not carried out; DB, double-blind; Aa, *Actinobacillus actinomycetemcomitans*; Pg, *Porphyromonas gingivalis*; Pi, *Prevotella intermedia*; P, placebo; PD, probing depth; AL, periodontal attachment loss; BL, radiographic bone loss.

(Courtesy of Rams TE, Slots J; *Compend Contin Educ Dent* 13:1130–1146, 1992.)

TABLE 2.—Clinical Studies of Locally Applied Antibiotics in Periodontitis Therapy

Study	No of Patients	Antibiotic and Delivery System	Concurrent Treatment	Control	Length of Follow-up	Outcome
Lazzaro & Bissada (1989)	12 AP	0.5% MET applied with syringe 7x in 14 d	-	Sc, P, F	6 wks	Sc improved clinic and microbial parameters better than MET alone.
Eckles et al (1990)	9 AP	40% TET in white petrolatum with syringe 1x	-	Sc, P, NT	3 mo	Sc improved clinical and microbial parameters better than TET alone.
Kimura et al (1991)	27 AP	10% OFLOX in soluble hydroxypropyl-cellulose and polymethacrylic inserts placed 6x in 42 d	Sc	Sc, P	1 wk	No significant adjunctive microbial benefits to OFLOX beyond that attained with Sc.
Linden & Newman (1991)	19 AP	0.5% MET in oral irrigator/28 d	Sc	P	3 mo	No significant clinical advantage of MET vs P. DB study.
Minabe et al (1991)	16 AP	TET in cross-linked resorbable collagen film 4x in 28 d	-	Sc, P, NT	2 mo	TET + Sc led to reduced AL, and significantly less bleeding on probing at 2 mo than Sc alone in class II furcation lesions.
Goodson et al (1991)	107 AP	25% TET in ethylene vinyl acetate copolymer monolithic fibers for 10 d	-	Sc, P, NT	2 mo	TET reduced PD, AL, and bleeding on probing better than Sc, although % of PD and AL reductions of ≥ 2 mm were similar for both groups (for PD: 21% of sites for TET vs 13% for Sc).

Reference	N/Group	Drug/Delivery		Control	Duration	Results
Nakagawa et al (1991)	11 R AP	2% MINO ointment applied 4 x in 28 d with syringe	-	P	3 mo	MINO + Sc significantly reduced PD, AL, bleeding on probing, motile organisms, total viable organisms, and *Pg* (but not *Aa* and *Pi*) better than Sc alone.
Abu Fanas et al (1991)	4 AP	40% AUG in acrylic strips placed for 7 d	-	NT	1 mo	AUG eliminated bleeding on probing up to 3 wks and reduced anaerobes and *Fusobacterium* spp up to 1 mo.
Yamagami et al (1992)	43 AP	10% OFLOX in soluble hydroxypropylcellulose and polymethacrylic inserts placed 4x in 28 d	-	P	1 mo	OFLOX improved clinical parameters better than P.
Wade et al (1992)	73 AP	50% TET or MET in acrylic strips placed for 7 d	-	Sc, NT, C	3 mo	No differences between TET, MET, and Sc in reduction of total viable counts or anaerobic/aerobic ratios. TET induced marked TET resistance in flora at 1 mo.
Giordano et al (1992)	54 R AP	20% MET in ethylcellulose films placed 2x in 14 d	-	C	?	MET reduced initially estimated surgical needs from 2.4 to 1.2 teeth/patient.
Okuda et al (1992)	30 AP	MINO powder microencapsulated in biodegradable polymer placed 1x with syringe	Sc	P	6 mo	MINO temporarily reduced microbial species better, but, no significant differences at 6 mo. compared to P.

(continued)

Table 2 *(continued)*

Jones et al (1992)	51 AP	2% MINO ointment applied with syringe	-	Sc, NT	6 mo	MINO+Sc temporarily reduced PD better than Sc alone, however, no significant differences were present by 6 mo.
Braswell et al (1992)	47 AP	2% MINO ointment applied with syringe	-	Sc, NT	6 mo	MINO+Sc tended to reduce PD and AL best, however, no significant differences were found as compared to Sc alone
Landry et al (1992)	35 AP	2% MINO ointment w/syringe	Sc	NT	12 mo	MINO+Sc improved clinical parameters better than NT.
van Steenberghe et al (1992)	101 AP	2% MINO ointment applied with syringe 4x in 42 d	Sc	Sc	3 mo	MINO+Sc improved clinical and microbial parameters better than Sc alone. DB study.

Abbreviations: AP, adult periodontitis with unknown disease activity rate; RAP, adult periodontitis with recent disease activity or refractory to previous treatment; MINO, minocycline; TET, tetracycline HCl; MET, metronidazole; AUG, Augmentin®; OFLOX, ofloxacin; Sc, subgingival débridement; – – –, not carried out; NT, no treatment; DB, double-blind; Aa, Actinobacillus actinomycetemcomitans; Pi, Prevotella intermedia; P, placebo; Pg, Porphyromonas gingivalis; PD, probing depth; AL, periodontal attachment loss; F, stannous fluoride; C, chlorhexidine.
(Courtesy of Rams TE, Slots J: Compend Contin Educ Dent 13:1130–1146, 1992.)

Calculus Removal From Multirooted Teeth With and Without Surgical Access: (I). Efficacy on External and Furcation Surfaces in Relation to Probing Depth

Parashis AO, Anagnou-Vareltzides A, Demetriou N (Univ of Athens, Greece)

J Clin Periodontol 20:63–68, 1993   105-94-9-14

Introduction.—Successful periodontal treatment includes removal of subgingival calculus. However, significant subgingival calculus can persist on the external root surfaces in moderate to advanced pockets, with greater amounts noted with increasing pocket depths. In multirooted teeth, access to the furcation area may be difficult if not impossible to achieve. Therefore, alternative methods of instrumenting the furcation, such as the use of diamonds and stones, have been proposed.

Methods.—The effectiveness of calculus removal from multirooted teeth using closed root planing, open root planing, and a rotary diamond for the furcation area, including the effect of pocket depth, was assessed. Thirty first and second lower molars scheduled for extraction were evaluated in 23 patients with moderate to advanced adult periodontitis. All teeth had a calculus index of 2 or more and degree II or III furcation involvement. Ten teeth were treated by open scaling and root planing, 10 by closed scaling and root planing, and 10 with open scaling and root planing with a rotary diamond for the removal of deposits in the furcation area. After extraction, the percentage of residual calculus

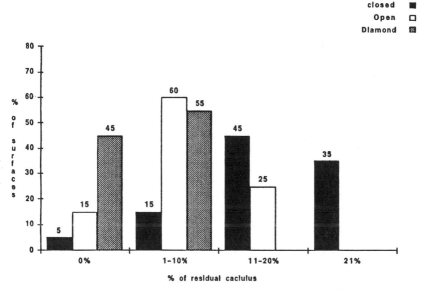

Fig 9–9.—Frequency distribution of furcation surfaces according to percent of residual calculus (0%, 1% to 10%, 11% to 20%, > 20%) for the three experimental groups. (Courtesy of Parashis AO, Anagnou-Variltzides A, Demetriou N: *J Clin Periodontol* 20:63–68, 1993.)

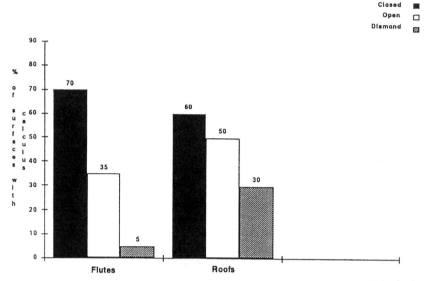

Fig 9–10.—Percentage of surfaces in the roof and flute of the furcation with residual calculus for the 3 experimental groups. (Courtesy of Parashis AO, Anagnou-Vareltzides A, Demetriou N: *J Clin Periodontol* 20:63–68, 1993.)

on the external and furcation surfaces was assessed stereomicroscopically.

Findings.—The external surfaces showed a significantly higher percentage of residual calculus with closed vs. open planing. In both internal and external scaling groups, more residual calculus was noted for pocket depths of 7 mm or more. Significant differences were noted in the percentage of residual calculus on furcation surfaces, with the most effective method being open root planing plus the use of the rotary diamond (Fig 9-9). Again, more calculus was noted with pocket depths of 7 mm or more, though the difference was only significant in the closed group. There was more residual calculus in the flute and roof of the furcation with closed than with open root planing; however, the most effective method in these areas was the use of the rotary diamond (Fig 9-10).

Conclusion.—Closed scaling and root planing rarely removes all calculus from furcation surfaces. Although more calculus can be removed by an open approach, total removal is still limited. The combination of open root planing and the use of the rotary diamond is the most effective method of calculus removal. Even so, many surfaces treated this way will still show small amounts of residual calculus.

▶ This study should give all of us reason to reassess what we expect to accomplish through scaling and root planing. We kid ourselves and our patients if we think that the dentist or the hygienist can adequately scale and débride the root where pocket depth exceeds 5 mm or where there is furcation involvement. The outcome described is not different even when scaling and root planing are carried out with curettes specially designed for deep pockets (1). The added benefit of using rotary instruments *after* surgical access should not be disregarded.—J.E. Kennedy, D.D.S., M.S.

Reference

1. Nagy J, et al: *J Periodontol* 63:954, 1992.

Outcomes of Therapy

A 4-Year Controlled Clinical Study Into the Use of a Ceramic Hydroxylapatite Implant Material for the Treatment of Periodontal Bone Defects
Galgut PN, Waite IM, Brookshaw JD, Kingston CP (Univ College, London; Natl Univ of Singapore)
J Clin Periodontol 19:570–577, 1992   105-94-9-15

Objective.—Ten patients with chronic adult periodontitis who had infrabony pockets associated with more than 1 tooth underwent periodontal flap procedures with and without implantation of hydroxylapatite particles.

Study Design.—The patients included 7 women and 3 men, aged 33 to 59 years. Fifty-eight defects were treated with hydroxylapatite, and 59 were treated without hydroxylapatite. Treatment was randomized between shallow sites of less than 3 mm, moderate defects of 3–6 mm, and deep pockets exceeding 6 mm in depth. Recession, probing pocket depth, and probing attachment level were estimated 6 months after treatment and yearly for 4 years.

Results.—Moderate and deep pockets exhibited significantly reduced probing depths and increased attachment levels during follow-up. At 4 years, initially deep pockets responded best when hydroxylapatite was implanted (table). The difference was just more than 1 mm. Initially shallow pockets exhibited postoperative losses in attachment level whether or not implant material had been used.

Conclusion.—There may be a role for using hydroxyapatite in treating deep infrabony defects. When pockets deeper than 6 mm are present, pocket depth is most reduced, and the probing attachment level is most increased when material is implanted at the time of periodontal flap surgery.

▶ Both the duration of observation in this study and the finding that the material is best suited to deeper defects are encouraging. The problem of recession must be noted and mentioned as part of the preoperative patient consul-

Mean and Standard Deviation for Change (Gain) in Attachment From Enamel-Cement Junction From Baseline for 10 Patients at the Various Intervals for Different Initial Depth of Pockets and for Test and Control Procedures

Pockets Time interval	Shallow initial <3 mm		Moderate initial 3–6 mm		Deep initial >6 mm	
	Test mean (SD)	Control mean (SD)	Test mean (SD)	Control mean (SD)	Test mean (SD)	Control mean (SD)
6 months	−0.56 (0.69)	−0.48 (0.65)	0.68 (0.62)	0.93 (0.55)	2.94 (1.60)	2.80 (1.17)
1 year	−0.68 (0.59)	−0.55 (0.88)	0.84 (0.52)	0.79 (0.59)	3.00 (1.12)	2.38 (0.88)
2 years	−0.52 (0.61)	−0.47 (0.59)	0.90 (0.53)	0.94 (0.51)	3.19 (1.33)	2.79 (1.43)
3 years	−0.77 (0.64)	−0.78 (0.80)	0.81 (0.60)	0.78 (0.63)	3.21 (0.82)	2.66 (1.05)
4 years	−0.90 (0.66)	−1.09 (1.35)	0.62 (0.58)	0.29 (0.90)	3.27 * (1.16)	2.24 (0.96)

* Approaching statistically significant difference ($P = .058$).
(Courtesy of Galgut PN, Waite IM, Brookshaw JD, et al: *J Clin Periodontol* 19:570–577, 1992.)

tation lest the patient not be aware of an outcome that is in large part predictable.—J.E. Kennedy, D.D.S., M.S.

Tissue Response to Biphasic Calcium Phosphate Ceramic With Different Ratios of HA/βTCP in Periodontal Osseous Defects
Nery EB, LeGeros RZ, Lynch KL, Lee K (VA Med Ctr, Milwaukee, Wis; New York Univ; Med College of Wisconsin, Milwaukee; et al)
J Periodontol 63:729–735, 1992   105-94-9–16

Background.—Hydroxyapatite (HA) and beta tricalcium phosphate (βTCP) are the most widely used calcium phosphate ceramics. When used in periodontal osseous defects, HA has shown no evidence of new periodontal tissue attachment, osteogenesis, or cementogenesis. Although βTCP forms new bone, there are questions about new periodontal attachment. With the development of biphasic calcium phosphate (BCP) ceramic it has become possible to control the resorbability of the material while maintaining its osteoconductive property. Although a ratio of about 60% HA to 40% βTCP seems to provide a bone conductive property, the optimum ratio is not known. A canine study attempted to determine the ideal ratio of HA to βTCP in a BCP ceramic for effective repair of periodontal osseous defects.

Mean Preoperative Probing Attachment Level and 6-Month Postoperative Gain

Treatment & Control Group HA/TCP Ratio	No. of Sites (teeth)	Preop. mean±SE	Gain mean±SE
100/0 (n=2)	16	10.3±0.6	3.9±0.5
85/15 (n=3)	22	11.3±0.5	5.3±0.4
65/35 (n=3)	20	10.8±0.4	5.4±0.5
50/50 (n=3)	21	10.0±0.6	4.0±0.6
35/65 (n=3)	20	9.2±0.7	4.2±0.7
15/85 (n=3)	23	10.3±0.5	4.5±0.4
0/100 (n=2)	16	8.8±0.5	3.3±0.5
0/0 (n=2)	16	10.6±0.8	1.8±0.3

(Courtesy of Nery EB, LeGeros RZ, Lynch KL, et al: *J Periodontol* 63:729–735, 1992.)

Methods.—Surgical defects were created in beagles, making them chronic to simulate periodontal disease. In 4 months, mucoperiosteal periodontal flaps were made, and the debridement of the osseous defects and root planing were done. Into these defects were placed BCP ceramic prepared with various HA/βTCP ratios ranging from 100/0 to 0/100; a control group had a ratio of 0/0. After 6 months of healing, including monthly scaling and polishing and probing of attachment levels, the animals were killed and histologic examination was performed.

Results.—According to Duncan's multiple range test, all ratios brought a significant gain in probing attachment levels compared with the control group. Significantly greater gains were noted with the HA/βTCP ratios of 65/35 and 85/15 than with ratios of 50/50, 100/0 or 0/100 (table). Except for the 100% HA group, the use of BCP with higher HA/βTCP ratios brought accelerated new bone formation and attachment levels.

Conclusion.—In the treatment of periodontal osseous defects, the HA/βTCP ratio of 85/15 appears to yield greatest gains in attachment level and bone regeneration, according to animal studies. Further studies in a larger sample are called for.

▶ The combination of compounds used in this study seeks to achieve both bone induction and resorbability. Attachment with 100% HA compares favorably to that reported in the previous study (105-94-9–15). Assuming that this provides a basis for comparison of efficacy in deeper defects, then the combination would seem to have a real advantage.—J.E. Kennedy, D.D.S., M.S.

Patient Preference Regarding 4 Types of Periodontal Therapy Following 3 Years of Maintenance Follow-Up
Kalkwarf KL, Kaldahl WB, Patil KD (Univ of Texas, San Antonio; Univ of Nebraska, Lincoln; Univ of Nebraska, Omaha)
J Clin Periodontol 19:788–793, 1992   105-94-9–17

Background.—Although several studies have attempted to evaluate the effectiveness of traditional periodontal therapy, none has addressed the question of patient preference. Some types of therapy can lead to increased posttherapy gingival recession, which may lead to maintenance complications. Patient preferences could be related to degree of gingival recession or other clinical differences.

Methods.—Patient perceptions of 4 types of periodontal therapy were studied after 3 years of maintenance. The subjects were 75 patients who had undergone split-mouth therapy with coronal scaling, root planing, modified Widman surgery, and flap with osseous resectional surgery. The patients were surveyed for their perceptions of each treatment in a variety of categories.

B. Sensitivity to Temperature

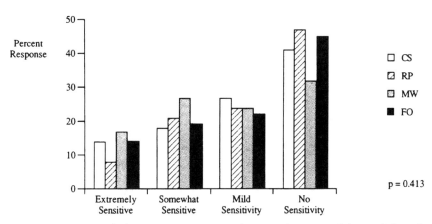

Fig 9–11.—Perception of sensitivity to temperature changes in the regions of the mouth for each therapy regimen. (Courtesy of Kalkwarf KL, Kaldahl WB, Patil KD: *J Clin Periodontol* 19:788-793, 1992.)

C. General "Feeling"

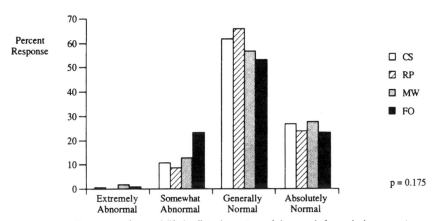

Fig 9–12.—Perception of general "feeling" in the regions of the mouth for each therapy regimen. (Courtesy of Kalkwarf KL, Kaldahl WB, Patil KD: *J Clin Periodontol* 19:788-793, 1992.)

G. **Repeat Therapy**

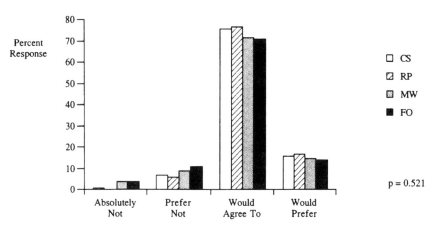

Fig 9–13.—Willingness to repeat the therapy for regions of the mouth treated by each therapy regimen. (Courtesy of Kalkwarf KL, Kaldahl WB, Patil KD: *J Clin Periodontol* 19:788–793, 1992.)

Results.—In terms of difficulty in cleaning, responses were similar for all 4 techniques, though regions treated by coronal scaling and root planing were rated somewhat easier to clean. Regions that underwent modified Widman surgery were rated somewhat more sensitive to temperature (Fig 9–11). With all techniques, most patients rated the overall feeling of the region as normal (Fig 9-12). Thirty percent to 40% of patients reported infrequent localized symptoms, with no differences among treatments. There were no significant differences in terms of food retention or comfort of oral examination. Finally, 80% to 90% of patients said they would be willing to repeat any of the 4 forms of therapy. Willingness to repeat therapy is outlined in Figure 9–13.

Conclusion.—After 3 years of maintenance therapy, most patients believed their mouths were normal, had few localized symptoms, and would repeat the treatment if necessary. Regions treated by flap with osseous resection appear to have somewhat less food retention but are more difficult to clean. The differences observed do not appear sufficient to warrant any modifications of current therapeutic approaches.

▶ The lack of a difference between nonsurgical and surgical therapy is encouraging given the established difficulty in thoroughly instrumenting root surfaces, especially those of multirooted teeth where deep (> 5-mm) pockets make surgical access necessary.—J.E. Kennedy, D.D.S., M.S.

Periodontal and Prosthodontic Treatment of Amelogenesis Imperfecta: A Clinical Report
Greenfield R, Iacono V, Zove S, Baer P (State Univ of New York, Stony Brook)
J Prosthet Dent 68:572–574, 1992   105-94-9-18

Background.—Amelogenesis imperfecta, an inherited disorder associated with defective ameloblasts, has a reported incidence of 1 person in every 16,000. Patients with this disorder have typically been treated by multiple extractions or construction of complete dentures. Overdenture therapy has been a successful alternative. A fixed prosthodontic treatment sequence for a patient with complete amelogenesis imperfecta was reported.

Case Report.—Woman, 45, with amelogenesis imperfecta, reported an inability to function with existing complete maxillary and mandibular overdentures. The patient had worn overdentures made for aesthetics, function, and dentinal hypersensitivity with simultaneous fluoride iontophoresis for many years. Other than the maxillary right third and left second molars, all teeth were accounted for. Localized mild to moderately advanced periodontitis, restricted to the mandibular molars, was seen via periapical radiographs and complete periodontal charting. Throughout the mouth, pocket depths ranging from 2 to 8 mm were seen, with the most significant depths seen in the mandibular molars. Mobility patterns ranging from type 1/2 to 1 were seen in the left mandibular posterior teeth; all other patterns were within normal limits. Throughout the dentition,

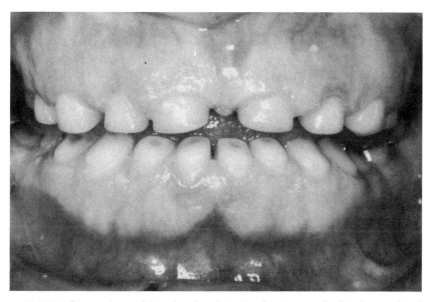

Fig 9–14.—Preoperative condition of teeth and gingivae showing generalized inadequate clinical crown length. (Courtesy of Greenfield R, Iacono V, Zove S, et al: *J Prosthet Dent* 68:572–574, 1992.)

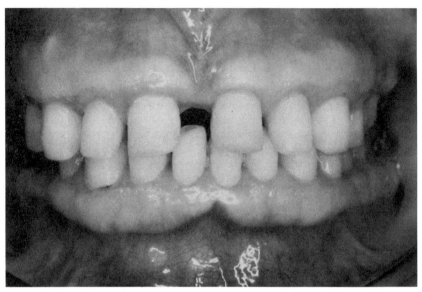

Fig 9–15.—Tissue healing 4 weeks after surgery. (Courtesy of Greenfield R, Iacono V, Zove S, et al: *J Prosthet Dent* 68:572-574, 1992.)

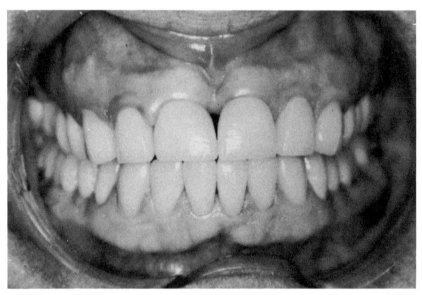

Fig 9–16.—Final restorations 5 years after placement. (Courtesy of Greenfield R, Iacono V, Zove S, et al: *J Prosthet Dent* 68:572-574, 1992.)

diastemas ranging from 1 to 3 mm were found. The gingivae appeared to be firm and healthy. However, the length of all clinical crowns was considered insufficient to permit restoration with fixed prostheses (Fig 9–14). Periodontal preparation, via scaling, root planing, and oral physiotherapy comprised the first treatment phase. Diagnostic casts, mounted on a fully adjustable articulator, were used to study soft tissue contours to determine the most favorable redevelopment of soft tissue and osseous and dental contours after surgery. Surgery was performed with both hand and high-speed rotary instruments, and included complete-mouth crown-lengthening by ostectomy and osteoplasty. After surgery, the patient was seen weekly, and healing was uneventful (Fig 9–15). At 12 postoperative weeks, the second phase of prosthodontic procedures was begun. During the provisionalization period, and throughout completion of the restoration, the vertical dimension of occlusion was carefully preserved. The patient has been regularly followed for 5 years on a 3–4-month appointment schedule, and has maintained periodontal health, function, and very acceptable aesthetics (Fig 9–16).

Conclusion.—This fixed prosthodontic technique provides restoration of aesthetics and function for patients with amelogenesis imperfecta, and it is an alternative to the dental destruction caused by this disorder.

▶ This paper serves as an excellent reminder that the best treatment outcome is often the result of a combination of therapies and therapists. That this patient maintained her dentition into the fourth decade of life is a significant accomplishment that should encourage others to take a similar approach in the treatment of patients with this developmental problem.—J.E. Kennedy, D.D.S., M.S.

Root Caries Susceptibility in Periodontally Treated Patients: Results After 12 Years
Ravald N, Birkhed D, Hamp S-E (The Specialist Dental Services, Linköping, Sweden; Univ of Göteborg, Sweden)
J Clin Periodontol 20:124–129, 1993   105-94-9-19

Objective.—The few longitudinal studies of root caries have found that they occurred to some degree in patients with good to excellent results after periodontal treatment. Risk factors varied between subjects, with no single variable being discriminative in all cases. Individual susceptibility to root caries in periodontal patients was studied after 12 years.

Methods.—The analysis included 27 patients, mean age 59 years, who had taken part in a clinical prospective study of root caries. All received periodontal treatment consisting of oral hygiene training, scaling and root planing, and selective surgery. The variables tested for their possible predictive value included age, plaque score, salivary counts of lactobacilli and mutans streptococci, salivary secretion rate and buffer effect, oral sugar clearance time, and dietary habit index.

Findings.—All but 3 of the patients had new root caries lesions develop during follow-up. Eight patients had 1 to 5 new decayed and filled surfaces (DFS), 7 had 6 to 9 DFS, and 9 had 12 or more DFS. However, the annual mean number of new DFS was low. Patients with more than 5 new DFS% during years 9 to 12 differed significantly from those with 5 or fewer new DFS% in terms of salivary mutans streptococcus counts, plaque scores, and new DFS% during years 5 to 8. At 8 years, the risk values among the tested variables were 3 times more common in patients with more than 5 new DFS% developing in years 9 to 12 than in those with 5 or less new DFS%. Throughout follow-up, root caries were significantly more common in smokers than nonsmokers.

Conclusion.—Root caries appears to be a minor problem among periodontal patients, although some patients have a high incidence of new lesions. Although some diagnostic tests and questionnaires can be useful in predicting the development of root caries, including salivary counts of mutans streptococci and lactobacilli and plaque scores, a history of root caries is the most valuable predictor.

▶ Some degree of root exposure is an almost inevitable sequela of the successful treatment of adult-onset periodontitis, but not all patients will have root caries develop. The importance of the information contained in this paper is that it can serve as a guide to identify those patients who may be at greater risk for caries and can also allow the institution of preventive measures as part of postsurgical therapy.—J.E. Kennedy, D.D.S., M.S.

Periodontal Healing in Teeth With Periapical Lesions: A Clinical Retrospective Study
Ehnevid H, Jansson L, Lindskog S, Blomlöf L (Public Dental Service at Skanstull, Sweden; Karolinska Institutet, Stockholm)
J Clin Periodontol 20:254–258, 1993   105-94-9–20

Background.—Periodontally involved teeth appear to develop significantly deeper pockets in the presence of root canal infection, although the prognosis of periodontal treatment for these teeth remains uncertain. Inflammation resulting from marginal plaque accumulation or root canal infection can contribute to the worsening of pocket depths.

Methods.—Periodontal healing of teeth with and without root canal infection was compared in a referral population. The analysis included 2,605 teeth in 163 patients with 2 pocket depth measurements made before and after an observation period, including an initial period of periodontal treatment. All patients received a full oral radiographic examination within 1 year of the first pocket depth measurement and had single-rooted teeth exhibiting either a periapical radiolucency or root

Multiple Regression Analysis After an Observation Period Exceeding 11 Months With Mean Pocket Depth Reduction for All Teeth Within Each Individual Patient With the Same Periapical Status as Dependent Variable After Stratifying the Material With Respect to Vertical Destructions and Surgical Treatment

Independant variable	Coefficient	SE	p
initial mean pocket depth (mm) per patient	−0.580	0.059	0.000
time (months)	0.013	0.006	0.035
periapical pathology	−0.321	0.172	0.060
periapical pathology × time	0.033	0.012	0.008
constant	1.230	0.209	0.000

(**B**) Non-surgical treatment of vertical marginal defects, number of teeth = 289

Independant variable	Coefficient	SE	p
initial mean pocket depth (mm) per patient	−0.593	0.069	0.000
time (months)	0.035	0.013	0.008
periapical pathology	0.097	0.210	0.644
constant	1.184	0.338	0.001

(**C**) Surgical treatment of horizontal and vertical marginal defects = 225

Independant variable	Coefficient	SE	p
initial mean pocket depth (mm) per patient	−0.886	0.053	0.000
time (months)	0.111	0.090	0.209
periapical pathology	0.089	0.118	0.454

(Courtesy of Ehnevid H, Jansson L, Lindskog S, et al: *J Clin Periodontol* 20:254–258, 1993.)

filling and at least 1 endodontically intact single-rooted tooth. Intraoral radiographic findings and periodontal conditions were recorded, and periapical conditions were scored for each tooth. Periapical conditions were correlated with periodontal healing patterns.

Findings.—On multiple regression analysis, there was a significant influence of initial mean pocket depth and time since treatment on change in pocket depth (table). There was significantly less reduction of pocket depths in teeth with periapical disease in patients receiving nonsurgical treatment of periodontal pockets more than 2.5 mm in teeth with horizontal marginal defects. Pocket depth reduction was unaffected by proximal restorations, abutments for fixed bridges, root fillings with and without dowels.

Conclusion.—Untreated root canal infection presenting as a periapical radiolucency may ultimately result in a retarded or impaired response to periodontal therapy. It is possible that periapical disease and the resulting root canal infection can, alone or in combination with a deep periodontal pocket induced by marginal plaque, impair periodontal healing and deepen angular bony defects (Fig 9-17). The effects of periapical

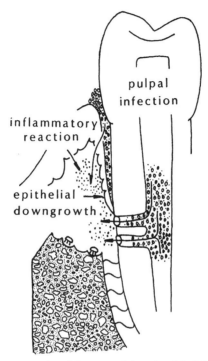

Fig 9–17.—Schematic representation of the proposed dynamics of the influence of pulp infection on periodontal status. (Courtesy of Ehnevid H, Jansson L, Lindskog S, et al: *J Clin Periodontol* 20:254–258, 1993.)

destruction on periodontal healing should be considered in treatment planning.

Relationship Between Periapical and Periodontal Status: A Clinical Retrospective Study
Jansson L, Ehnevid H, Lindskog S, Blomlöf L (Public Dental Service at Skanstull, Sweden; Karolinska Institutet, Stockholm)
J Clin Periodontol 20:117–123, 1993   105-94-9–21

Purpose.—Although the influence of endodontic infection on periodontal disease is apparent in traumatized young teeth with necrosis of the periodontal membrane, this relationship is more difficult to assess in older, nontraumatized teeth with marginal periodontitis. Endodontic infection cannot initiate the development of marginal lesions without the presence of additional factors such as primary dental plaque. The associations between clinical periodontal status in periodontally involved teeth with and without endodontic infection were explored.

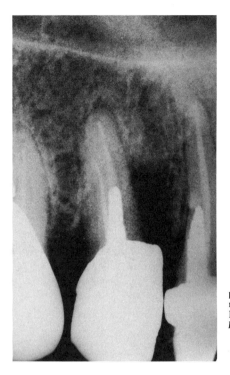

Fig 9–18.—Intraoral radiograph of a premolar (15) exhibiting a periapical radiolucency of score 1. (Courtesy of Jansson L, Ehnevid H, Linkskog S, et al: *J Clin Periodontol* 20:117–123, 1993.)

Methods.—The retrospective study included 163 patients referred for periodontal treatment. All had single-rooted teeth with either a periapical radiolucency or root filling and at least 1 endodontically intact single rooted tooth. Intraoral radiographic findings, periodontal conditions, and periapical conditions were evaluated in each tooth. Teeth were assigned a score of 1 for periapical destruction (Fig 9–18), 0 if intact (Fig 9–19), and .5 if the examiners disagreed (Fig 9–20).

Findings.—A significant correlation was noted between periapical pathology and vertical bony destruction in extant teeth. The distributions of mean pocket depths for both horizonal and marginal destruction were different, depending on the periapical conditions. Teeth with periapical disease tended to have deeper pockets, and the relative frequency of angular bony defects increased along with periapical score. In the absence of vertical bony destruction, periapical disease was significantly related to increased pocket depth in 3 of 4 tooth groups (table).

Conclusion.—The presence of endodontic infection, appearing as a periapical radiolucency, promotes the formation of periodontal pockets on instrumented marginal root surfaces. Endodontic infection thus appears to be a risk factor for the progression of periodontitis. Even though the recorded mean difference of .5 to 1.00 mm may seem clini-

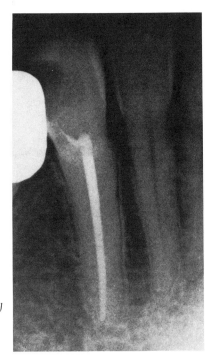

Fig 9–19.—Intraoral radiograph of a canine (43) exhibiting a periapical radiolucency of score 0. (Courtesy of Jansson L, Ehnevid H, Linkskog S, et al: *J Clin Periodontol* 20:117–123, 1993.)

cally negligible, it should be taken into account during treatment planning.

▶ The preceding papers by the same group of investigators (Abstracts 105-94-9–20 and 105-94-9–21) cover both aspects of the relationship between pulpal disease and adult-onset periodontitis. The large number of patients involved and the design of the retrospective study add credibility to the results. It would not be unreasonable to suggest that a comprehensive assessment of pulpal status should be part of any evaluation of a patient with adult-onset periodontitis.—J.E. Kennedy, D.D.S., M.S.

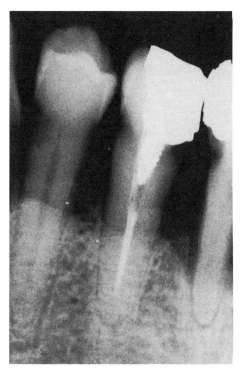

Fig 9–20.—Intraoral radiograph of a premolar (35) exhibiting a periapical radiolucency of score .5. (Courtesy of Jansson L, Ehnevid H, Linkskog S, et al: *J Clin Periodontol* 20:117-123, 1993.)

Analysis of Intra-Individual Comparisons Between Teeth With and Without Periapical Pathology

Tooth group	n	Angular bony destruction	Difference MPD (mm)	p
13–23	39	—	0.66	0.020
13–23	9	+	0.51	0.650
14–15, 24–25	15	—	0.27	0.200
14–15, 24–25	4	+	0.32	0.270
33–43*	17	—	0.98	0.008
34–35, 44–45*	30	—	0.50	0.006

* "Difference MPD" denotes the difference in mean pocket depth between teeth in each tooth group with periapical scores 1 and 0, respectively.

† The number of teeth with angular bony destructions in each tooth group in the lower jaw was 1. They were, consequently, excluded because they provided no basis for statistical analysis.

(Courtesy of Jansson L, Ehnevid H, Linkskog S, et al: *J Clin Periodontol* 20:117-123, 1993.)

10 Oral Medicine and Diagnosis

Introduction

The articles in this chapter of the 1994 YEAR BOOK OF DENTISTRY were selected with 2 primary objectives in mind. The first was to fulfill the traditional concept of the YEAR BOOK to provide current information in a readily digestible form with commentary relating to the significance of the information to the current practice of dentistry. The second was to encourage the practitioner to think about oral medicine not solely as an academic discipline that primarily resides within the organization of schools of dental medicine, but as a dynamic and rapidly growing discipline that should be playing an ever-increasing role in the everyday practice of dentistry. For example, the implications for oral health care for the patient who is medically compromised will always be an essential element of oral medicine. A new dimension is rapidly increasing needs for the treatment of oral diseases other than dental caries or the periodontal diseases, and for the management of side effects of treatment for a patient with a systemic disease that are expressed in oral or perioral structures. There is a growing awareness that many of these problems can either be prevented or their severity lessened if the dentist is involved early in the course of treatment.

Another dimension of oral medicine in which the dentist may be the first point of contact or asked to accept referral is the patient with a disorder of taste, smell, or oral malodor. These are very real problems that dental practitioners, by virtue of their education and training, are well qualified to evaluate, diagnose and, in many instances, treat. The conscientious and progressive general practitioner continually assesses his or her practice with a view to providing for all of the oral health-care needs of most of their patients. In reviewing the articles contained in this chapter, the practitioner should keep in mind the question of whether the problems described and the approaches to treatment offered might serve as the basis for adding a new dimension to his or her practice.

James E. Kennedy, D.D.S., M.S.

AIDS and Related Issues

Efficacy of Preprocedural Rinsing With an Antiseptic in Reducing Viable Bacteria in Dental Aerosols

Fine DH, Mendieta C, Barnett ML, Furgang D, Meyers R, Olshan A, Vincent J (Columbia Univ, New York; Warner-Lambert Co, Morris Plains, NJ)
J Periodontol 63:821–824, 1992   105-94-10–1

Background.—During dental procedures, oral microbes are aerosolized, carrying the potential for cross-contamination of the operatory and transmission of pathogens to dental professionals as well as patients. Use of an antiseptic mouthrinse before procedures has been shown to reduce the bacteria level in the backspray from a handpiece and to reduce salivary bacteria. The efficacy of using a preprocedural antiseptic mouthrinse in reducing the level of bacteria in aerosols generated by ultrasonic scaling was evaluated.

Methods.—The double-blind, controlled, crossover study included 18 healthy adult patients, all of whom underwent a supragingival scaling and rubber cup prophylaxis and returned 1 week later, after having abstained from all oral hygiene procedures for 24 hours. Half of the mouth was randomly selected for a 10-minute ultrasonic scaling as the unrinsed

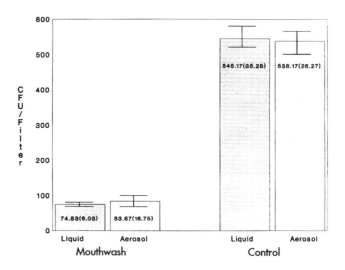

Fig 10–1.—Effect of impaction on cell viability. The mean (SD) recoverable counts of S. *sanguis* after exposure to mouthwash or control, either delivered to the filter gently by liquid or impacted from an aerosolized mist. (Courtesy of Fine DH, Mendieta C, Barnett ML, et al: *J Periodontol* 63:821–824, 1992.)

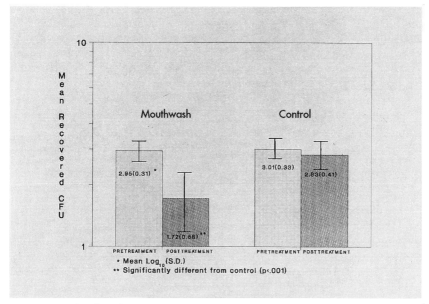

Fig 10–2.—The effect of mouthwash carryover on cell viability. The mean (SD) recoverable counts of presented *S. sanguis* after exposure to aerosols generated by ultrasound scaling after rinsing with either mouthwash or control. (Courtesy of Fine DH, Mendieta C, Barnett ML, et al: *J Periodontol* 63:821-824, 1992.)

control. After the patients used either an antiseptic mouthrinse or a control rinse, 20 mL/30 sec, the other half of the mouth was ultrasonically scaled. During each scaling period, aerosolized bacteria were collected using a modified vacuum air-sampling device. Then the filters of the device were incubated, and the number of resulting colony forming units (CFUs) were counted.

Results.—The number of viable bacteria on the filter was unaffected by the collection method or by the aerosolized antiseptic mouthrinse in preliminary experiments (Fig 10-1). Compared with the unrinsed control, use of antiseptic mouthrinse reduced the number of CFUs by 94%. The control rinse yielded a reduction of 34%. Both differences were significant (Fig 10-2).

Conclusion.—Rinsing with an antiseptic mouthwash before ultrasonic scaling can significantly reduce the number of viable bacteria in the aerosols generated. Although no conclusions can be drawn about the effect on the risk of cross-contamination, preprocedural rinsing may play an important part in the dental office infection control regimen.

▶ Many dental procedures generate an aerosol. This fact is part of the rationale for the universal precautions and other strategies used in the dental office that are directed at preventing the spread of blood-borne pathogens. Although the assay method used in this study did not measure all of the possible micro-organisms in an aerosol, it is reasonable to assume that all were affected in a similar way. Although this study is not absolutely conclusive, the use of a preprocedural rinse should be considered. In choosing a rinse, a compound such as chlorhexidine, which has been shown to be effective against oral micro-organisms and which possesses significant substantivity, may be preferable.—J.E. Kennedy, D.D.S., M.S.

Latex Glove Allergy: A Survey of the US Army Dental Corps
Berky ZT, Luciano WJ, James WD (Craven Dental Clinic, Fort Knox, Ky; USA Dental Clinic, Fort Ritchie, Md; Walter Reed Army Med Ctr, Washington, DC)
JAMA 268:2695–2697, 1992   105-94-10-2

Introduction.—With the growing use of gloves by health professionals has come an increase in the incidence of allergic reactions to latex gloves. These reactions include the commonly reported delayed allergic contact dermatitis or the more serious contact urticaria. The prevalence of allergies to rubber gloves in dentists was studied in a survey of 1,628 active-duty officers of the U.S. Army Dental Corps.

Findings.—The overall response rate was 64%, of which 14% of the responses were consistent with a history of latex glove allergy. Assuming that all nonrespondents were nonallergic, the overall prevalence of latex glove allergy would be 9%. Fifty-nine percent of the respondents reported wearing latex gloves for all clinical procedures, 96% changed their gloves after each patient contact, and 76% washed their hands each

Results of Latex Glove Allergy Survey ($n = 1,043$)

	No. Positive (%)	95% Confidence Interval
Latex glove allergy	143 (13.7)	11.6-15.8
Delayed allergy	54	. . .
Localized contact urticaria	20	. . .
Generalized urticarial reactions	20	. . .
Type not identifiable by history	49	. . .
100% glove use for all clinical procedures	955 (91.6)	89.9-93.2
Change gloves after contact with each patient	997 (95.6)	94.4-96.9
Wash hands each time after removing gloves	795 (76.2)	73.6-78.8

(Courtesy of Berky ZT, Luciano WJ, James WD: JAMA 268:2695-2697, 1992.)

time they removed their gloves (table). Thirty-five percent of the 40 respondents who reported contact urticaria were atopic by history. Only about a fourth of the dentists with latex allergy had been diagnosed as such by a physician. Fifty-six percent had found another latex glove they could use without a reaction, 8% used medications before wearing latex gloves, and 6% used vinyl undergloves.

Conclusion.—Latex glove allergy is a common problem among practicing dentists. Most dentists do not seek testing and diagnosis by a physician. Instead, they try different brands of gloves until they find one they can tolerate. There is a need for heightened awareness of the potential for serious allergic events and protection against them.

▶ The universal use of gloves as part of barrier techniques makes the occurrence of allergy to latex a genuine concern for dental practitioners. The practitioner must be aware that the reaction can go well beyond a local response.—J.E. Kennedy, D.D.S., M.S.

Periodontal Changes by HIV Serostatus in a Cohort of Homosexual and Bisexual Men
Barr C, Lopez MR, Rua-Dobles A (Beth Israel Med Ctr, New York)
J Clin Periodontol 19:794–801, 1992   105-94-10–3

Objective.—Important questions remain about the relationship between periodontal health and HIV-1 infection. Some studies have suggested that patients with HIV infection or compromised immune systems are more susceptible to periodontal disease, whereas others have suggested that immunocompromised patients cannot mount an inflammatory response to local factors such as plaque or calculus. Still other studies showed no difference in periodontal status between immunosuppressed and nonimmunosuppressed patients.

Methods.—A cohort of 114 homosexual or bisexual men was followed for 20 months to examine the relationship of periodontal attachment levels, oral indices, immune status, and HIV serologic status. Eighty-six of the men were HIV positive, and 28 were HIV negative. The investigators measured gingival index (GI), plaque index (PI), and relative attachment levels (RAL) at 4-month intervals using the computerized Florida disk probe. The association of GI with PI, HIV status, CD4 lymphocyte counts, and salivary flow rates was examined, as were possible confounding variables.

Findings.—Subjects with T4 cell counts under 200 were more than 6 times more likely to have a significant RAL of 3 mm or more. Subjects 35 years of age and older with T4 cell counts under 200 had a 33% incidence of significant RAL, compared with 5% for subjects of the same age who had less immunosuppression (Tables 1 and 2). Such an association was nonsignificant in younger subjects. Seventy-eight men com-

TABLE 1.—Percentage of Subjects With Relative Attachment Loss (RAL) Greater Than or Equal to 1 mm, 2 mm, or 3 mm in 1 or More Mesiobuccal Sites by HIV Serostatus, Immune Status, Age, and Race

Variable *	N †	RAL≥1 mm	RAL≥2 mm	RAL≥3 mm
All	114	77%	30%	10%
HIV status:				
seropositive	86	78%	33%	14%*
seronegative	28	75%	21%	0
T4 Count/mm³:				
T4 < 200	26	85%	42%	27%**
T4 ≥ 200	86	74%	26%	6%
T4 < 400	49	84%	35%	18%
T4 ≥ 400	63	71%	25%	5%
Age group:				
< 35	56	79%	23%	7%
≥ 35	58	76%	36%	14%
Race:				
white	96	77%	31%	10%
black/hispanic	18	78%	22%	11%

Note: Relative attachment loss at last visit relative to baseline.
* For each variable, the difference between group categories was analyzed using the χ^2 statistic; * P < .05; ** P < .01.
Abbreviation: N, total number of subjects in each category. Subtotals may not add up to totals because of missing data.
(Courtesy of Barr C, Lopez MR, Rua-Dobles A: J Clin Periodontol 19:794–801, 1992.)

pleted all of the follow-up visits. Although the average GI increased significantly more in seropositive subjects, there was no association between GI and T4 cell counts. Linear regression analyses suggested that men in the seropositive group were more sensitive to plaque.

Conclusion.—The HIV serologic status and immunosuppression appear to be significantly related to short-term periodontal changes. Immunosuppression may be a risk factor for RAL and HIV seropositivity for GI, particularly in older subjects. When these risk factors are present, the patient should be advised to practice good oral hygiene and seek more frequent preventive dental treatment.

▶ Immunosuppression, like several other factors, such as hormones, is not by itself a cause of any of the various periodontal diseases, but it can modify the expression of the disease. An aggressive approach to the control of local factors becomes increasingly important as immune status becomes less favorable.—J.E. Kennedy, D.D.S., M.S.

TABLE 2.—Means ($\pm$ the Standard Error of the Mean) of Age, Plaque Index (PI), Gingival Index (GI), and T-Cell Counts by Relative Attachment Loss (RAL) Above and Below a Threshold of 3 mm

Variable *	RAL $\geq$ 3 mm ($N=12$)	RAL $<$ 3 mm ($N=102$)	P †
Age	39.5 ± 2.1	36.1 ± 0.7	0.10
Plaque Index	1.7 ± 0.3	1.3 ± 0.1	0.09
Gingival Index	1.2 ± 0.2	0.7 ± 0.04	0.02
T4 count/mm³	222 ± 63	497 ± 31	0.003
T8 count/mm³	891 ± 90	742 ± 37	0.07
T4:T8 Ratio	0.3 ± 0.1	0.9 ± 0.1	0.0007

Note: Relative attachment loss at last visit relative to baseline.
* The baseline mean values for all variables except age. Age coincides with RAL measures at last visit.
† Wilcoxon 2-sample rank sum W-test, 2-tailed P-value.
(Courtesy of Barr C, Lopez MR, Rua-Dobles A: *J Clin Periodontol* 19:794–801, 1992.)

The Simultaneous Occurrence of Oral Herpes Simplex Virus, Cytomegalovirus, and Histoplasmosis in an HIV-Infected Patient

Jones AC, Migliorati CA, Baughman RA (Univ of Florida, Gainesville)
Oral Surg Oral Med Oral Pathol 74:334–339, 1992   105-94-10-4

Background.—The proper diagnosis and management of oral diseases in patients infected with HIV can maintain the health and prolong the lives of these patients. However, the oral diseases may be difficult to diagnose because of unusual clinical manifestations. Because of HIV status, the oral disease may be refractory to conventional therapy. Oral ulcerations of a viral and fungal nature can be the only clinical manifestations of HIV infection.

Case Report.—Man, 51, was evaluated for oral ulcerations of 7 months' duration. The patient was infected with HIV, but there were no clinical manifestations of the disease. The oral ulcerations first appeared after extraction of a periodontally involved upper left first molar. Systemic acyclovir and cyphalexin provided no improvement. During the next several months, several extractions were performed because of extensive periodontal disease and gingival ulcerations. Biopsy of the ulcer revealed nonspecific inflammation, but laboratory and clinical tests remained negative or noncontributory. The initial ulcer enlarged to include the right hard and soft palates and the upper left buccal vestibule. The patient was treated with metronidazole and ketoconazole when the ulcer displayed a somewhat granular appearance and white pseudomembranous plaques were observed on the oral mucosa. The drug regimen was effective but was changed when the patient developed steroid-induced diabetes. Intraoral biopsy specimens confirmed cytomegalovirus (CMV) infection and histoplasmosis with herpes simplex virus (HSV) ulceration. The patient died, and autopsy revealed a disseminated CMV infection.

Conclusion.—This is the first reported case of an HIV-infected patient with the simultaneous occurrence of oral HSV, CMV, and histoplasmosis. The extensive oral ulcerations were the only clinical manifestations of AIDS. This case fulfilled the Centers for Disease Control surveillance case definition for AIDS. Disseminated CMV infection was determined to be the primary cause of death. To establish a definitive diagnosis of oral ulcerations, a biopsy specimen, culture, or cytologic smear of the involved area should be examined and appropriate serum titers should be performed.

▶ We tend to think of patients as having one or another infection. This case report serves to heighten the awareness that patients with AIDS may have multiple concurrent oral infections.—J.E. Kennedy, D.D.S., M.S.

Natural History of HIV-Associated Salivary Gland Disease
Schiødt M, Dodd CL, Greenspan D, Daniels TE, Chernoff D, Hollander H, Wara D, Greenspan JS (Hillerød Central Hosp, Denmark; Univ of California, San Francisco)
Oral Surg Oral Med Oral Pathol 74:326–331, 1992   105-94-10-5

Purpose.—The salivary glands may be affected by HIV infection in a variety of ways, including neoplasms and a less well-defined involvement called HIV-associated salivary gland disease (HIV-SGD). This term describes the diffuse enlargement of the major salivary glands or xerostomia in HIV-infected patients. The clinical, pathologic, and immune characteristics of such patients have been previously reported; this study describes the natural history of HIV-SGD.

Patients.—The study included 22 patients, 21 adult men and 1 11-year-old girl, who were followed for a median of 15 months (Table 1). Bilateral parotid gland enlargement (PGE) was present in three fourths of the patients. It remained stable in 10 of the patients, progressed in 2, and regressed during zidovudine or steroid treatment in 4. Seventeen patients had xerostomia, and 11 had both PGE and xerostomia. The mean stimulated parotid flow rate was .27 mL/min/gland in the patients with PGE vs. .48 mL/min/gland in a control group of HIV-positive patients without PGE. There was no significant difference in mean unstimulated whole salivary flow rates, which did not change during follow-up. Twenty-three percent of the patients had AIDS at the time of the diagnosis of HIV-SGD, whereas 46% had AIDS at follow-up (Table 2). Of the latter, 7 had Kaposi's sarcoma. Their mean peripheral blood CD4 cell count increased from 280 m^3 at the initial examination to 225 mm^3 at follow-up, and the CD8 counts decreased from 1138 to 900.

TABLE 1.—Data on 22 Patients With HIV-Associated Salivary Gland Disease at the Time of Diagnosis

Patient No.	Sex	Age	CDC group	Duration, PGE	Dry mouth*	Dry eyes*	Arthralgia*	Other conditions
1	F	4	AIDS, IVE	24 mo	+	−	−	LIP
2	M	27	III	10 yrs	+	+	+	HL, EC
3	M	54	IVC2	6 mo	+	−	+	ITP (1985)
4	M	41	IVE	30 mo	+	+	+	HL, EC, GP
5	M	57	IVC2	1 mo	+	+	+	EC
6	M	42	III	24 mo	+	−	−	KS, HL, GP
7	M	36	AIDS, IVD	1 mo	−	−	−	EC
8	M	32	III	5 mo	+	−	+	KS, HL, GP
9	M	37	IVC2	−	+	−	−	EC
10	M	45	IVC2	4 mo	+	+	+	HL, GP
11	M	45	IVB, C2	−	+	+	−	Neuro-pathy, HL, GP, KCS
12	M	34	IVC2	−	+	−	−	EC, GP
13	M	51	IVC2	24 mo	+	+	−	LIP
14	M	41	AIDS, IVD	−	+	−	+	Cryptococcosis, KS, CNS involvement
15	M	31	III	−	+	−	−	HL
16	M	38	IVC2	−	+	+	+	KS
17	M	43	AIDS, IVD	8 mo	−	−	−	KS, EC
18	M	29	AIDS, IVD	3 mo	−	−	−	HL, EC
19	M	31	IVC2	1 mo	−	−	+	
20	M	39	III	8 mo	+	+	−	
21	M	44	III	1 mo	−	+	−	Oral ulcer
22	M	60	III	36 mo	+	−	−	EC

Abbreviations: PGE, parotid gland enlargement; LIP, lymphoid interstitial pneumonitis; HL, hairy leukoplakia; EC, erythematous oral candidiasis; GP, gingivitis/periodontitis (not necrotizing gingivitis); ITP, idiopathic thrombocytopenic purpura; KS, Kaposi's sarcoma; KCS, keratoconjunctivitis sicca. * = Symptoms.
(Courtesy of Schiødt M, Dodd CL, Greenspan D, et al: Oral Surg Oral Med Oral Pathol 74:326–331, 1992.)

TABLE 2.—Change in Status of Patients With HIV-SGD During Observation

	Baseline	Follow-up examination
No. with AIDS	5/22 (23%)	10/22 (45%)
No. with parotid gland enlargement	16/22	13/22
CD4 cells/mm^3, mean (range)	280 (37-800)	225 (0-768)
CD8 cells/mm^3, mean (range)	1138 (259-3333)	900 (268-1512)
CD4/CD8 ratio, mean (range)	0.41 (0.06-1.1)	0.26 (0-0.8)

(Courtesy of Schiødt M, Dodd CL, Greenspan D, et al: Oral Surg Oral Med Oral Pathol 74:326-331, 1992.)

Conclusion.—The prognosis for HIV-SGD appears to be rather favorable, but this must be confirmed by case control studies. Intraparotid lymphoid tissue hyperplasia may be part of the pathogenesis of HIV-SGD, and patients have many of the clinical features of Sjögren's syndrome. Therefore, HIV infection should be included in the differential diagnosis of bilateral PGE.

▶ This paper and the preceding paper provide a good reminder that patients with AIDS can have several other problems that affect structures that fall within the normal purview of the dentist.—J.E. Kennedy, D.D.S., M.S.

Painful Gingivitis May Be an Early Sign of Infection With Human Immunodeficiency Virus

Rowland RW, Escobar MR, Friedman RB, Kaplowitz LG (Virginia Commonwealth Univ, Richmond)
Clin Infect Dis 16:233–236, 1993   105-94-10-6

Introduction.—Patients with HIV infection often experience painful severe gingival conditions requiring emergency treatment. These gingival problems usually include either periodontal abscesses or necrotizing ulcerative gingivitis (NUG). The incidence of NUG or NUG-like (NUGL) lesions and the preliminary CD4 and CD8 T-lymphocyte profiles were investigated in patients with HIV infections.

Methods.—Patients seen in the emergency department with gum pain were diagnosed with NUG if they had painful gingiva, ulcerated papillae, and bleeding. The diagnosis of NUGL included those with similar symptoms, but without the bleeding.

Results.—Over 24 months, 24 patients received a diagnosis of NUG or NUGL. Twenty of the 24 agreed to participate in the study. Of these 20, 7 tested positive for HIV. Four of the 7 knew they were HIV positive. The seropositive patients had a mean age of 31.4 years, whereas the seronegative group had a mean age of 24 years, a significant difference. All seronegative individuals and 2 of the HIV-positive patients had typical NUG lesions in the interdental spaces of the anterior teeth regions. All subjects with pain and all HIV-seropositive individuals smoked cigarettes, whereas none of the HIV-seronegative individuals did. Two of the 7 HIV-positive subjects lacked enough T lymphocytes for testing. The HIV-seropositive group had a significantly lower percentage and lower count of CD4 lymphocytes than did the HIV-seronegative group. All patients had a severely depressed mitogenic response when compared to control subjects without gingivitis. The HIV-positive individuals had significantly lower CD4/CD8 lymphocyte ratios than did the HIV-seronegative participants.

Conclusion.—Although only 20 subjects participated in this study, 7 (35%) were HIV positive. Because of this much greater incidence of gingivitis in HIV-positive individuals, health-care providers should consider testing for HIV infection in patients seeking treatment for gum pain and other gingivitis symptoms.

▶ The 35% incidence found in this study requires the practitioner to consider HIV infection in every patient with NUG. It is more difficult to exclude HIV infection as an etiologic factor based on earlier definitions of high-risk groups. Thus, through one mechanism or another, it is highly advisable to rule out HIV infection for all patients with NUG.—J.E. Kennedy, D.D.S., M.S.

A Comparison of T4:T8 Lymphocyte Ratio in the Periodontal Lesion of Healthy and HIV-Positive Patients

Steidley KE, Thompson SH, McQuade MJ, Strong SL, Scheidt MJ, Van Dyke TE (US Army, Ft Gordon, Ga; Baylor College of Dentistry, Dallas; Univ of Rochester, NY)

J Periodontol 63:753–756, 1992   105-94-10-7

Introduction.—Human immunodeficiency virus attacks the T4 lymphocyte and is associated with a rapidly progressive form of periodontitis. Therefore, HIV infection might affect local gingival immunoregulation.

Methods.—The gingival and serum T4:T8 lymphocyte ratios in HIV-negative and HIV-positive patients with periodontitis were compared. Flow cytometry was used to measure T cell subsets in the peripheral blood. Papillary gingival tissue from 8 HIV-positive patients and 6 healthy controls was taken during gingival surgery. Specimens were labeled with monoclonal antibodies developed by an avidin-biotin-peroxidase technique, and T4:T8 lymphocyte ratio for each specimen was evaluated by histologic examination.

Findings.—The mean serum T4:T8 ratio was 2.07 for controls vs. 0.58 for the HIV-positive patients. In controls, mean T4:T8 lymphocyte ratio was highly variable, with a mean of 2.70. The HIV-positive patients showed almost complete absence of T cells in their gingival specimens (table).

Conclusion.—Patients who are HIV positive with periodontal disease lack local immune effector and regulator cells in their gingiva, which might contribute to the characteristic and rapidly progressive periodon-

Relationship Between Periodontal Status, Walter Reed Staging (WRS), Absolute T4 Count, Serum T4:T8 Ratio, and Gingival T4:T8

HIV + Patient	Periodontal Status	WRS	ABS T4	Serum T4:T8	Gingival T4:T8
1	Moderate	IV	392	0.520	N.D.*
2	HIV-P	V	30	0.095	N.D.
3	HIV-P	V	32	0.777	N.D.
4	Moderate	II	419	0.095	N.D.
5	Moderate	II	1055	1.210	0.425
6	Moderate	III	244	0.579	N.D.
7	Severe	II	799	0.737	N.D.
8	Gingivitis	II	472	0.600	N.D.

Note: The data suggest a relationship between periodontal disease status and local T4 count and T4/T8.
* No T cells detected in the biopsy specimen.
(Courtesy of Steidley KE, Thompson SH, McQuade MJ, et al: *J Periodontol* 63:753–756, 1992.)

tal disease in these patients. The number of serum T4 cells in the serum appears to be related to the presence of T lymphocytes in the gingiva.

▶ The existence of local immune reactions in the gingiva has long been considered one of the important elements in the defense against the progression of periodontitis. Knowing that the gingival tissues of HIV-positive patients are devoid of T cells not only provides some explanation for the rapid progression of adult-onset periodontitis, but requires that the approach to therapy be aggressive and monitored frequently, e.g., every 3 months.—J.E. Kennedy, D.D.S., M.S.

Systemic/Oral Relationships

Non-Oral Etiologies of Oral Malodor and Altered Chemosensation

Preti G, Clark L, Cowart BJ, Feldman RS, Lowry LD, Weber E, Young IM (Monell Chemical Senses Ctr, Philadelphia; Jefferson Med College, Philadelphia; Univ of Pennsylvania, Philadelphia)
J Periodontol 63:790–796, 1992   105-94-10–8

Background.—Oral malodor may have several nonoral causes that may be indicative of systemic disease (Table 1). The potential severity of these diseases necessitates early diagnosis and treatment. Several metabolic and transport errors that may also produce oral malodor were examined.

Methods.—Patients examined in this study were seen by referral, typically after previous clinical examination had failed to discover the etiology of the complaint. Gas chromatography and mass spectrometry were used to examine the expired air of 20 patients with idiopathic malodor,

TABLE 1.—Oral Volatiles Identified in Patients With
Systemic Pathologies

Pathology

Diabetes mellitus: (ketonic breath) acetone
and other ketones

Uremia/kidney failure: (fishy odor)
dimethylamine $[(CH_3)_2NH$; trimethylamine $(CH_3)_3N]$

Cirrhosis of the liver: (*Fetor Hepaticus*)
C_2-C_5 aliphatic acids, methylmercaptan
(CH_3SH), ethanethiol (CH_3CH_2SH), and
dimethylsulfide $(CH_3S\ CH_3)$

(Courtesy of Preti G, Clark L, Cowart BJ, et al: *J Periodontol* 63:790–796, 1992.)

TABLE 2.—Persistent, Idiopathis Malodor Producers ($n = 20$)

Group (N)	Presenting Symptoms	Cause
1 (2)	Foul smell/taste* persistent, long-standing; may vary with diet	Excess trimethylamine caused by trimethylaminuria (TMAU)
2 (11)	Long-standing oral malodor and/or nasal odor†	High levels volatile sulfur compounds in mouth air/saliva and/or expired breath
3 (4)	Oral malodor, bad breath*	No apparent elevation in the components analyzed
4 (3)	Axillary, genital, and/or general body odor‡	

* The odors may or may not be apparent to individuals near the patient because they are episodic and vary in intensity. Spouses, children, and/or those intimate with the patient often corroborate the complaint of malodor.
† As with the individuals with TMAU, those close to the patient would corroborate the malodor complaint, although many in this group suggested the malodor could be transient. In the clinic, these patients were seen most often with detectable oral malodor.
‡ These patients are seen in collaboration with colleagues in the Department of Dermatology, Obstetrics/Gynecology, and/or Metabolic Disorders, University of Pennsylvania.
(Courtesy of Preti G, Clark L, Cowart BJ, et al: J Periodontol 63:790–796, 1992.)

55 patients with altered chemosensation, and 18 normal controls. All patients also underwent clinical sensory examinations.

Results.—Patients reporting dysgeusia and/or dysosmia had a wide a variety of complaints without any correlating anatomical disease. Interestingly, 4 volatile compounds were shown to be 95% efficient in distinguishing between this patient group and normal controls. In addition, patients within this group were characterized by elevated levels of dimethyltrisulfide and aniline, and lowered levels of acetoin and 1-octen-3-ol.

Patients with idiopathic malodor were separated into 4 groups (Table 2). Trimethylaminuria was identified in 2 patients. Although this defect is known to be an autosomal recessive trait, it may also result from excessive trimethylamine production by bacteria within the gastrointestinal tract. Several other patients also had high levels of H_2S and CH_3SH. Two patients with the highest levels of these gases also had elevated cysteine or cystathionine levels.

Conclusion.—Because subtle metabolic disorders may be responsible for oral malodor, patients with long-standing oral malodor problems should not be dismissed by the physician or dentist, even after consultation with specialists proves unsuccessful.

Biochemical and Clinical Factors Influencing Oral Malodor in Periodontal Patients

Yaegaki K, Sanada K (Nippon Dental Univ, Niigata, Japan)
J Periodontol 63:783–789, 1992   105-94-10–9

Background.—Pathologic oral malodor, caused primarily by volatile sulfur compounds (VSC), including hydrogen sulfide, methyl mercaptan, and dimethyl sulfide, is frequently associated with periodontal disease. To develop treatment for this condition, the factors that influence pathologic oral malodor must first be discerned. Further understanding of the pathology of halitosis associated with periodontal disease was obtained.

Study Design.—The clinical and biomechanical factors that accelerate the production of VSC were examined via comparison between 17 patients with periodontal disease and 14 control participants.

Results.—In patients with periodontal disease, the VSC amounts and methylmercaptan/hydrogen sulfide ratio in mouth air were 8 times higher than those of control participants (Fig 10-3). Patients with periodontal disease also demonstrated increased disulfide concentrations in proportion to the total pocket depth (Fig 10-4). The disulfide content (which is converted to VSC) of saliva correlated significantly with periodontal disease. Within this patient group, 60% of the VSC was produced from the tongue surface, and the amount of tongue coating was 4

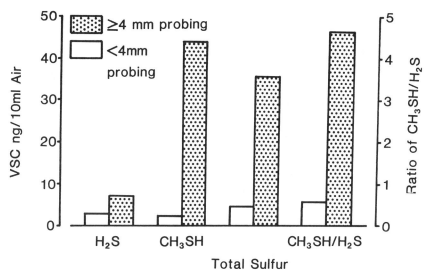

Fig 10-3.—Volatile sulfur compound (VSC) production in mouth air from subjects ($n = 17$) with a gingival probing depth of 4 mm or more. In comparison with subjects ($n = 14$) with a probing depth of less than 4 mm, a large amount of VSC production was observed, and the methyl mercaptan/hydrogen sulfide ratio was markedly increased. (Courtesy of Yaegaki K, Sanada K: *J Periodontol* 63:783–789, 1992.)

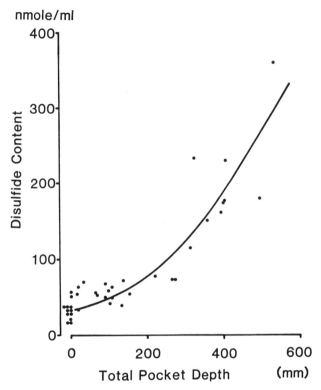

nmole/ml

Fig 10–4.—Disulfide in saliva and periodontal disease. Disulfide content (nmol/mL) in saliva was increased with total pocket depth in each patient. A regression curve was obtained, Y = 40.5275 + .0299X + .0009X², with a coefficient of determination of .8407 (P < .01). (Courtesy of Yaegaki K, Sanada K: J Periodontol 63:783–789, 1992.)

times greater in patients with periodontal disease as compared with controls. An increase in VSC production and methyl mercaptan/hydrogen sulfide ratio of the tongue coating were also seen in patients with periodontal involvement. The periodontal group also displayed greater amounts of 2-ketobutyrate, a byproduct of the metabolism of methionine to methylmercaptan, in their saliva. Therefore, in the oral cavities of patients with periodontal pockets, an increase in metabolism of methionine to methylmercaptan is seen. Because free L-methionine is the main source for methylmercaptan, the methionine supply from the gingival fluid into the oral cavity of patients with periodontal involvement was estimated. The ratio of methionine to whole free amino acids was significantly greater as compared to cysteine.

Conclusion.—In patients with periodontal disease, VSC production is enhanced not only by micro-organisms, but by the tongue coating and gingival fluid as well.

▶ The preceding 2 articles give a comprehensive picture of the range of clinical problems that can result in malodor for the patient who has the courage to ask or the individual who is concerned about a family member. In such situations, the information reported can be the basis of a search for the cause, and even if therapy is not possible, then at least there can be an understanding of the problem. Those interested in additional information should refer to the article by Kleinberg and Westbay (1), which describes the role of saliva in this clinical problem. (The reader may obtain copies of this and other articles featured in the YEAR BOOK by accessing Mosby's Document Express.)—J.E. Kennedy, D.D.S., M.S.

Reference

1. Kleinberg I, Westbay GJ: *J Periodontol* 63:768, 1992.

Oral Cancer

Regression of Oral Leukoplakia With α-Tocopherol: A Community Clinical Oncology Program Chemoprevention Study

Benner SE, Winn RJ, Lippman SM, Poland J, Hansen KS, Luna MA, Hong WK (Univ of Texas, M. D. Anderson Cancer Ctr, Houston; Methodist Hosp of Indiana, Indianapolis; Columbia River Community Clinical Oncology Program, Portland, Ore)

J Natl Cancer Inst 85:44–47, 1993   105-94-10-10

Background.—Lesions in the upper aerodigestive tract can result from carcinogen exposure, including tobacco and alcohol, and may precede invasive cancer development. Oral leukoplakia can serve as an important model for the development of chemoprevention treatment approaches.

Clinical and Histologic Responses to Treatment With α-Tocopherol for Oral Leukoplakia

	Clinical response		Histologic response	
	No. of patients	%	No. of patients	%
Complete response	10	23	0	0
Partial response	10	23	9	21
No change	8	19	16	37
Progressive disease	3	7	7	16
Not assessable	12	28	11	26
Total	43	100	43	100

Note: Complete clinical response: disappearance of lesion for 1 month or more. Partial clinical response: 50% or more decrease in the product of the two longest diameters of a single lesion or in the sum of these figures for all lesions. Complete histologic response: complete reversal of dysplasia; reversion to normal epithelium. Partial histologic response: improvement in the degree of dysplasia; persistent, abnormal maturation of the epithelium. Clinically not assessable: lesion measurements not recorded during baseline visit, 24-week visit, and one of the interim follow-up visits. Histologically not assessable: biopsy specimens not obtained at both the baseline and 24-week visits.

(Courtesy of Benner SE, Winn RJ, Lippman SM, et al: *J Natl Cancer Inst* 85:44–47, 1993.)

In animal models, α-tocopherol (vitamin E), a powerful antioxidant, has prevented oral cavity cancer development. The toxicity and efficacy of α-tocopherol in patients with oral leukoplakia were assessed in a single-arm phase II study. In addition, the practicality of performing chemoprevention trials via the Community Clinical Oncology Program (CCOP) network was evaluated. Seven institutions affiliated with the CCOP through the University of Texas M.D. Anderson Cancer Center participated.

Patients and Methods.—A total of 43 patients with symptomatic leukoplakia or dysplasia were included in this study. All patients were treated with 400 IU of oral α-tocopherol 2 times per day for 24 weeks. The follow-up evaluations were conducted at 6, 12, and 24 weeks after initiation of treatment. Serum α-tocopherol levels were determined at baseline and at 6 and 24 weeks.

Results.—After completing 24 weeks of treatment, clinical responses were noted in 20 patients, and histologic responses were seen in 9 (table). At baseline, the mean serum α-tocopherol levels were 16.1 μg/mL, which increased to 34.29 μg/mL after 24 weeks of treatment. Excellent patient compliance was demonstrated via patient-recorded drug calendars and serum drug levels. In fact, 95% of the prescribed pills were taken. No grade 3 or 4 toxic effects were reported during the study. Overall, treatment was tolerated well in all participants.

Conclusion.—Both clinical and histologic responses in premalignant leukoplakia lesions were noted after administration of α-tocopherol. Chemoprevention trials can be conducted through the CCOP, although limited participation within the CCOP network was noted. Future trials for evaluation of α-tocopherol alone and in combination with other chemopreventive agents for carcinogenesis in the upper aerodigestive tract are recommended.

▶ Although the results of this study are described as interim, the evidence is strong enough to seriously consider this approach to the management of oral leukoplakia. A note of caution: there is no substitute for an accurate diagnosis by means of exfoliative cytology or biopsy.—J.E. Kennedy, D.D.S., M.S.

Cytobrush and Wooden Spatula for Oral Exfoliative Cytology: A Comparison
Ogden GR, Cowpe JG, Green M (Dundee Univ, Scotland)
Acta Cytol 36:706–710, 1992   105-94-10–11

Background.—The wooden tongue spatula often is used to obtain oral musocal smears, but clumping of cells make the smear unsuitable for cytomorphologic evaluation. The Cytobrush has been developed for use in the uterine cervix; its potential value in oral cytology is uncertain.

Comparison of Cell Yield Using the Wooden Spatula and Cytobrush for Each Oral Site Smeared

Cell yield grade	Dorsal tongue				Buccal mucosa				Ventral tongue				Hard palate			
	W		C		W		C		W		C		W		C	
	Good	Poor	Good	Poor	Good	Poor	Good	Poor	Good	Poor	Good	Poor	Good	Poor	Good	Poor
0	2	0	0	0	2	0	0	0	11	3	0	0	6	8	2	12
1	6	3	1	1	2	5	1	0	3	3	0	4	2	7	0	5
2	13	2	23	1	16	1	23	2	4	2	15	7	1	2	2	4
Total	21	5	24	2	20	6	24	2	18	8	15	11	9	17	4	22

Abbreviations: W, wooden spatula; C, cytobrush.
(Courtesy of Ogden GR, Cowpe JG, Greene M: *Acta Cytol* 36:706–710, 1992.)

Objective.—Smears were collected with both a wooden spatula and the Cytobrush from 4 clinically normal sites (dorsal tongue, ventral tongue, hard palate, buccal mucosa) in 26 patients. Each of the instruments was scraped firmly across the mucosa 10 times before transfer to a glass slide. Smears were examined independently by 2 observers.

Results.—The Cytobrush yielded nearly twice as many grade 2 smears, indicating better dispersion and cell yield than were obtained using the wooden spatula. The 2 methods gave comparable cell yields when used in the buccal mucosa and hard palate, but the Cytobrush was superior for the tongue surfaces (table). Cell dispersion was significantly better with the Cytobrush for the tongue surfaces and the buccal mucosa. The 2 instruments gave comparable results for the hard palate.

Conclusion.—The Cytobrush is an effective means of obtaining cytologic samples of the normal oral mucosa.

▶ The selection of this article is intended to remind the practitioner that there is another method for obtaining cells, which may be preferable in some situations. The need to repeat this study with other than normal mucosa must be emphasized.—J.E. Kennedy, D.D.S., M.S.

Comparison of Low-Dose Isotretinoin With Beta Carotene to Prevent Oral Carcinogenesis
Lippman SM, Batsakis JG, Toth BB, Weber RS, Lee JJ, Martin JW, Hays GL, Goepfert H, Hong WK (Univ of Texas M. D. Anderson Cancer Ctr, Houston)
N Engl J Med 328:15–20, 1993   105-94-10–12

Background.—The high risk of transformation of dysplastic leukoplakia into invasive cancer suggests the need for systemic treatment. Isotretinoin in high dosage has proved to be an effective treatment, but relapses and toxic reactions are frequent. In this study, a high dose of isotretinoin was used in the induction phase only, followed by either a low dose of isotretinoin or β-carotene as maintenance therapy.

Study Design.—Seventy patients with measurable premalignant oral lesions received isotretinoin, 1.5 mg/kg daily, for 3 months (Table 1). All but 4 patients were evaluable. Subsequently, 26 patients were maintained on isotretinoin, .5 mg/kg daily, for 9 months and 33 others received 30 mg of β-carotene daily.

Results.—Substantial toxicity accompanied induction treatment. One patient withdrew because of gastrointestinal toxicity, but there was no major hepatic toxicity. Disease progression occurred at a significantly lower rate in patients maintained on isotretinoin than in those given β-carotene. Invasive carcinoma occurred in 5 patients in the β-carotene group, and in situ cancer occurred in 1 patient in each group. All 7 of these patients had curative wide excision. Toxicity in the maintenance phase was relatively mild (Table 2).

TABLE 1.—Major Characteristics of the Patients

CHARACTERISTIC	INDUCTION PHASE (N = 70)	MAINTENANCE PHASE*	
		ISOTRET-INOIN (N = 26)	BETA CAROTENE (N = 33)
Median age (range) — yr	59 (24–83)	60 (34–83)	61 (31–80)
		no. of patients (%)†	
Sex			
Female	37 (53)	13 (50)	19 (58)
Male	33 (47)	13 (50)	14 (42)
Histologic type			
Dysplasia, mild	32 (46)	14 (54)	15 (45)
Dysplasia, moderate	8 (11)	3 (12)	4 (12)
Dysplasia, severe	2 (3)	1 (4)	1 (3)
Hyperplasia	28 (40)	8 (31)	13 (39)
Carcinogens currently used			
Tobacco	39 (56)	15 (58)	18 (55)
Alcohol	45 (64)	16 (62)	22 (67)
Both	31 (44)	12 (46)	15 (45)

* Of the 70 patients enrolled, 59 had responses or stable lesions after completing high-dose isotretinoin induction therapy and were eligible for low-dose isotretinoin or β-carotene maintenance therapy.
† Because of rounding, not all percentages equal 100.
(Courtesy of Lippman SM, Batsakis JG, Toth BB, et al: N Engl J Med 328:15–20, 1993.)

Conclusion.—After induction treatment of leukoplakia with high-dose isotretinoin, the same agent in low dosage is significantly more active than is β-carotene, and it is adequately tolerated.

▶ The occurrence of squamous cell carcinoma in 5 patients receiving β-carotene should be reason for caution. These results call into question whether β-carotene is an effective agent for the maintenance of areas of leukoplakia. The combination of both clinical and microscopic evaluation adds credibility to the results. The β-carotene dosing error reported is very likely to have been a factor in the outcome of the study.—J.E. Kennedy, D.D.S., M.S.

TABLE 2.—Final Clinical Results of
Maintenance Therapy

RESULT	ISOTRETINOIN (N = 24)	BETA CAROTENE (N = 29)
	no. of patients (%)	
Positive outcome	22 (92)	13 (45)
Further response	8	3
Stable lesions	14	10
Disease progression	2 (8)*	16 (55)

* *P* < .001 for the comparison between treatment groups.
(Courtesy of Lippman SM, Batsakis JG, Toth BB, et al: N Engl J Med 328:15-20, 1993.)

Dry Mouth

Burning Mouth Syndrome: Evaluation of Multiple Variables Among 85 Patients

Maresky LS, van der Bijl P, Gird I (Univ of Stellenbosch, Tygerberg, South Africa)
Oral Surg Oral Med Oral Pathol 75:303–307, 1993   105-94-10–13

Introduction.—Burning mouth syndrome (BMS), a type of atypical facial pain affecting postmenopausal women, has been associated with a wide variety of local and systemic causative factors. Associations between BMS and 48 variables were investigated in a retrospective study of clinic patients.

Methods and Results.—The records of 241 patients 45 years of age and older attending an oral medicine clinic over 4 years were reviewed. A diagnosis of BMS, defined as the complaint of a burning sensation of the oral mucosa, was made in 85 patients. Three fourths of these patients were women, 86% of them postmenopausal. Compared with controls, both men and women with BMS showed significant associations with self-medication, xerostomia, and other salivary disturbances. In the women, further associations were noted with anemia, dietary inadequacy, chronic infection, hormone therapy, ulcerative or erosive lesions, and atrophy. In men, associations were also noted with prescription medications, central nervous system disorders, gingivitis, and denture problems. Other variables significantly associated with BMS included psychogenic factors, regurgitation, flatulence, and periodontitis (table).

Conclusion.—In reviewing the variables associated with BMS, climacteric changes appear to be responsible for only a small percentage of cases, whereas drugs, xerostomia, and other salivary disorders play an important role. Although the cause of the condition remains unclear,

Variables With Statistically Significant Differences Between BMS and Control Groups

Variables	Women			Men		
	BMS (n = 65) %	Control (n = 89) %	p-value	BMS (n = 20) %	Control (n = 67) %	p-value
Prescribed medication	83	78	0.396	90	66	0.035*
Self-medication	60	40	0.011*	75	30	0.000*
CNS disturbance	23	25	0.814	35	7	0.005*
Anemia	20	7	0.013*	10	5	0.324
Inadequate diet	23	7	0.004*	15	6	0.196
Chronic infection	18	3	0.002*	15	15	0.619
Hormone therapy	28	12	0.016*	5	4	0.656
Gingivitis	35	30	0.509	60	33	0.029*
Denture-related problems	55	67	0.128	40	66	0.040*
Ulcerative/erosive lesions	37	65	0.001*	60	69	0.471
Atrophy	40	25	0.043*	45	27	0.124
Xerostomia	34	9	0.000*	35	4	0.000*
Other salivary disturbances	18	7	0.025*	15	1	0.011*

* Statistically significant (P < .05).
(Courtesy of Maresky JL, van der Bijl P, Gird I: Oral Surg Oral Med Oral Pathol 75:303–307, 1993.)

management requires careful initial investigation, elimination or reduction of possible contributing factors, and regular monitoring and reevaluation.

▶ This study has 2 advantages over previous reports. The number of patients allows for rigorous statistical analysis, and the number of variables assessed was extensive. The results provide a practitioner with a good basis from which to sort through a patient's complaint of burning mouth and provide a logical approach to the identification of possible cause.—J.E. Kennedy, D.D.S., M.S.

Mucin-Containing Lozenges in the Treatment of Intraoral Problems Associated With Sjögren's Syndrome: A Double-Blind Crossover Study in 42 Patients
's-Gravenmade EJ, Vissink A (Univ Hosp Groningen, The Netherlands)
Oral Surg Oral Med Oral Pathol 75:466–471, 1993   105-94-10–14

Background.—The chronic inflammation of the exocrine glands that characterizes Sjögren's syndrome can cause irreversible hyposalivation and xerostomia. The efficacy and therapeutic value were evaluated in high-molecular-weight glycoproteins given in the form of mucin-containing lozenges for diminishing the symptoms of hyposalivation.

Patients.—Forty-one women and 1 man with Sjögren's syndrome who complained of moderate-to-severe xerostomia were enrolled in the study. After a 2-week washout period, 21 patients were given mucin-con-

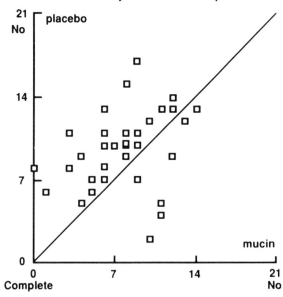

Fig 10–5.—Relief of dryness-related complaints after using mucin and placebo lozenges. The sum scores of the variables, "general pattern of complaints," "extent of oral dryness," "dryness during daytime," "dryness at night," "oral functioning," and "taste of lozenges," are indicated. The X and Y axis range from 0 (complete relief) to 28 (no relief). *Straight line* means equal scores. Only patients who answered all questions are included. (Courtesy of 's-Gravenmade EJ, Vissink A: *Oral Surg Oral Med Oral Pathol* 75:466–471, 1993.)

taining lozenges for 2 weeks, and 20 received placebo lozenges. After 2 weeks, the patients were crossed over to the alternate medication for another 2 weeks. All patients were asked to complete a questionnaire at baseline and every 2 weeks thereafter, yielding 4 completed questionnaires for each patient.

Results.—Thirty-two patients (76%) preferred the mucin lozenge, 4 patients (10%) preferred the placebo lozenge, and 6 patients (14%) had no preference. Compared with the placebo lozenge, the mucin lozenge more effectively improved the total range of dryness-related complaints and moistened the oral cavity longer (Fig 10–5). However, the placebo lozenge more effectively improved oral functioning and the sensation of bad taste. Patients with the most complaints at the start of the study appeared to have benefited the most from the mucin lozenge.

Conclusion.—Mucin-containing lozenges appear to be useful in reducing the oral discomfort associated with the hyposalivation of Sjögren's syndrome.

▶ The design of this study and the results provide the practitioner with ample evidence that the use of mucin lozenges as a first approach to treatment should receive serious consideration.—J.E. Kennedy, D.D.S., M.S.

Management of the Medically Compromised

The Relationship Between Reduction in Periodontal Inflammation and Diabetes Control: A Report of 9 Cases

Miller LS, Manwell MA, Newbold D, Reding ME, Rasheed A, Blodgett J, Kornman KS (Univ of Texas, San Antonio)
J Periodontol 63:843–848, 1992   105-94-10–15

Background.—Periodontists are likely to see an increasing number of diabetic patients. Some of the host defects seen in diabetics are risk factors for periodontal disease, and diabetic patients ar relatively susceptible to infection. Although it has been taught that controlling periodontal disease will benefit diabetic control and may lower insulin requirements, there is minimal evidence that this is true.

Objective.—The effects of eliminating gingival inflammation on blood glucose levels were examined in 9 poorly controlled diabetics with periodontitis.

Management.—Scaling and root planing were done in conjunction with oral hygiene instruction. The patients were placed on home monitoring and given doxycycline for 2 weeks and a chlorhexidine rinse. They were reassessed 4 and 8 weeks after treatment.

Findings.—Treatment reduced bleeding on probing (Fig 10–6) and decreased probing depth. The mean glycated hemoglobin decreased from 9.4 to 9.0 following treatment. Glycated albumin values did not

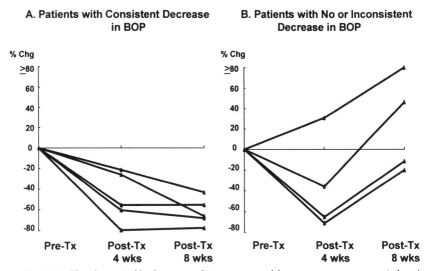

Fig 10–6.—The change in bleeding on probing as measured by a constant-pressure periodontal probe is shown for each of the post-treatment (Post-Tx) monitoring periods for each patient. Bleeding scores for patients who had a consistent decrease at both 4 and 8 weeks after therapy are shown in **A**, with the remaining patients presented in **B**. (Courtesy of Miller LS, Manwell MA, Newbold D, et al: *J Periodontol* 63:843–848, 1992.)

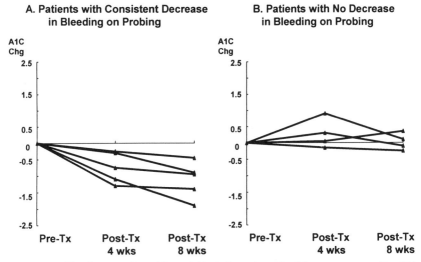

Fig 10–7.—The change in glycated hemoglobin is shown for each of the post-treatment (Post-Tx) monitoring periods for each patient. The patients are grouped according to the bleeding response patterns in Figure 10-6. (Courtesy of Miller LS, Manwell MA, Newbold D, et al: *J Periodontol* 63:843–848, 1992.)

change significantly. All 5 patients who consistently had less bleeding had a reduction in glycated hemoglobin after treatment (Fig 10-7).

Discussion.—Some connection was found between lessened periodontal bleeding and improved metabolic control in diabetic patients with periodontitis. Periodontal disease, however, is only 1 of many factors in metabolic control, and it may be relatively minor. It may not be possible to limit periodontal disease in all poorly controlled diabetics.

▶ Most studies evaluating the relationship between diabetes and periodontal diseases have focused on the effect of the severity of disease on adult-onset periodontitis. This study adds a new and very important dimension to our understanding of that relationship. The successful elimination of multiple foci of oral infection may well warrant reevaluation of insulin dosage. For such patients, the dentist would be well advised to establish a close working relationship with the physician managing the patient's diabetes.—J.E. Kennedy, D.D.S., M.S.

Contraindications to Vasoconstrictors in Dentistry: Part I. Cardiovascular Diseases
Pérusse R, Goulet J-P, Turcotte J-Y (Université Laval, Ste-Foy, PQ)
Oral Surg Oral Med Oral Pathol 74:679–686, 1992   105-94-10–16

Introduction.—Epinephrine and levonordefrin are widely used in dental practice to enhance anesthesia, promote hemostasis, and prevent toxic reactions to local anesthetics by limiting their absorption into the blood. There are a number of absolute and relative contraindications to using vasoconstrictors in dentistry (table). Epinephrine and its congeners are capable of producing significant hemodynamic changes and even life-threatening complications.

Coronary Heart Disease.—Serious hemodynamic effects have been described in patients with unstable angina who receive intravenous epinephrine. Low infusion rates lead to increased cardiac output and myocardial oxygen consumption. Often patients with recent myocardial infarction are advised to defer dental treatment for at least 3-6 months. The myocardium may remain electrically unstable for months after infarction, making epinephrine and other vasoconstrictors strictly contraindicated. There are no clear guidelines to the management of patients who have recently undergone coronary bypass surgery.

Arrhythmias.—Refractory arrhythmias that fail to respond adequately to medical measures place patients at high medical risk and are a major contraindication to using vasoconstrictors. A history of infarction or the use of new antiarrhythmic agents should alert the practitioner to the possibility of resistant arrhythmia.

Hypertension.—There is concern over a sudden, dramatic rise in blood pressure when a vasoconstrictor is administered. Vasoconstrictors

Contraindications to Using Vasoconstrictors in Dentistry

Absolute contraindications
  Heart diseases
    a. Unstable angina
    b. Recent myocardial infarction
    c. Recent coronary artery bypass surgery
    d. Refractory arrhythmias
    e. Untreated or uncontrolled severe hypertension
    f. Untreated or uncontrolled congestive heart failure
  Uncontrolled hyperthyroidism
  Uncontrolled diabetes
  Sulfite sensitivity; steroid-dependent asthma
  Pheochromocytoma
Relative contraindications
  Patients taking tricyclic antidepressants
  Patients taking phenothiazine compounds
  Patients taking monoamine oxidase inhibitors
  Patients taking nonselective β-blockers
  Cocaine abuser

(Courtesy of Pérusse R, Goulet J-P, Turcotte J-Y: *Oral Surg Oral Med Oral Pathol* 74:679–686, 1992.)

may, however, counter the massive release of endogenous catecholamines that often results from anxiety and stress in the dental setting. Epinephrine produces a dose-dependent change in systolic blood pressure. Vasoconstrictors probably should be avoided in patients whose blood pressure is 180/100 mm Hg or higher.

Heart Failure.—Uncontrolled congestive heart failure is a major contraindication to any dental treatment. There is a high risk of sudden death from ventricular arrhythmia. The myocardium is electrically unstable in these patients, and the cardiac reserve is significantly reduced.

Contraindications to Vasoconstrictors in Dentistry: Part II. Hyperthyroidism, Diabetes, Sulfite Sensitivity, Cortico-Dependent Asthma, and Pheochromocytoma

Pérusse R, Goulet J-P, Turcotte J-Y (Université Laval, Ste-Foy, PQ)

Oral Surg Oral Med Oral Pathol 74:687–691, 1992   105-94-10–17

Background.—The absolute and relative contraindications to the use of vasoconstrictors in dentistry depend on the potential risk of cardiovascular and metabolic complications. The focus in the literature has been primarily on patients with cardiovascular diseases, but other noncardiac conditions should also be carefully assessed. Patients with a history of hyperthyroidism, diabetes, sulfite allergy, asthma, or pheochromocytoma should be carefully assessed before the use of vasoconstrictors.

Absolute Contraindications to Vasoconstrictors.—Hyperthyroidism is characterized by a constellation of symptoms reflecting an increased metabolic activity of the body tissues. Vasoconstrictors should be avoided in patients with hyperthyroidism because of the possibility that sympathomimetic amines could potentiate the vascular effect of thyroid hormone. In patients with diabetes treated by diet or hypoglycemic agents, vasconstrictors may be used safely if their condition is under medical control. However, patients with labile or unbalanced diabetes are at risk for serious complications if vasoconstrictors are used. Local anesthetics with vasoconstrictor contain sulfites as antioxidant agents. Therefore, vasoconstrictors should be avoided in patients with sulfite sensitivity. It has been reported that a substantial proportion of patients with asthma are potentially sulfite-sensitive. As a conservative strategy, local anesthetics with vasoconstrictors should be avoided in cortico-dependent asthma patients because of the higher risk of sulfite allergy. Patients with pheochromocytoma have catecholamine-producing tumors. Vasoconstrictors are contraindicated in these patients because of the high risk for lethal cardiac or cerebrovascular complications.

Conclusion.—Serious medical complications after the use of local anesthetics with vasoconstrictor or epinephrine-impregnated retraction cords may occur in patients with certain noncardiac conditions. These conditions include hyperthyroidism, diabetes, sulfite sensitivity, cortico-dependent asthma, and pheochromocytoma. A thorough medical history for every dental patient allows the dentist to evaluate the use of vasoconstrictors in patients who are medically compromised.

Contraindications to Vasoconstrictors in Dentistry: Part III. Pharmacologic Interactions
Goulet J-P, Pérusse R, Turcotte J-Y (Université Laval, Ste-Foy, PQ)
Oral Surg Oral Med Oral Pathol 74:692–697, 1992   105-94-10–18

Background.—The dentist must evaluate the prescription and illicit drug use of patients to avoid medical complications with the concomitant use of vasoconstrictors. In particular, patients medicated with tricyclic antidepressants, monoamine oxidase inhibitors, phenothiazines, and β-blockers should be carefully evaluated before vasoconstrictors are used. The epinephrine in local anesthetics may have harmful interactions with these drugs. The dentist should always use the lowest dose of vasoconstrictor compatible with effective pain control of sufficient duration. As a routine procedure, the local anesthetic solution should be injected slowly with frequent aspiration to minimize the potential hazard of an accidental intravascular injection.

Use of Vasoconstrictors in Medicated Patients.—In patients treated with tricyclic antidepressants (TCAs), there is the potential for enhancement of the cardiovascular effects associated with exogenously administered catecholamines. These patients may receive reduced doses of vasoconstrictors. The monoamine oxidase inhibitors (MAOIs) are also used to treat major depression. Vasoconstrictors have been contraindicated in patients taking MAOIs because of the possibility that serious potentiation of exogenously administered catecholamines lead to hypertensive crisis. This finding, however, has not been confirmed in human studies and there is no theoretical basis for restricting the use of a local anesthetic with vasoconstrictor other than phenylephrine in patients currently treated with MAOIs. In patients treated with phenothiazine drugs, dentists should administer the smallest amount of anesthetic solution required for the desired anesthetic effect. Vasoconstrictors appear to be safe for patients treated with cardioselective β-blockers, but there is a potential risk for patients taking nonselective β-blockers. To avoid drug interaction, vasoconstrictors should not be used in patients taking nonselective β-blockers. Patients who are using cocaine are at very high risk for cardiovascular complications. The patient should be cocaine or crack-free for at least 24 hours before the use of local anesthetic with epinephrine or epinephrine-impregnated retraction cords.

Conclusion.—A thorough understanding of the potential pharmacologic interactions between exogenously administered adrenergic drugs and vasoconstrictors is essential for the dentist. Vasoconstrictors should not be administered to patients using psychotropic drugs, nonselective β-blockers, or illicit drugs such as cocaine.

▶ These 3 articles provide a comprehensive, current, and authoritative discussion of the question that is invariably raised when a practitioner is faced with the need to use a local anesthetic for a patient with a systemic disease that alters the normal ability to tolerate a vasoconstrictor. At the same time, inadequate anesthesia might result in the production of more endogenous epinephrine than that contained in the anesthetic. Physician consultation is essential in most circumstances. Armed with the information contained in these papers, the dentist should be a well-prepared participant in such a dialogue.—J.E. Kennedy, D.D.S., M.S.

Oral Medicine

Triamcinolone Acetonide Versus Chlorhexidine for Treatment of Recurrent Stomatitis
Miles DA, Bricker SL, Razmus TF, Potter RH (Indiana Univ, Indianapolis)
Oral Surg Oral Med Oral Pathol 75:397–402, 1993   105-94-10–19

Background.—The exact cause of recurrent aphthous stomatitis (RAS) is still unknown. Because there is increasing evidence for an immunodeficiency, some are treating RAS on an immune basis. The

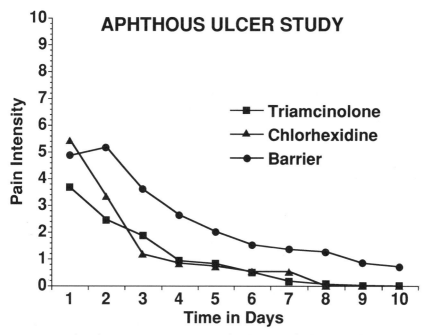

Fig 10–8.—Chart plotting pain intensity vs. time in days. (Courtesy of Miles DA, Bricker SL, Razmus TF, et al: *Oral Surg Oral Med Oral Pathol* 75:397–402, 1993.)

amount of pain relief obtained from 2 agents widely used in the treatment of RAS was compared by using a locally applied isobutyl cyanoacrylate barrier to promote ulcer healing.

Patients.—Ten of 30 patients with RAS were randomized to topical application of triamcinolone acetonide .025% followed by application of a drop of Iso-Dent for coverage, 10 received topical chlorhexidine digluconate .12% covered by Iso-Dent, and 10 were given Iso-Dent barrier only. All patients were asked to keep a record of pain intensity as estimated on a 10-point visual analogue scale. The duration of the study was 12 weeks.

Results.—The data from 19 patients who experienced a total of 35 episodes of RAS during the 12-week study were evaluated. A significant reduction in mean pain intensity occurred almost immediately after application of either chlorhexidine or triamcinolone, acetonide, compared with physical barrier alone. Analysis of the data revealed a highly significant difference in pain intensity and pain perception over time (Fig 10–8). No significant difference was found between the effect of triamcinolone acetonide and that of chlorhexidine digluconate.

Conclusion.—The application of a physical barrier over topically applied triamcinolone acetonide or chlorhexidine digluconate in the treatment of RAS appears to significantly shorten the duration of pain and to improve patient compliance.

▶ This study provides an alternative treatment that has the advantage of controlling dental plaque at a time when conventional oral hygiene may be difficult for the patient. It is especially worth considering as an alternative in those patients in whom ulcerations are particularly numerous or large or in areas where they are subject to trauma by conventional oral hygiene measures.—J.E. Kennedy, D.D.S., M.S.

Gustatory and Olfactory Considerations: Examination and Treatment in General Practice
Ship JA (Univ of Michigan, Ann Arbor)
J Am Dent Assoc 124(6):55–61, 1993   105-94-10-20

Objective.—Taste and smell are vital physiologic functions, disorders of which have deleterious consequences for systemic health, nutritional status, and quality of life. Many patients with gustatory and olfactory problems will initially consult their dentist, because taste and smell are intimately associated with the orofacial region. The literature on chemosensory dysfunction has been reviewed to help dentists familiarize themselves with these problems.

Taste.—Gustatory dysfunction may arise from a variety of conditions, ranging from local to systemic (Table 1). It is especially common in the elderly. The common oral sources, such as burns and lacerations, can be evaluated by the dentist. Burning mouth syndrome, a poorly understood condition occurring mainly in postmenopausal women, may be associated with taste dysfunction. Salivary dysfunction, including that associated with drugs, may alter taste sensitivity. Impairment of smell must also be evaluated in the patient complaining of taste dysfunction. Many neurologic and systemic diseases may cause taste and smell dysfunction, as may the treatments used against them, such as radiation therapy.

Assessment of the patient with taste dysfunction begins with a thorough history or the problem, including medical history and treatment. Specific questions about both taste and smell must be asked (Table 2). The history may often identify an etiologic agent, such as an anesthetic. Topical anesthetics can be used to determine if dysgeusia, a distortion of taste or unexplained taste, is associated with peripheral mechanisms in the mouth. Orofacial sources of taste dysfunction may be treated and followed up by the dentist. Patients with apparent nervous problems may be referred to a neurologist, and those with systemic causes should be referred to their primary care physician. If no cause can be identified, the patient may be referred to a multidisciplinary taste and smell center.

Smell.—The main causes of olfactory dysfunction are upper respiratory infections, head trauma, and chronic nasal and paranasal sinus dis-

TABLE 1.—Etiologic Categories of Gustatory and
Olfactory Dysfunction

---Oral causes

Trauma

Burns, lacerations, chemical damage

Anesthetic, surgical

Oral mouthrinses, gels and dentifrices

Periodontal diseases

Dental-alveolar and other infections

Soft tissue lesions

Candidiasis, denture stomatitis

Removable prosthodontic appliances

Burning mouth syndrome

Salivary dysfunction, drugs in saliva

Galvanism

---Upper respiratory tract problems

Lesions of the nose/airway

Viral and bacterial infections

Exposure to toxic airborne contaminants

---Peripheral or central nervous system pathologies

Head trauma

Tumors, lesions

Neurological diseases

(*Continued.*)

Table 1   *(continued)*

---Systemic complications

Systemic diseases

Nutritional deficiencies

Prescription and non-prescription medications

Chemotherapy and radiation therapy

Psychiatric disorders

---Others

Aging

Circadian variation

Menses and pregnancy

Idiopathic

(Courtesy of Ship JA: *J Am Dent Assoc* 124(6):55–61, 1993.)

TABLE 2.—Questions in the Evaluation of Altered Gustation and Olfaction

Can you taste the bitterness of coffee?*

Can you taste the sweetness of icecream?*

Can you taste the saltiness of potato chips?*

Can you taste the sourness of lemons?*

Have you lost your taste for steak?

*   Negative response may denote taste dysfunction. If there is a positive response with an addition al reply that the patient can't taste anything else, it may denote smell dysfunction.

Positive response may denote smell dysfunction.

(Courtesy of Ship JA: *J Am Dent Assoc* 124(6):55–61, 1993.)

ease. A number of other medical problems and their treatments, as well as environmental factors, may cause smell dysfunction. Oral pathologic conditions may also play a role, such as poor oral hygiene. Evaluation is much the same as for the taste dysfunction. Objective assessment may be done by using the University of Pennsylvania Smell Identification Test, a standardized "scratch-and-sniff" test; it may be especially helpful in following the patient. Bad breath is harder to evaluate and may be improved by better oral hygiene. Otherwise, treatment and referral are much the same as for gustatory disorders. It must be remembered, however, that olfactory function diminishes progressively with age.

Summary.—The dentist may see many patients with disorders of taste and smell. These disorders are especially likely in the elderly. Although many chemosensory problems are difficult to diagnose, the dentist can assess function, identify and treat orofacial causes, and refer as appropriate.

▶ Problems related to taste and smell are appropriate for inclusion in the scope of a general dental practice. A practitioner who is in the process of evaluating his or her practice with a view to adding new dimensions might well consider addressing these clinical problems.—J.E. Kennedy, D.D.S., M.S.

Call Mosby Document Express at **1 (800) 55-MOSBY** to obtain copies of the original source documents of articles featured or referenced in the YEAR BOOK series.

11 Radiology

Introduction

The discipline or oral and maxillofacial radiology is rapidly changing. In the private dental office, direct digital imaging represents one of the most significant technological advances since the introduction of panoramic machines in the early 1960s. In institutional settings, the increasing use of advanced imaging modalities continues to directly impact patient care in the diagnosis of such conditions as TMJ disorders, traumatic injuries, developmental anomalies, and implant site assessment. Consistently, these and other changes are driven by the need to continually enhance the diagnostic accuracy of imaging systems, a desire to reduce the amount of radiation delivered to patients during diagnostic imaging procedures, and by efforts to use technological advances that simplify existing techniques.

Denise K. Kassebaum, D.D.S., M.S.

Validation of a Specific Selection Criterion for Dental Periapical Radiography
Brooks SL, Cho SY (Univ of Michigan, Ann Arbor)
Oral Surg Oral Med Oral Pathol 75:383–386, 1993   105-94-11–1

TABLE 1.—Relationship Between Periapical Pathosis and Presence or Absence of Restoration in Nonemergency Patients

Periapical pathosis	Restoration		
	Present	*Absent*	*Totals*
No	2082	1250	3332
Yes	187	56	243
Total	2269	1306	3575

Note: $\chi^2 = 20.452$; $P < .001$; $n = 209$ subjects with 2,269 restored teeth and 100 subjects with 1,306 nonrestored teeth.
(Courtesy of Brooks SL, Cho SY: *Oral Surg Oral Med Oral Pathol* 75:383-386, 1993.)

TABLE 2.—Relationship Between Periapical Pathosis
and Depth of Restoration in Nonemergency Patients

Periapical pathosis	Depth of Restoration		
	Shallow	*Deep*	*Totals*
No	768	1314	2082
Yes	45	142	187
Total	813	1456	2269

Note: $\chi^2 = 12.272$; $P < .001$; $n = 209$ subjects with 2,269 restored teeth.

(Courtesy of Brooks SL, Cho SY: *Oral Surg Oral Med Oral Pathol* 75:383–386, 1993.)

Background.—Prescription of dental radiography is based on a series of selection criteria, one of which specifies the presence of large or deep restorations. The frequency of periapical pathosis on teeth with large or deep restorations was studied. Also determined was whether the presence of extensive restoration presents a valid high yield or selection criteria for periapical radiography.

Method.—Patients undergoing routine examinations and intraoral radiographs were questioned about pain or sensitivity to cold, heat, sweets, or pressure for all restored teeth. Their radiographs were evaluated for depth of restoration and presence or absence of periapical pathosis. The same procedure was carried out in a control group.

Results.—Although there was no significant difference in the frequency of periapical pathosis in teeth with shallow restorations compared with teeth with no restorations, chi-square tests showed marked differences between no restorations and any type of restoration and between shallow and deep restorations (Tables 1 and 2). A significant relationship was also seen between severity of pain symptoms and presence or periapical pathosis in restored teeth. Teeth with deep restorations more commonly had periapical changes than those with no restorations, regardless of the radiographic criteria used. Restored teeth with moderate or severe symptoms showed periapical pathosis more often than those with mild or no symptoms. When symptomatic teeth with deep restorations were compared with asymptomatic teeth and shallow restorations, a threefold to fivefold increase in the incidence of periapical change was seen.

Discussion.—The radiographic yield of positive periapical changes in restored teeth is low, especially in shallow restorations. It may not be useful to use random radiography on all teeth containing large or deep restorations. However, the radiographic yield should be increased if other factors, such as pain, sensitivity, or integrity of the restoration, are also taken into consideration.

▶ Currently accepted guidelines for prescribing dental radiographs categorize patients by the type of dental visit, their dental status, and a risk identification based on the presence or absence of certain conditions. This article investigates whether the presence of large or deep restorations has a significant risk for periapical pathology to justify exposure of a periapical radiograph. The authors conclude that although it may not be useful to perform a periapical radiograph of all teeth with large restorations, factors such as pain, sensitivity, integrity of the restoration, and the use of the tooth as an abutment are important reasons to expose periapical radiographs on restored teeth.—D.K. Kassebaum, D.D.S., M.S.

Clinical Correlation of Oral-Dental Findings With Radiographs and With Total Body Bone Scans
Laga EA Jr, Toth BB, Podoloff DA, Keene HJ (Univ of Texas MD Anderson Cancer Ctr, Houston)
Oral Surg Oral Med Oral Pathol 75:253–263, 1993   105-94-11-2

Background.—Processes that cause an increase in osteoblastic activity may result in increased radionuclide uptake. On a bone scan this increase could be interpreted as a positive finding, and distant bony metastasis suspected in patients with malignant neoplastic disease. Because various dental conditions cause areas in the jaws to have increased uptake of radiopharmaceuticals, metastatic disease could be misinterpreted as oral-dental disease or vice versa. This potential problem was examined by correlating oral-dental findings on panoramic radiographs with those on bone scans in a group of 30 cancer patients.

Methods.—The study subjects had a median age of 51 years; 24 were women. All had total body scans to check for bony metastasis. Patients were selected so that all scan intensities in the maxilla and mandible would be represented (Table 1). The scans were performed 2–3 hours after patients received 20–30 mCi of ^{99m}Tc-labeled methylene diphosphate. In addition, the patients had a panoramic radiograph made and evaluated and underwent a thorough dental/oral examination.

TABLE 1.—Scale of Bone Scan Intensity (Radionuclide Uptake) in Maxilla and Mandible

Intensity	Definition
0	Same intensity as normal bone
I	Slightly greater intensity than normal bone
II	Greater intensity than I, less intensity than III
III	Equal to intensity of bladder and kidney

(Courtesy of Laga EA Jr, Toth BB, Podoloff DA, et al: *Oral Surg Oral Med Oral Pathol* 75:253-263, 1993.)

TABLE 2.—Distribution of Bone Scan Intensities in the
Jaws of 30 Patients with Cancer

Scan intensity	Maxilla*		Mandible*	
	Number	%	Number	%
0	11	36.7	6	20.0
I	16	53.3	14	46.7
II	2	6.7	5	16.7
III	1	3.3	5	16.7
Totals	30	100.0	30	100.1

* Chi-square = 5.48; DF = 3; $P > .05$. No significant difference in the frequency of different scan intensities between the maxilla and mandible.
(Courtesy of Laga EA Jr, Toth BB, Podoloff DA, et al: *Oral Surg Oral Med Oral Pathol* 75:253–263, 1993.)

Results.—There was no significant difference in the frequency of the different scan intensities between the maxilla and the mandible (Table 2). No correlation was found between the intensity of radionuclide uptake in the jaws on bone scans and the number of teeth in each jaw, patient age, the degree of periodontal disease, or the number of dental pathoses per jaw. The frequency and intensity of positive scan results were related to the presence or absence of intrabony lesions of the maxilla and mandible. Intrabony defects were either radiopaque or radiolucent and tooth related or non-tooth related. Three patients, all women with breast cancer, had a metastatic lesion in the mandible. The intensities of the mandibular bone scans were I, diffuse in 2 patients, and III, focal in the third.

Conclusion.—In this small series of patients, dental disease did not appear to mask metastatic disease in the jaws. Distant metastasis to the mandible and maxilla is rare and has a grave prognosis. Patients may experience pain or numbness and swelling. Radiographic changes, when present, are usually osteolytic. When metastatic disease is suspected in the jaws, radiographs should be taken to rule out dental disease.

▶ Several other articles have suggested that various types of dental pathology may cause an increased radionucleotide uptake in the jaws during bone scans. In this small study, the authors seem to dispute this, concluding that dental disease does not mask the presentation of metastatic disease to the jaws.—D.K. Kassebaum, D.D.S., M.S.

A Comparison of Flow and Kodak Dental X-Ray Films by Means of Perceptibility Curves

Svenson B, Petersson A (Postgraduate Dental Education Center, Örebro,

Sweden; Univ of Lund, Malmö, Sweden)
Acta Odontol Scand 51:123–128, 1993   105-94-11-3

Introduction.—Faster film materials have allowed the exposure time required for a full-mouth examination to be substantially reduced. The first consideration, however, must be the diagnostic usefulness of a film imaging system. The recently introduced Flow dental x-ray films of speed groups D and E were compared with Kodak Ultraspeed and Ektaspeed, the predominant film brands.

Methods.—A test object consisting of a rectangular block of aluminum with 10 cylindrical holes was radiographed using Kodak Ultraspeed and Ektaspeed and Flow DX-58 and EX-58. Four series, each containing 6 radiographs, were exposed. The films were developed in an automatic processor and the radiographs mounted in frames. Eleven dentists were given the radiographs in random order for evaluation under ideal viewing conditions (Fig 11-1). Perceptibility curves were constructed for each film. This psychometric method establishes the minimum perceptible exposure difference at different exposure levels.

Results.—The average number of perceptible images of holes was highest for Ektaspeed and lowest for EX-58. Differences between films were not, however, statistically significant. Perceptibility curves for the films indicated that EX-58 was most sensitive to radiation and had the lowest subjective contrast (Fig 11-2). Flow EX-58 also had the highest speed of the compared films. Exposure for EX-58 had to be lowered by

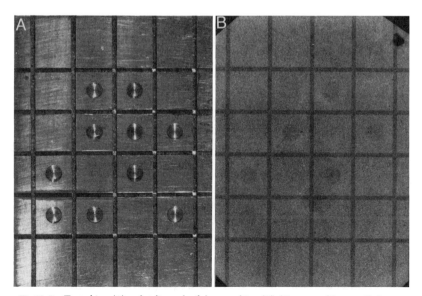

Fig 11–1.—Test object (**A**) and radiograph of the test object (**B**). (Courtesy of Svenson B, Petersson A: *Acta Odontol Scand* 51:123–128, 1993.)

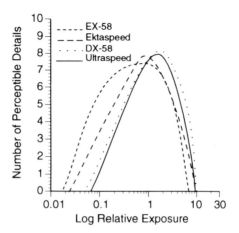

Fig 11–2.—Perceptibility curves for Kodak Ultraspeed and Ektaspeed films and for Flow x-ray DX-58 and EX-58 films. (Courtesy of Svenson B, Petersson A: *Acta Odontol Scand* 51:123–128, 1993.)

66% and Ektaspeed by 39% compared with Ultraspeed film to obtain the same density. Ultraspeed and DX-58 had the same sensitivity.

Conclusion.—There is concern that improvements in film speed may result in poorer film quality. The films evaluated exhibited no apparent difference in their ability to display small contrast differences, using perceptibility curves to describe the films' diagnostic potentials. The use of faster films is encouraged as the most important means of lowering the radiation dose to patients.

▶ The diagnostic accuracy of D-speed and E-speed films has been compared in many studies and has been found to be similar for specified tasks. However, few practicing dentists use the faster film. In this article, Flow DX-58 and Flow EX-58 were compared with Kodak Ultraspeed and Kodak Ektaspeed. The authors determined that no statistically significant differences were found with respect to contrast and the subjectively assessed perceptibility measures. An important feature to note about Flow EX-58 is that it is fast enough to be put in film speed group F. Although more extensive studies will need to be performed on this film, it allows exposure reductions of 66% when compared to the commonly used D speed film. As current attention focuses on direct digital imaging systems because of their patient dose reductions, it should be remembered that faster film speeds also allow for substantial reductions in patient radiation dose if only practitioners would use them.—D.K. Kassebaum, D.D.S., M.S.

Observer Variation in Interpretation of Magnetic Resonance Images of the Temporomandibular Joint

Tasaki MM, Westesson P-L, Raubertas RF (State Univ of New York, Buffalo;

Univ of Rochester, NY)
Oral Surg Oral Med Oral Pathol 76:231–234, 1993   105-94-11–4

Introduction.—Magnetic resonance imaging is reported to have an accuracy of 73% to 95% in diagnosing internal derangement and osseous changes of the TMJ. Observer performance is an important factor in the validity and reliability of an imaging technique. Interobserver and intraobserver variability in reporting MR images of the TMJ was measured.

Methods.—The study was based on MR images of 149 TMJs, 55 from frozen cadaver specimens and 94 from patients referred because of TMJ pain and dysfunction. The mean age of the cadaver specimen donors was 75 years; the mean age of TMJ patients was 31 years. Images were interpreted independently by 2 observers on 2 occasions, 2–4 weeks apart. These observers had worked together in the interpretation of MR images of the TMJ for 7 months before the study. Image quality was similar in patient and cadaver joints. The MR images were interpreted for configuration of the disk and osseous changes. Ten categories of disk position were recognized (Table 1).

TABLE 1.—Categories of
Disk Position

Superior
Anterior
Anterior in the lateral third of joint ∗
Anterior in the medial third of joint †
Anterior and lateral ‡
Anterior and medial §
Lateral
Medial
Posterior
Indeterminate

∗ Partial anterior disk displacement when the disk is anteriorly displaced in the lateral part of the joint but remains in a superior position in the medial part of the joint. There is no associated medial or lateral displacement.

† Partial anterior disk displacement when the disk is anteriorly displaced in the medial part of the joint but remains in a superior position in the lateral part of the joint. There is no associated medial or lateral displacement.

‡ Anterior and lateral disk displacement. This is a combination in which the disk is both anteriorly and laterally displaced.

§ Anterior and medial disk displacement. This is a combination in which the disk is anteriorly and medially displaced.

(Courtesy of Tasaki MM, Westesson P-L, Raubertas RF: *Oral Surg Oral Med Oral Pathol* 76:231-234, 1993.)

TABLE 2.—Intraobserver Agreement in Reporting of MR Images of the TMJ

	Observer 1	Observer 2
Disk position	95% ($\kappa = 0.93$)	95% ($\kappa = 0.93$)
	Standard error for $\kappa = 0.024$	Standard error for $\kappa = 0.023$
Disk form	91% ($\kappa = 0.79$)	89% ($\kappa = 0.76$)
	Standard error for $\kappa = 0.055$	Standard error for $\kappa = 0.056$
Osseous changes	99% ($\kappa = 0.95$)	95% ($\kappa = 0.86$)
	Standard error for $\kappa = 0.036$	Standard error for $\kappa = 0.053$

Note: K values are given in parentheses; $n = 149$ joints.
(Courtesy of Tasaki MM, Westesson P-L, Raubertas RF: Oral Surg Oral Med Oral Pathol 76:231-234, 1993.)

Results.—Intraobserver agreement for assessment of position and configuration of the disk and osseous changes ranged from 89% and 99% (Table 2). Agreement was highest for osseous changes and lowest for disk configuration. Interobserver agreement ranged from 85% to 95%, was highest for osseous changes, and was lowest for configuration of the disk.

Conclusion.—With high-quality images, well-defined criteria for interpretation, and suitable training of observers, MRI of the TMJ should exhibit a low level of inter- and intraobserver variation. The level of observer performance in this study was well within acceptable limits. Magnetic resonance imaging is a reliable and valid imaging technique for assessment of the TMJ.

▶ Few studies to date have examined interobserver and intraobserver variation in reporting MR images of the TMJ. In this study, the authors concluded that interobserver and intraobserver variation can be kept at a low level with high-quality images, suitable training of the observers, and well-defined criteria for interpretation. The 2 observers in this study trained together for about 7 months before the project. It is interesting to speculate how the results may have been influenced if observers from 2 different institutions were compared.—D.K. Kassebaum, D.D.S., M.S.

Direct Digital Dental X-Ray Imaging With Visualix/VIXA
Molteni R (Gendex Dental Systems, Monza, Italy)
Oral Surg Oral Med Oral Pathol 76:235–243, 1993   105-94-11–5

Introduction.—The exposure and processing of the dental x-ray film is time-consuming and often a source of mistakes. Visualix (marketed as

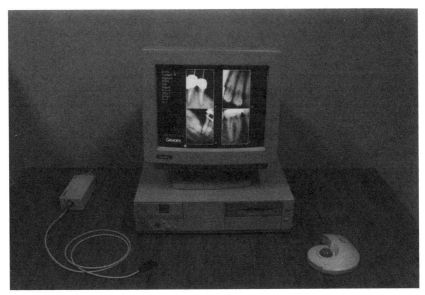

Fig 11-3.—Gendex Visualix system. (Courtesy of Molteni R: *Oral Surg Oral Med Oral Pathol* 76:235-243, 1993.)

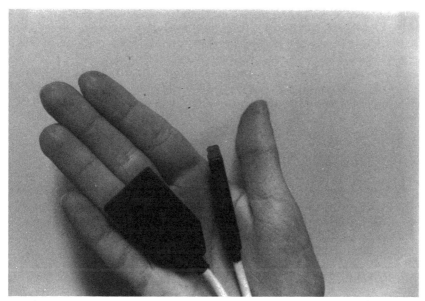

Fig 11-4.—An x-ray image sensor, front and side view. (Courtesy of Molteni R: *Oral Surg Oral Med Oral Pathol* 76:235-243, 1993.)

VIXA in North America), a new device for direct capture of dental intraoral radiographic images as digital files by means of a special radiographic image sensor in real time and without intercession of radiographic film or optics, was studied.

System Description.—The VIXA is composed of an intraoral radiographic image sensor, a main image processor and control unit based on a standard compatible personal computer platform and peripherals, special hardware and software to control it, a high-resolution color monitor, and application software VIXA for interfacing with the operator and controlling the display, processing, storage, and retrieval of image files (Fig 11-3). The radiographic image sensor (Fig 11-4) is engineered for oral use and designed for disposable covers to prevent cross-contamination.

Application Software.—The VIXA application software is able to take full advantage from the real-time availability of the radiographic images. This feature is of particular value in endodontics and implantology when immediacy and simplicity are important. Modification of the gray-scale parameters can make the visual appearance of the images more suitable for the observer. Images can be saved and subsequently retrieved in various standard file formats. It is also possible to transmit the images to an external video printer to prepare a hard copy.

System Performance.—The exposure time required with the Visualix/VIXA sensor is at least 6 times less than that with a D-type film and 3 times less than that with an E-type film. Absorbed doses are expected to reflect the same relationship. The performance limits in signal-to-noise (SNR) ratio with high-sensitivity electronic radiographic image sensors arise essentially from the quantitized nature of the information. Actual diagnostic needs should determine the tradeoff among resolution or modulation transfer function, minimal imparted dose, and SNR.

▶ One of the most important advantages of using direct digital image receptors instead of film is the reduction in patient radiation dose. In considering this reduction, it should be emphasized that the image capture area for the digital receptor is considerably smaller than that for a standard no. 2 size intraoral film, and it takes more digital images to describe the areas of interest. Direct digital imaging systems have many potential benefits, but the practitioner must look closely at all of the features and potential disadvantages before incorporating one into his or her practice.—D.K. Kassebaum, D.D.S., M.S.

Panoramic Radiographs: Necessary for Edentulous Patients?
Seals RR Jr, Williams EO, Jones JD (Univ of Texas, San Antonio)
J Am Dent Assoc 123(11):74–78, 1992   105-94-11–6

Comparison of Present Study With Previous Panoramic Study of Edentulous Patients

RADIOGRAPHIC ENTITIES	NO.	PREVIOUS STUDY PATIENTS (%)	ENTITIES (%)	NO.	PRESENT STUDY PATIENTS (%)	ENTITIES (%)
ROOT FRAGMENTS	14	12.3	37.8	5	1.1	9.6
RETAINED TEETH	1	0.9	2.7	15	3.3	28.8
RADIOPACITIES	12	10.5	32.4	15	3.3	28.8
FOREIGN BODIES	10	8.8	27.0	17	3.8	32.7
TOTAL	37			52		
EDENTULOUS PATIENTS	114			448		

(Courtesy of Seals RR Jr, Williams EO, Jones JD: *J Am Dent Assoc* 123(11):74-78, 1992.)

Introduction.—Panoramic radiographs are often the first means of screening edentulous patients before complete dentures are made, but concerns about safety and cost have raised questions about this practice. Panoramic radiographs from 448 edentulous patients requiring complete denture treatment were reviewed. The mean age of patients was 60 years. The patients reported no relevant symptoms and had no clinical evidence of pathosis.

Findings.—Abnormalities were found in 11.6% of patients. They included root fragments, unerupted teeth, radiopacities, and foreign bodies. In 42 patients (9.4%), 1 or both mental foramina were present at or near the crest of residual ridge.

Discussion.—These results are compared with those obtained at the same school 8 years earlier (table). Positive findings were less frequent in the current series, but newly edentulous adults still should have a panoramic examination. Routine radiographs are not necessary in edentulous patients who seek replacement dentures.

▶ Although the incidence of positive findings is relatively low, it is more than sufficient to justify a panoramic radiographic examination for all new patients, but not for those who seek replacement of a prosthesis previously fabricated.—J.E. Kennedy, D.D.S., M.S.

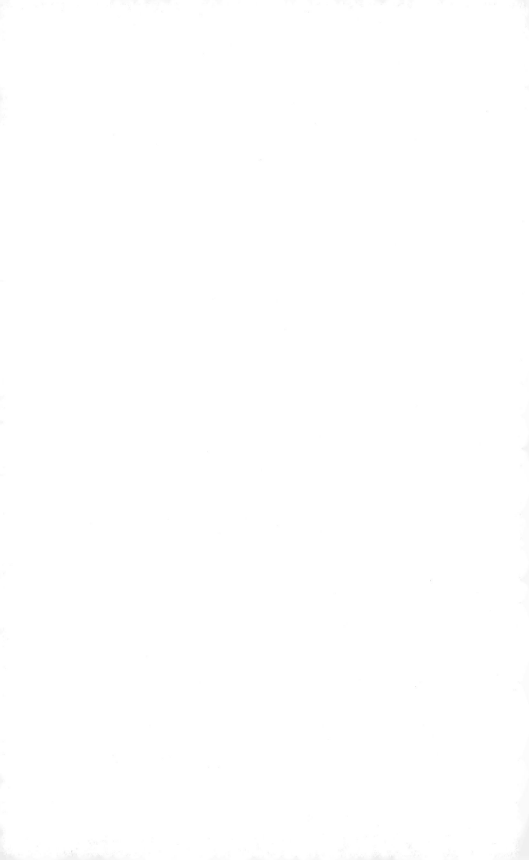

12 Restorative and General Dentistry

Introduction

Each year brings significant advances in the diagnostic devices we use, the medications we prescribe, the treatments we perform, the materials we place, and the instruments we use. The clinician has sometimes viewed the researcher as being too removed from the "real" world. It is now obvious that the advances we enjoy and that benefit our patients are the result of the painstaking work of the scientists in the laboratory and the research clinicians in the operatory. It is important that dentists incorporate these advances in practice, but only after research has validated them.

Restorative dentistry has been altered a great deal by bonding and adhesion procedures. They allow more conservative preparations, less marginal leakage, protection from future development of caries, better retention of the restoration, and better esthetic quality. As luting agents are developed that have adhesion to all the materials used in dentistry and that possess a small film thickness, tooth preparation and material selection will be very radically altered.

Implants are bringing about great changes in prosthodontics. The use of implants has become routine and has a very high success rate. The long-span fixed partial denture and the distal extension removable partial denture may someday become treatments of the past.

Infection control still presents a problem. It adds significant time and cost to dental care. Unfortunately, methods of disinfecting and sterilizing impressions are still of limited effectiveness, and there is a risk of distortion of the cast poured in those impressions. Development of a better method of disinfecting impressions and casts is much needed.

Although there are many areas of dentistry that have questions yet unanswered, it is obvious that treatment is becoming easier, faster, and better for our patients. We need to continue to support efforts in meaningful research and then apply what is learned from those efforts.

Thomas G. Berry, D.D.S., M.A.

Composite Resin, Glass Ionomer Cement, Bonding, and Esthetics

Evaluation of Subsurface Defects Created During the Finishing of Composites

Ferracane JL, Condon JR, Mitchem JC (Oregon Health Sciences Univ, Portland)
J Dent Res 71:1628–1632, 1992   105-94-12–1

Introduction.—One cause of the accelerated wear of certain posterior composites during the first 6 months may be related to a degraded surface layer produced during finishing. Whether a degraded subsurface layer containing microcracks is produced in dental composites as a consequence of finishing products was studied.

Methods and Findings.—Various composites in rectangular bars were finished with a 12-fluted carbide bur or a fine diamond within minutes of light-curing. These bars were then stained with silver nitrate. Microscopic assessment showed that significant penetration of stain occurred in both the unfinished and finished surfaces. The extent of dye penetration directly attributable to a damaged layer produced by the finishing procedure was less than 10 μm. It was greatest for a microfill composite, Silux Plus, and a hybrid composite, P-50. The effects of the finishing instruments did not differ. There were no cracks on SEM analysis of the subsurface. However, there was occasional disruption of the interface between the prepolymerized resin fillers and the matrix in the microfill material (table; Figs 12–1 and 12–2).

	Average Depth (mm) of Material Removed During the Finishing Procedures	
	Carbide	Diamond
1 Q	0.62 ± 0.19	0.63 ± 0.25
1/8 Q	0.30 ± 0.05	0.72 ± 0.15
SIL	0.19 ± 0.09	0.56 ± 0.16
HERC	0.59 ± 0.08	0.89 ± 0.10
P-50	0.74 ± 0.13	1.10 ± 0.16

The values represent means $\pm$ 1 standard deviation ($n = 6$).
(Courtesy of Ferracane JL, Condon JR, Mitchem JC: *J Dent Res* 71:1628–1632, 1992.)

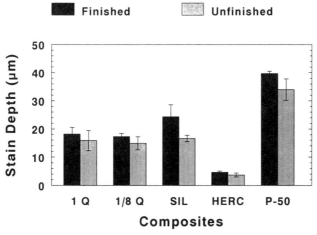

Fig 12–1.—Stain depths for the 5 composites on the surfaces finished with the fine diamond and on the unfinished surfaces. (Courtesy of Ferracane JL, Condon JR, Mitchem JC: *J Dent Res* 71:1628-1632, 1992.)

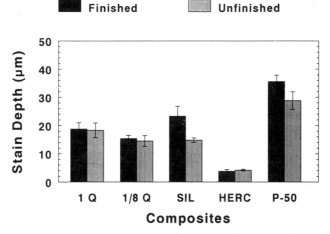

Fig 12–2.—Stain depths for the 5 composites on the surfaces finished with the 12-fluted carbide and on the unfinished surfaces. (Courtesy of Ferracane JL, Condon JR, Mitchem JC: *J Dent Res* 71:1628-1632, 1992.)

Conclusion.—The subsurface damage created in certain composites during initial contouring of a restoration may be very limited. Silver nitrate is absorbed by dental composites before and after finishing.

▶ Wear of composite resins in posterior teeth that are subjected to occlusal contact is well known, but the reasons for this wear may be a bit more obscure. Some investigators have suggested that it is the result of effects of the finishing process, which tends to produce microcracks in the composite subsurface. These microcracks would then lead to the loss of portions of the material. It is interesting that this study does not bear out that contention. The use of the usual array of finishing instruments and techniques did not disturb the integrity of the material. This would indicate that the occlusal function is of greater concern than the finishing process. Newer materials have displayed greater resistance to wear, so the premature wear exhibited by earlier generations of composite resins is no longer considered a major problem.—T.G. Berry, D.D.S., M.A.

Microleakage of Composite Resin and Glass Ionomer Cement Restorations in Retentive and Nonretentive Cervical Cavity Preparations
Kaplan I, Mincer HH, Harris EF, Cloyd JS (Univ of Tennessee, Memphis)
J Prosthet Dent 68:616–623, 1992   105-94-12–2

Background.—Composite resin and glass ionomer cement (GIC) restorations, used for dental cervical lesions, are capable of bonding to tooth structure but are also subject to microleakage. The microleakage of GIC and a bonded composite resin restoration in retentive and nonretentive cavity preparations of cervical cavities was determined.

Methods.—Ketac Fil GIC and Scotchbond 2 dentinal bonding agent (DBA)/Silux Plus composite resin restorations were placed in cervical cavity preparations in extracted teeth. The specimens were thermocycled, invested, and sectioned longitudinally and horizontally through the restoration center. The ratio of the extent of penetration of methylene blue dye at the tooth-restoration interface was used as an assessment of microleakage (Fig 12–3).

Findings.—All restorations displayed leakage. However, the GIC and bonded composite resin restorations had less leakage in retentive than in nonretentive cavity preparations. Compared with the GIC restorations, composite resin restorations in nonretentive cavity preparations had significantly more dye penetration toward the pulpal chamber. Ketac Fil GIC restorations placed without a matrix strip showed less leakage than those with a matrix strip. The most durable results were obtained with Scotchbond 2 DBA/Silux Plus composite resin restorations in retentive preparations (Figs 12–4 and 12–5).

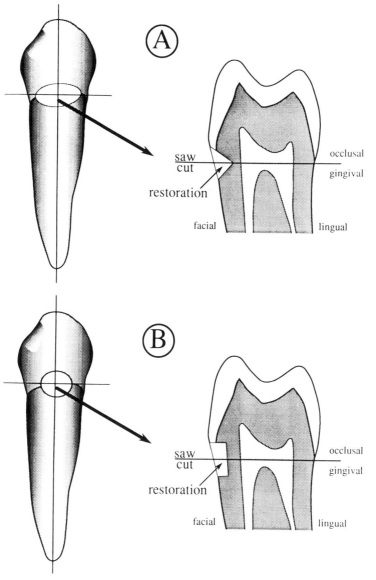

Fig 12–3.—Positions of restorations in nonretentive (**A**) and retentive (**B**) preparations and orientation of 2 saw cuts. (Courtesy of Kaplan I, Mincer HH, Harris EF, et al: *J Prosthet Dent* 68:616-623, 1992.)

Conclusion.—Both the GIC and bonded composite resin restorations used in this study showed some leakage. However, both types had substantially less overall leakage in retentive than in nonretentive cavity preparations.

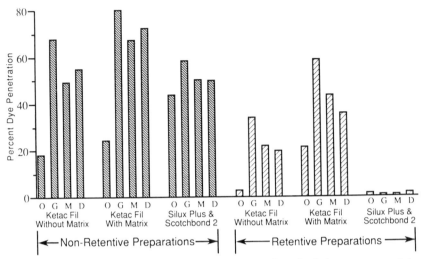

Fig 12–4.—*Abbreviations:* O, occlusal; G, gingival; M, mesial; D, distal. Average percent of dye penetration by type of restoration and form of preparation for each cavity wall. (Courtesy of Kaplan I, Mincer HH, Harris EF, et al: *J Prosthet Dent* 68:616–623, 1992.)

▶ Composite resin and GIC each have their own distinct attributes as a restorative material. Microleakage and detachment of the restoration from cervical preparations have been noted for both materials. This study supports others that note that a more conventional preparation with retentive features

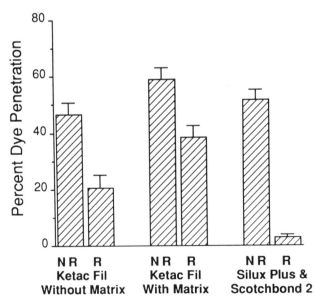

Fig 12–5.—Average percent of dye penetration of restorations in nonretentive (NR) and retentive (R) preparations. (Courtesy of Kaplan I, Mincer HH, Harris EF, et al: *J Prosthet Dent* 68:616–623, 1992.)

decreases the microleakage of both the composite resins and the GICs used in this study. These retentive features compensate for some of the polymerization shrinkage of the composite resin, which pulls the material away from the cavity wall as it cures. The benefit to the GIC possibly results from the greater axial depth of the preparation creating a greater thickness of the cement to compensate somewhat for any cracking or crazing caused by dehydration of the material. Improved dentin bonding agents for composite resin and the introduction of photocured GICs offer great promise in minimizing the microleakage problems.—T.G. Berry, D.D.S., M.A.

Microleakage of Glass Ionomer/Composite Resin Restorations: A Laboratory Study: Part 2. The Influence of Bonding Systems
Martin FE, Smith EDK, Andrews N (Univ of Sydney, Surry Hills, New South Wales, Australia)
Aust Dent J 37:172–177, 1992   105-94-12-3

Background.—Acid-etching and bonding of composite resin to beveled enamel margins produces reliable seals. It is more difficult to achieve a seal with dentine and cementum margins.

Methods and Findings.—Four different dentine bonding systems were combined with Silux composite resin to restore 80 prepared cervical cav-

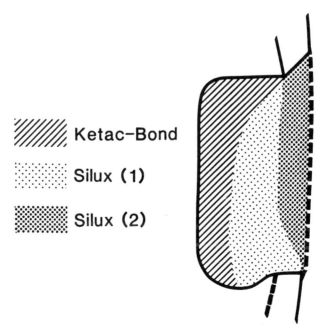

Fig 12–6.—Buccolingual, longitudinal section showing a finished restoration. (Courtesy of Martin FE, Smith EDK, Andrews N: *Aust Dent J* 37:172-177, 1992.)

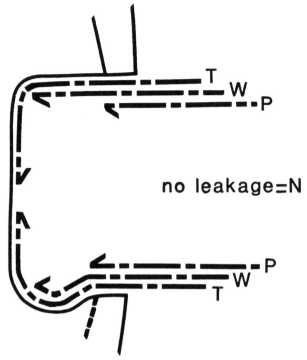

Fig 12–7.—The system used to score dye penetration. *Grade* N: no dye penetration. *Grade* P: partial dye penetration along the occlusal or gingival wall. *Grade* W: dye penetration along the cavity wall, but not including the axial wall. *Grade* T: total dye penetration along the cavity walls extending onto the axial wall. (Courtesy of Martin FE, Smith EDK, Andrews N: *Aust Dent J* 37:172–177, 1992.)

ities in vitro. The bonding systems tested were light-cured Scotchbond, Scotchbond 2, GLUMA, and Tenure. Manufacturers' directions were followed in all cases. Silux was placed into cavities in 2 oblique layers after the dentine and enamel bonding agents were placed (Fig 12–6). A grading system was used to assess dye penetration (Fig 12–7). None of the bonding systems tested were found to completely seal the occlusal or gingival margins (Fig 12–8 and 12–9). The GLUMA system provided the best seal among the systems assessed, at both the occlusal and gingival margins.

Conclusion.—None of the systems tested completely sealed the occlusal enamel margins or the gingival dentine margins. The gingival margin had an inferior seal compared with the occlusal margin in all cases. The combination of GLUMA and Silux provided the highest number of restorations with a complete seal at both occlusal and gingival margins.

▶ Microleakage is not considered a major problem for composite resin restoration margins placed in enamel. The problem increases significantly, however, when 1 or more of the margins are in dentin. Although the results of

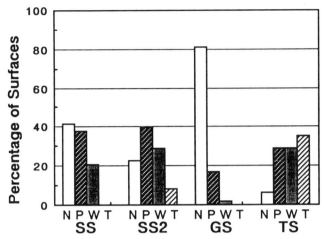

Fig 12–8.—Microleakage results for the occlusal margins. (Courtesy of Martin FE, Smith EDK, Andrews N: *Aust Dent J* 37:172–177, 1992.)

different studies vary considerably, it is safe to say that some microleakage always occurs at the interface between the composite resin and the dentin at the gingival margin. Polymerization shrinkage detaches the composite resin from its comparatively weaker bond to dentin more than from enamel, so greater microleakage is the result. Careful placement techniques minimize this shrinkage. It is important to note that a newer generation of bonding agents has been developed since the introduction of those used in this study. The newer generation appears to provide greater bond strength, so microleakage should be significantly lessened.—T.G. Berry, D.D.S., M.A.

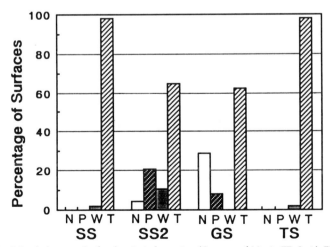

Fig 12–9.—Microleakage results for the gingival margins. (Courtesy of Martin FE, Smith EDK, Andrews N: *Aust Dent J* 37:172–177, 1992.)

Factors Affecting Cure at Depths Within Light-Activated Resin Composites

Rueggeberg FA, Caughman WF, Curtis JW Jr, Davis HC (Med College of Georgia, Augusta)
Am J Dent 6:91–95, 1993   105-94-12-4

Objective.—In maximizing the cure of light-activated resin composites, several factors play important roles, including filler type, light source intensity, duration of exposure, and resin shade. Data on the relative importance of these parameters at specific depths in the light-activated resin were sought.

Methods.—A study examined the relative impact on extent of cure of hybrid vs. microfill filler type; universal vs. gray composite shade; 20-, 40-, 60-, or 80-second exposure duration; and 800, 578, 400, and 233 mW/cm² light source intensity. The depths studied were top surface and 1, 2, and 3 mm on a simulated restoration. Thin wafers were made of P-50 and Silux Plus composite between a cured composite underlay and various thicknesses of cured overlay. The resulting wafer reproduced the curing environment within a cylinder of composite. Infrared spectroscopy was used to determine the monomer conversion of each specimen.

Results.—At depths of 2 mm and greater, lower source intensities produced increasingly lower percentages of monomer conversion (Fig 12-10). At a depth of 2 or 3 mm, duration of exposure was somewhat more important than source intensity (Fig 12-11). Independently, the variables did not seem to produce great differences in cure at each composite depth. According to analysis of variance, however, filler type was

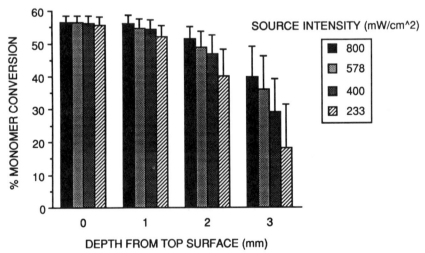

Fig 12–10.—Resin cure as a function of composite depth and source intensity only. (*Bar* = standard deviation). (Courtesy of Rueggeberg FA, Caughman WF, Curtis JW Jr, et al: *Am J Dent* 6:91-95, 1993.)

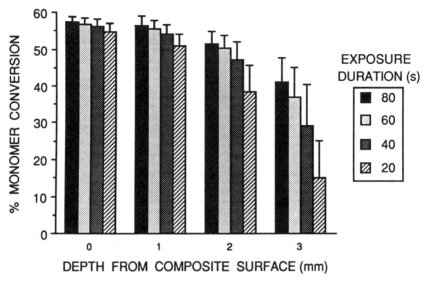

Fig 12–11.—Resin cure as a function of composite depth and exposure duration only. (*Bar* = standard deviation). (Courtesy of Rueggeberg FA, Caughman WF, Curtis JW Jr, et al: *Am J Dent* 6:91-95, 1993.)

the most important variable at the top surface, followed by exposure duration and resin shade. Duration of exposure was the most important at a depth of 1 mm, followed by filler type and source intensity. At 2 mm and more, cure was overwhelmingly determined by source intensity and

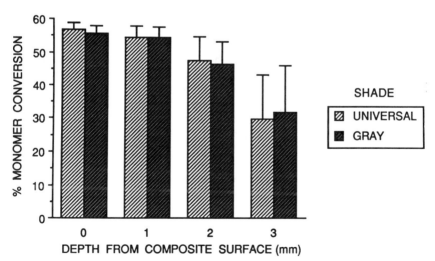

Fig 12–12.—Resin cure as a function of composite depth and resin shade only. (*Bar* = standard deviation). (Courtesy of Rueggeberg FA, Caughman WF, Curtis JW Jr, et al: *Am J Dent* 6:91-95, 1993.)

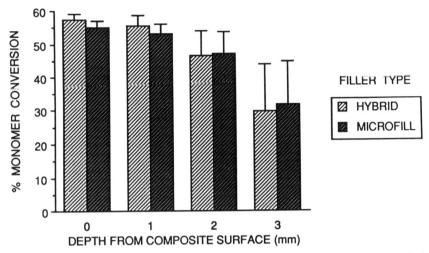

Fig 12–13.—Resin cure as a function of composite depth and filler type only. (Bar = standard deviation). (Courtesy of Rueggeberg FA, Caughman WF, Curtis JW Jr, et al: *Am J Dent* 6:91–95, 1993.)

exposure duration, with resin shade (Fig 12–12) and filler type (Fig 12–13) having little influence.

Conclusion.—Different factors vary in importance with depth in the curing of light-activated resin composites. At 2 mm or more, the important factors are source intensity and exposure duration, much more than filler type or resin shade. Composite should be placed in increments no more than 1 mm thick, approaching 2 mm only if source intensity and exposure duration are adequate.

▶ Curing light-activated composite resin appears to be a very straightforward task. Simply expose the material to the light until the buzzer/beeper sounds, and that is enough. There are, however, many factors that have an important effect on the degree of polymerization achieved. This study clearly identifies the factors that have the strongest impact. Variations in depth of the material not only affect the degree of polymerization, but they also change the impact of other factors. Exposure duration is always the most influential factor no matter the depth of the material. As depth increases, the importance of the light intensity also increases. This information reminds us to guard against placing large increments of composite resin at one time to prevent having a layer that is not completely polymerized. It is difficult to determine the hardness of the inner layers. Inadequate polymerization can lead to discoloration, increased microleakage, loss of strength, and possible premature loss of the restoration. The use of a radiometer will ensure that the light intensity is sufficient.—T.G. Berry, D.D.S., M.A.

Precision of Hand-Held Dental Radiometers

Rueggeberg FA (Med College of Georgia, Augusta)
Quintessence Int 24:391–396, 1993   105-94-12–5

Background.—When light curing is used for composite resins, the intensity of the radiant source has been shown to affect both the degree of cure at the surface closest to the light source and the depth to which polymerization occurs. Several causes may affect the intensity of the light source, such as bulb aging, filter degradation, optical guide wear, fluctuation in the line voltage, and breakdown of electric components in the power supply. The curing of resins 2 mm beneath the surface can be adversely affected by as little as a 10% decrease in intensity at the surface of a composite resin. Thus, knowledge of the light intensity of a dental curing unit is crucial.

Methods.—The precision of 2 newly marketed hand-held radiometers, the Demetron model 100 and the EFOS model 800, were compared. A light source fixture that simulated a typical dental curing unit was used.

Results.—A linear response was obtained for each instrument. Both units responded to a given amount of reduction in light source intensity with a corresponding decrement in measured intensity value. Both instruments yielded precise results. The pass band of intensity readings was limited to between 400 and 515 mm. However, the Demetron unit did indicate significantly higher intensity values for a given radiant energy, compared to the EFOS model.

Conclusion.—Even though the Demetron unit had superior intensity values, both units were judged to be useful clinical instruments.

▶ Dr. Rueggeberg, as well as others, has effectively documented that successful polymerization of composite resin depends on curing light supplying an adequate intensity of light in the correct range. The intensity cannot be determined by simply viewing the light. Two relatively simple methods of checking the intensity output are available for in-office use. A disk of composite resin of a specific thickness can be cured, and then the side of the resin opposite the side exposed to the light can be tested for hardness by comparing it with a surface with a Knoop Hardness value equal to fully polymerized composite resin. The other method uses a radiometer to determine the output. The radiometer is simple, quick to administer, and very accurate. Because full polymerization is critical to the success of composite resin and other photocured materials, it is imperative that the unit deliver adequate light. One recent study reported that almost 30% of the lights checked in the survey delivered inadequate light to affect maximum polymerization. The periodic use of a radiometer is a very effective and rapid way to ensure that the curing unit is doing its job. At least 1 manufacturer now includes a built-in radiometer on the curing unit itself.—T.G. Berry, D.D.S., M.A.

Saucer-Shaped Cavity Preparation for Composite Resin Restorations in Class II Carious Lesions: Three-Year Results

Nordbo H, Leirskar J, von der Fehr FR (Univ of Oslo, Norway)
J Prosthet Dent 69:155–159, 1993   105-94-12–6

Purpose.—The conventional box-shaped cavity preparation for amalgam restorations and gold inlays is inappropriate for class II composite resin restorations. Use of a saucer-shaped cavity preparation for class II composite resin restorations was investigated.

Methods.—Thirty-nine saucer-shaped cavity preparations in small proximal incipient carious lesions of premolars and mesial lesions of first molars were completed with composite resin (Fig 12–14 and 12–15). Ful-fil composite resin was used in 23 restorations and Occlusin composite resin in 16 restorations. The patients ranged in age from 13–17 years at the time of restoration. Clinical, radiographic, and replica cast evaluations were performed after 6, 18, and 36 months. The overall results at 3 years were rated as acceptable or nonacceptable.

Results.—One restoration had to be replaced after 6 months because of marginal voids identified on radiographs. An additional 4 restorations had to be replaced after 18 months because of recurrent caries, excessive gingival extension beyond the dentoenamel junction, and voids created during composite resin insertion. At the 3-year follow-up, 2 more restorations were replaced because of recurrent gingival caries and poor marginal adaptation. Two restorations showed slight but distinctive occlusal wear. At the end of the 3-year follow-up, 32 restorations (82%) were rated acceptable; none of the restorations had been lost or dislodged.

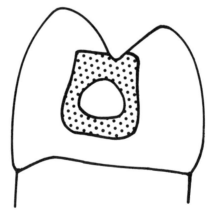

Fig 12–14.—Outline form of saucer cavity. The *dotted area* represents prepared enamel. (Courtesy of Nordbo H, Leirskar J, von der Fehr FR: *J Prosthet Dent* 69:155–159, 1993.)

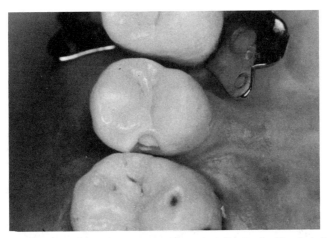

Fig 12–15.—Convenience form of saucer cavity. The cavity is lined and acid etched. (Courtesy of Nordbo H, Leirskar J, von der Fehr FR: *J Prosthet Dent* 69:155–159, 1993.)

Conclusion.—A saucer-shaped cavity preparation for restoring class II carious lesions with composite resin provides acceptable early retention, resistance form, and wear resistance. Long-term durability remains to be determined.

▶ Current cavity preparation designs often owe more to the influence of G.V. Black and to the demands of older restorative materials than to the physical properties of the materials, methods of retention, and caries prevention modalities now available. Although composite resin is a very different restorative material than amalgam in many ways other than color, many dentists prepare cavities for composite resin as if they were for amalgam. No longer are dovetails, retention grooves, etc., necessary. It is not necessary to extend the restoration into the uninvolved grooves of the occlusal surface if a sealant is used. The preparation design advocated follows the principle of tooth conservation while providing adequate retention. The reduced occlusal contacts allowed by this design lessen the occlusal stress, which should improve the restoration's length of service. It is time for dentists to fashion their preparations to take advantage of the new technology.—T.G. Berry, D.D.S., M.A.

Tunnel Restorations Versus Class II Restorations for Small Proximal Lesions: A Comparison of Tooth Strengths
Papa J, Cain C, Messer HH, Wilson PR (Univ of Melbourne, Australia)
Quintessence Int 24:93–98, 1993   105-94-12-7

Background.—Concepts of cavity preparation have shifted toward an emphasis on the preservation of tooth structure. For early proximal caries, a more conservative approach to class II cavity preparation is now possible, although removal of the marginal ridge is still required. The

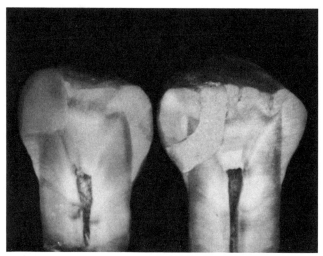

Fig 12–16.—Cross section through the tunnel-restored and mesio-occlusal composite resin-restored teeth. (Courtesy of Papa J, Cain C, Messer HH, et al: *Quintessence Int* 24:93–98, 1993.)

tunnel restoration can preserve the marginal ridge, but it may leave it with little or no underlying dentin.

Methods.—Tooth strength with minimal mesio-occlusal class II cavity restorations was compared with that of tunnel restorations in 21 extracted, noncarious, single-rooted maxillary premolars (Fig 12–16). Sequential testing at physiologic loads was conducted using nondestructive techniques with strain gauges and closed-loop servohydraulics. After loading to fracture, the teeth were cross-sectioned to measure how close the restoration was to the pulp and how much dentin remained in the marginal ridge.

Results.—Both preparations reduced stiffness by approximately 10% compared with the intact tooth. After restoration, the relative stiffness of the tooth was significantly greater with the conservative cavity restoration, 99% vs. 81%. Loads to fracture were 2,650 N for intact teeth, 2,013 N for restored class II preparations, and 1,177 N for teeth with tunnel restorations. Most teeth in both groups failed by mesiodistal vertical fracture.

Conclusion.—Both destructive and nondestructive testing show that minimal class II composite resin restorations are stronger than glass-ionomer cement tunnel restorations. The tunnel restoration is also more difficult to prepare as well as being more damaging, as shown by the stiffness, load to fracture, and the proximity of the restoration to the pulp.

▶ The emphasis on conservation of tooth structure has been strengthened by new bur designs, new materials, and new techniques to allow new preparation designs. This allows the preservation of such important features as occlusal stops, proximal relationships, and the overall strength of the cusps. The tunnel preparation has been credited by some lecturers and authors as doing this. This study would indicate that the tunnel preparation does not preserve as much of the tooth's resistance to fracture as does a conservative conventional preparation. Additional research is needed to fully settle this point. Furthermore, the tunnel preparation approaches nearer the pulp than does the conservative conventional class II preparation. Dentists need to perform a careful review of the research literature on any preparation design to determine whether the treatment to be rendered *is* conservative in effect rather than simply appearing to be so.—T.G. Berry, D.D.S., M.A.

Current Concepts in Dentin Bonding: Focusing on Dentinal Adhesion Factors
Heymann HO, Bayne SC (Univ of North Carolina, Chapel Hill)
J Am Dent Assoc 124(5):27–36, 1993   105-94-12–8

Introduction.—As the need for root surface treatments increases, dentinal adhesives are in greater demand. Research efforts on adhesives have focused primarily on materials and product comparisons. Although differences in materials affect adhesion, other important co-variables, including dentin, tooth, and patient factors, must also be considered for successful treatment.

Dentin.—Three dentin factors influence adhesive properties. The first factor is the smear layer produced by rotary instruments during cavity preparation. The smear layer, generally 1–5 μm thick, reduces postoperative sensitivity and provides a dry adhesive surface. Unfortunately, the smear layer is only weakly attached to underlying dentin. Thus, newer techniques either penetrate or remove this layer. Dentin tubules affect adhesion by controlling the wetness of the dentin. Tubule density is distributed in a radially concentric fashion with the highest density near the pulp. Tubule density is also high in the inner third of the cusps and lowest at the outer third of the cervical dentin. Newer bonding agents penetrate the surface moisture to mitigate this problem. Finally, dentinal sclerosis, caused by trauma or other factors, also affects adhesion. An opaque, whitish, or light yellow dentin indicates no sclerosis and is designated as category 1 on the dentin sclerosis scale. Category 4 dentin, typical of lesions in older patients, is glassy or significantly translucent and dark yellow to a brownish discoloration.

Teeth.—Four tooth factors also significantly affect dentin adhesion. Recent research has indicated that lesion size and shape may significantly affect restoration retention. Shallow, saucer-shaped lesions are less adhesive sites than notch-shaped regions with incisal and gingival wall angles less than 135 degrees. Another contributing factor is the variation in enamel and dentin structure. Cervical regions have thin, aprismatic enamel with brittle dentin. Tooth flexure may affect adhesion by contributing to both lateral and vertical tooth deformation. Tooth location must also be considered. Research has indicated increased cervical failure occurs in mandibular teeth.

Patients.—Patient variables such as occlusal stress and age may affect adhesion. Greater stress and advanced age are both linked to greater restoration losses.

Materials.—Newer dentin bonding systems use hydrophilic monomers to penetrate intertubular dentin and attach to the superficial dentin. The hybrid layer formed is the primary site of dentinal adhesion. An effective hybrid layer requires that the remaining collagen within the penetrated intertubular layer remains structurally intact.

Conclusion.—Dentin, tooth, patient, and material factors must be included to determine the overall "bonding equation."

▶ Dentin bonding agents, when introduced, appeared to offer the solution to problems of microleakage and of attaching restorative materials to cervical areas of the tooth. Dentists followed the manufacturers' directions, only to have them fail. The first and second generations of bonding agents were definitely faulty, sometimes even in their concept. It is good news that the current generation of bonding agents works well, but only if correctly applied to a well-chosen dentin surface. The authors have addressed the problems well by reviewing those factors that affect the success of the bonding process. Dentin bonding works as well as advertised but not in every situation.—T.G. Berry, D.D.S., M.A.

Efficacy of Vital Home Bleaching
Simon JF, Allen H, Woodson RG, Eilers AS (Univ of the Pacific School of Dentistry, San Francisco)
J Calif Dent Assoc 21(1):72–75, 1993   105-94-12–9

Background.—The nightguard vital bleaching technique has become a popular and well-accepted dental procedure. Although the history, safety, and efficacy of this technique are well-documented, little has been done to quantify specific coloration changes. A numerical value was given to teeth coloration changes in a group of volunteer patients.

Patients and Methods.—Twenty-five volunteers aged 25–50 years participated in the study. All participants had a baseline examination, including oral prophylaxis and pretreatment photographs. All were then instructed to apply the bleaching material to maxillary teeth for 2 hours each morning and 2 hours each afternoon or evening for 4 weeks. Each patient's own mandibular teeth were used as controls. Follow-up examinations were performed weekly and included evaluation for hard or soft tissue sensitivity, or both, and photographic documentation. To obtain an objective, numerical value for color differences, a light transmisson densitometer was used with the photographic slides from each patient.

On the linear scale used by the densitometer a change of .30 corresponded to a 100% difference in light transmission, a change from shade tab color A1 to A4 or C1 to C4 was roughly .28, and a change from B1 to B4 was .25.

Results.—Two patients did not exhibit any change, and 1 patient had very little change. A change value of .20 or higher was noted in 9 patients. The overall group average was .158. No patients discontinued use of the bleach because of sensitivity. Patient compliance for total wearing time was a problem.

Conclusion.—Vital home bleaching is not always effective. However, for most patients it appears to be a useful procedure with limited adverse side effects.

▶ With the increasing emphasis on appearance, bleaching has become a very popular procedure that is much in demand by patients. A body of research has shown the process to be relatively harmless to the patient. The degree to which it is effective has not been so well documented. Simon and associates have quantified the effectiveness to allow some predictability of the results for patients in general. They do not differentiate among different problems involving shade or discoloration. It has been reported that some problems (e.g., tetracycline stain) are more difficult to effectively alter than are others. Patients must be informed that the results of home bleaching are not completely predictable.—T.G. Berry, D.D.S., M.A.

Leaching of Hydrogen Peroxide From Bleached Bovine Enamel

Adibfar A, Steele A, Torneck CD, Titley KC, Ruse D (Univ of Toronto; Univ of British Columbia, Vancouver)
J Endodont 18:488–491, 1992   105-94-12–10

Background.—Discolored teeth most frequently are bleached with 30% to 35% hydrogen peroxide (HP) solution. In previous studies, it was shown that the attachment of a light-cured resin to bovine enamel was compromised by previous exposure to 30% HP for longer than 5 minutes. This effect was ascribed to peroxide-resin interactions at the enamel surface. Other studies have suggested that adequate attachment may be restored by immersing peroxide-treated enamel in water for 1 week before applying resin.

Objective and Methods.—An attempt was made to identify and quantify the peroxide released from bleached bovine enamel on immersion. Slabs of bovine enamel were immersed in 35% HP for 1, 3, 5, 30, or 60 minutes or in saline for 60 minutes. The samples were acid-etched with 37% phosphoric acid for 1 minute before leaching in doubly distilled water for periods of 1, 5, 10, or 20 minutes or 7 days. In 1 group, the samples were leached a second time for 1 minute. Hydrogen peroxide was identified spectrophotometrically and quantified by the oxidation reaction of leuco-crystal violet buffer solution, a reaction catalyzed by horseradish peroxidase.

Results.—The quantity of peroxide leached from the enamel samples differed significantly between the bleached and saline-treated groups. Releached samples did not differ from saline-treated control samples.

Conclusion.—Peroxide is rapidly leached from bleached enamel on immersion in water. Immersion, however, is a relatively stable setting that could be more conducive to ionic transport than is rinsing.

▶ Because teeth are sometimes bleached with a hydrogen peroxide solution before bonding of composite resin to the enamel, it is important to know what effect the peroxide has on the bond. Polymerization is inhibited by oxygen, so an excess of oxygen in the enamel could be highly detrimental to the bond established. This is especially important when bonding porcelain or metal to the prepared tooth. The bleaching process does deposit oxygen into the permeable enamel surface that is released over time. The regimen described in this article will remove this oxygen by leaching if the surfaces are immersed. Merely spraying with water does not leach enough of the oxygen to permit a good bond. Previous studies have shown that within a few days, excess oxygen is also eliminated from human teeth. Dentists should take heed to avoid attempting bonding within a short time after bleaching, but they should be reassured that a few days of immersion in oral fluids should eliminate any problem.—T.G. Berry, D.D.S., M.A.

Bleaching: Is It Safe and Effective?
Goldstein GR, Kiremidjian-Schumacher L (New York Univ)
J Prosthet Dent 69:325–328, 1993   105-94-12–11

Predictability.—Teeth may be effectively bleached with hydrogen peroxide, but the process is not a predictable one. In one study, only one third of the subjects exhibited substantial change. It is difficult to predict the exact shade that will be achieved, and uncertainty about the extent of bleaching may be a cause of patient dissatisfaction.

Side Effects.—External cervical resorption is well documented in connection with the bleaching of nonvital teeth. Pulpal responses to bleaching may be extensive but probably are reversible. Most practitioners have described some post-treatment sensitivity, which tends to decrease over time. Ledoux et al. found that bleaching with 30% peroxide produced extensive structural changes in rat dentin and enamel. Torneck et al. reported a decrease in the bond strength between composite resin and bovine enamel bleached with 30% hydrogen peroxide. Oral ulcerations have been described in patients after the use of 3% peroxide for 1–2 minutes from 3 to 5 times a day. Edematous changes have been produced in animal studies using 1% hydrogen peroxide.

Conclusion.—Bleaching of teeth, although effective, is unpredictable and produces enough adverse effects to warrant professional concern. In addition to its effects on teeth, hydrogen peroxide can produce changes in the oral soft tissues after prolonged contact, and there also is a risk of aspirating or inhaling peroxide and its byproducts.

▶ The high profile the popular press has given to bleaching has stimulated patients to request to have their teeth "whitened." This process, which has existed for many decades, is now a very popular one. Both in-office and home bleaching regimens are routinely used with varying success and, very occasionally, with some side effects. Careful control of the in-office bleaching procedure is both necessary and possible. Home bleaching is not under the dentist's control, but good patient education and careful observation will help to achieve the desired results and avoid the side effects. If the directions are carefully followed and the precautions all observed, bleaching is safe and effective. Patients must be warned that the degree of color change is not always absolutely predictable, and the tooth is likely to redarken somewhat over a period of time. The dentist must also inform the patient that some discoloration, such as a tetracycline stain, may be somewhat resistant to the bleaching process, so limited improvement should be expected.—T.G. Berry, D.D.S., M.A.

Triclosan/Copolymer/NaF Dentifrice Prophylaxis, Reduced Etching Time and Shear Bond Strength of a Resin Composite to Enamel
Garcia-Godoy F (Univ of Texas Health Science Ctr, San Antonio)
Am J Dent 5:312–314, 1992   105-94-12-12

Objective.—The effects of prophylaxis with a new triclosan/copolymer/NaF dentifrice and a reduced etching time with 37% phosphoric acid gel on the shear bond strength of a resin composite to enamel were assessed. Sixty human extracted permanent molars were included in this study.

Methods.—A 600 grit SiC paper was used to obtain a flat enamel surface on each tooth. Each tooth was next cleaned with a rubber cup and a water slurry of fine flour of pumice. The teeth were then randomly divided into 4 equal groups. Group 1 received a pumice prophylaxis with a rubber cup and 30 seconds of etching. Group 2 was treated with a pumice prophylaxis and 60 seconds of etching. Groups 3 and 4 received Triclosan/copolymer/NaF dentifrice prophylaxis, with 30 and 60 seconds of etching, respectively. All teeth were then rinsed in distilled water and dried with oil-free compressed air for 20 seconds. An unfilled resin was thinly applied with a brush. After curing for 30 seconds, a nylon ring was positioned over the area and filled with a light-cured composite resin. All teeth were thermocycled for 500 cycles and then sheared with a knife-edged blade in an Instron set at a crosshead speed of 1 mm/min.

Shear Bond Strength (in MPA) for Different Groups

Group	N	Etch time	Mean (MPa)	S.D.	Range
Pumice					
	15 *	30 s	18.84	7.08	3.88 - 30.19
	15 †	60 s	22.65	4.37	12.11 - 29.15
Triclosan/copolymer/ NaF dentifrice					
	15 *	30 s	18.79	5.77	7.47 - 28.55
	15 ‡	60 s	19.62	6.13	10.31 - 29.90

* Three specimens fractured enamel during shear bond testing.
† Eight specimens fractured enamel during shear bond testing.
‡ Seven specimens fractured enamel during shear bond testing.
(Courtesy of Garcia-Godoy F: Am J Dent 5:312–314, 1992.)

Results.—Comparable bond strengths were noted for the groups treated with triclosan/copolymer/NaF dentifrice and pumice prophylaxis. No statistically significant differences were seen among the 4 groups (table). After shear bond testing, enamel fractures were noted in 20% of group 1, 53% of group 2, 20% of group 3, and 47% of group 4.

Conclusion.—Before bonding resin composites to enamel, prophylactic treatment using triclosan/copolymer/NaF dentifrice with a reduced etching time of 30 seconds is recommended.

▶ Many factors can affect the bond strength of composite resin to etched enamel. These factors may include moisture contamination, surface coatings, inadequate etch time, and high fluoride content of the enamel. It is common practice to ensure the enamel is free of surface contaminants by cleaning it with a rubber cup and pumice. Because many prophylactic pastes contain fluoride, there is concern that the deposition of the fluoride on the enamel surface may interfere with the etching process and, ultimately, decrease the bond strength achieved. The results of this study are reassuring. There was no adverse effect. In fact, it is not even necessary to increase the etch time to compensate for the fluoride on the enamel.—T.G. Berry, D.D.S., M.A.

A Clinical Evaluation of Ceramic Laminate Veneers

Karlsson S, Landahl I, Stegersjö G, Milleding P (Univ of Göteborg, Sweden)
Int J Prosthodont 5:447–451, 1992   105-94-12–13

Background.—Complete-coverage tooth preparation can result in pulpal involvement, especially when used in young patients. The use of bonding resin composite to etched enamel has improved treatment for

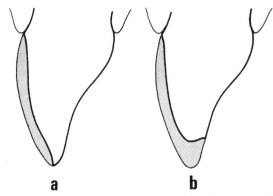

Fig 12–17.—Two tooth-preparation designs evaluated in this study; **a,** prepared labial surface is terminated at the incisal edge; **b,** incisal edge is included. (Courtesy of Karlsson S, Landahl I, Stegersjö G, et al: *Int J Prosthodont* 5:447–451, 1992.)

young patients, but acrylic resin and resin composite veneers can wear and discolor with time, making their longevity limited. The use of ceramic veneers has become more common in the past decade. The clinical quality of resin-bonded ceramic veneers was assessed in a general practice.

Methods and Findings.—Four independent examiners assessed ceramic veneers using the California Dental Association (CDA) guidelines for evaluation of dental care (Fig 12–17). Bleeding, margin index, and mode of tooth preparation were also documented. One hundred nineteen veneer restorations in 36 patients were evaluated. At assessment, the restorations had been in place an average of 18 months. Almost all veneers were rated satisfactory for surface, color, and margin integrity, and more than half had a satisfactory anatomical form. None of the veneers had been replaced. Only 2 had fractured. The bleeding index was similar to that of other types of crowns. The most common margin was an equigingival or subgingival one (Fig 12–18; Tables 1 and 2).

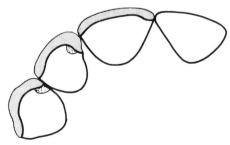

Fig 12–18.—Relationship of veneer to existing resin composite restoration. *Canine:* finishing line crosses an existing restoration. *Lateral incisor:* existing restoration is included within extension of the veneer. *Central incisor:* no preexisting restoration. (Courtesy of Karlsson S, Landahl I, Stegersjö G, et al: *Int J Prosthodont* 5:447–451, 1992.)

TABLE 1.—Frequency Distribution (%) of Ratings in 119 Ceramic Veneers According to the CDA Quality Evaluation System

	Satisfactory		Not acceptable	
	Excellent (R)	Acceptable (S)	Replace/correct (T)	Replace (V)
Surface	87	8	3	2
Color	62	38	0	0
Margin integrity	31	68	1	0
Anatomic form	69	26	5	0

(Courtesy of Karlsson S, Landahl I, Stegersjö G, et al: *Int J Prosthodont* 5:447–451, 1992.)

Conclusion.—In this series, 87% of the surface and 62% of the color assessments were rated as excellent. One third of the veneers were rated as having excellent margin integrity. The most common reason for a rating less than excellent for anatomical form was overcontour.

▶ Ceramic veneers have become very popular because they require a relatively conservative preparation and often offer a dramatic improvement in appearance for patients. However, many of the past concerns about the long-term results seem to have been answered to a large degree by better preparation design, improvement in porcelain materials, development of better luting resin, and a better understanding of the bonding process. Certainly, this study indicates that the initial results are quite good. A median interval of 1½ years postinsertion is not enough time to truly assess the success of ceramic laminate veneers, however. Longer term studies are needed to fully assess the incidence of marginal staining, fracture, debonding, and periodontal problems. It is anticipated that subsequent recall examinations will show the porcelain laminate veneers still doing well many years later.—T.G. Berry, D.D.S., M.A.

TABLE 2.—Frequency Distribution (%) of the Margin Index

Margin Index	n (%)
0	0
1	12
2	56
3	32

0, veneer margin greater than 2 mm supragingivally; 1, veneer margin between 2 mm supragingivally and the gingival margin; 2, veneer margin level with gingival margin; 3, veneer margin placed subgingivally.
(Courtesy of Karlsson S, Landahl I, Stegersjö G, et al: *Int J Prosthodont* 5:447–451, 1992.)

Care and Repair of Porcelain Veneers

McIntyre FM (State Univ of New York, Buffalo)
Compend Contin Educ Dent 14:374–377, 1993   105-94-12–14

Introduction.—The porcelain veneer restoration is a conservative esthetic procedure that has been used as an alternative to direct composite veneering. It also may be used as an alternative to placement of a metal-ceramic crown.

Proper Care.—Scaling a tooth bearing a porcelain veneer is best done by using curets. The ultrasonic scaler and air polisher should be avoided because they may debond the veneer or remove color and glaze from its surface, particularly when the color of the veneer has been added to the tooth surface. It is best to use low-abrasive prophylaxis paste. If a diamond polishing paste is used, care is needed not to abrade the glaze. Neutral 2% sodium fluoride solution should be used in prophylaxis. Acidulated fluoride may etch the porcelain, and a stannous fluoride product may stain or darken the veneer.

Conclusion.—The porcelain veneer can be a superior restorative alternative. When damage does occur, techniques are available to remedy the flaws or failure. Good communication among the dentist, patient, laboratory technician, and hygienist can ensure that the procedure will be successful over the long term.

▶ The popularity of laminate veneers has grown tremendously during the past decade because the materials and techniques for fabrication and luting the laminates have improved considerably. When appropriately prescribed and correctly placed, they provide truly superior esthetic results. Although durable, they can be fractured or debonded so care to preserve them is critical. It is important that the hygienist recognizes the laminate veneer and then exercises the necessary caution when scaling and polishing the teeth. Ultrasonic scalers can fracture or debond the teeth, and air-polishers can dull the surface finish and remove any extrinsic stain added to the veneer. This article presents several methods of correcting problems with the bonded veneer. As more and more patients receive veneers, it will become more and more important to know how to handle the problems that will occur.—T.G. Berry, D.D.S., M.A.

Porcelain Laminate Veneers for Discolored Teeth Using Complementary Colors

Yamada. K (Cusp Dental Supply Co, Ltd, Aichi, Japan)
Int J Prosthodont 6:242–247, 1993   105-94-12–15

Background.—Restoration of teeth discolored by tetracycline can be challenging. Conventional porcelain laminate veneer restorations are popular, but they may leave the teeth with an artificially white appear-

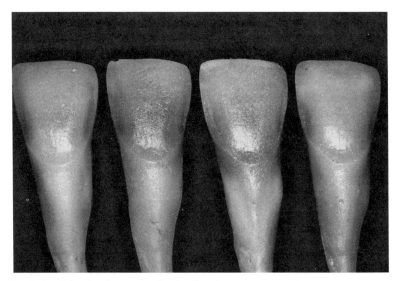

Fig 12–19.—Color classification for discolored teeth. **From left:** orange, brown, blue-purple, and reddish gray base colors in artificial teeth made using resin composite. (Courtesy of Yamada K: *Int J Prosthodont* 6:242–247, 1993.)

ance. A technique using the tooth's discoloration to achieve a more harmonious restoration was examined.

Technique.—The discoloration is first classified as either orange, brown, blue-purple, or reddish gray base (Fig 12-19). To achieve harmony with the untreated teeth, complementary color theory is used. A complementary porcelain color is chosen that neutralizes the abutment tooth color. Complementary color porcelain is a mixture of body and modifier porcelains. The complementary color porcelain is applied in the same manner as masking porcelain with a .3 mm cervical

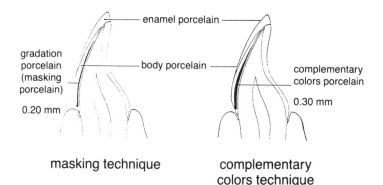

Fig 12–20.—Layering technique for base layer of porcelain laminate veneer. **Left:** masking porcelain technique (conventional technique). **Right:** complementary color porcelain technique. (Courtesy of Yamada K: *Int J Prosthodont* 6:242–247, 1993.)

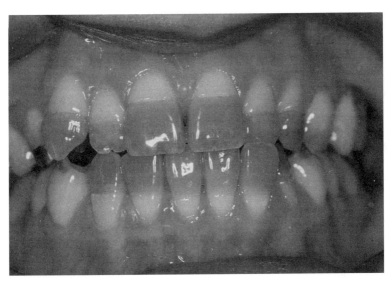

Fig 12–21.—Brown-based, moderately discolored teeth before treatment. (Courtesy of Yamada K: *Int J Prosthodont* 6:242-247, 1993.)

thickness tapering at the incisal edge (Fig 12–20). The selected color should produce a grayish tone, to which a white modifier is added, followed by a translucent cover. The base layer is fired, and then the body and enamel porcelains are applied.

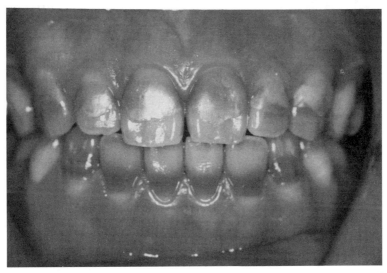

Fig 12–22.—Blue-purple-based, severely discolored teeth before treatment. (Courtesy of Yamada K: *Int J Prosthodont* 6:242-247, 1993.)

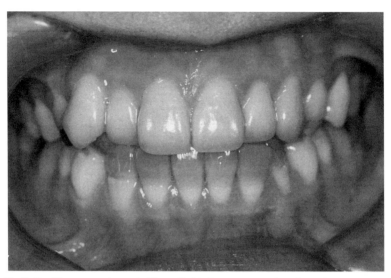

Fig 12–23.—The same patient as in Figure 12-21 after treatment. The color and shape of the teeth were improved. A more gentle facial appearance is expected. (Courtesy of Yamada K: *Int J Prosthodont* 6:242–247, 1993.)

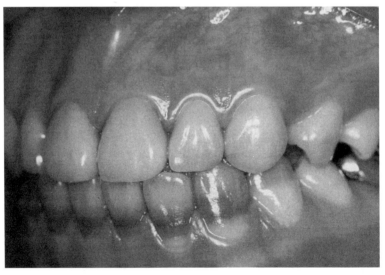

Fig 12–24.—The same patient as in Figure 12-22 after treatment. Note the color harmony with the posterior teeth. (Courtesy of Yamada K: *Int J Prosthodont* 6:242–247, 1993.)

Results.—Complementary color porcelain produces a less dramatic whitening but a more natural appearance. Moderately discolored brown-based and severely discolored blue-purple based teeth were treated with this technique (Figs 12–21 and 12–22). This restoration resulted in a harmonious and esthetically pleasing appearance (Figs 12–23 and 12–24).

Conclusion.—Complementary color porcelain produces a less dramatic, but more natural, appearance than conventional porcelain laminate veneer restorations.

▶ Porcelain laminate veneers offer marvelous esthetic results if the underlying color of the tooth is reasonably acceptable. Distinct discoloration of the tooth presents a much more difficult challenge because the translucency of the porcelain makes it harder to conceal the underlying discoloration. Bleaching the teeth offers some answer to the problem, but some stains (such as tetracycline stain) are very difficult to remove. Resorting to the use of an opaque porcelain or strong dentin masking defeats the natural translucency of the veneer, which is its chief esthetic benefit. The author suggests a way to overcome the problem of severe discoloration without blocking out all the light transmission. It is logical to use the complementary colors to neutralize the undesirable colors of the tooth. This seems to be a practical solution to achieve the esthetic results desired. It does require precise communication with the laboratory.—T.G. Berry, D.D.S., M.A.

The Effect of Polishing Porcelain Laminates on Induced I-Bar Wear
Tietge JD, Dixon DL, Breeding LC (Med Univ of South Carolina, Charleston; Univ of Alabama, Birmingham; Univ of Kentucky, Lexington)
Int J Prosthodont 5:523–526, 1992   105-94-12–16

Objective.—Undercuts for removable partial denture (RPD) abutment teeth may be produced by means of partial-coverage porcelain laminate restorations. Recontouring of these restorations, if needed, would require surface polishing before fabrication of the RPD. The wear of polished-surface porcelain-laminate restorations with I-bar clasps was studied during a simulated 2-year period, including placement and removal of the RPD.

TABLE 1.—Calculated Wear Data for the I-Bar Specimens

I-bar group	N	Mean (μm)	SD	SEM	Variance	CV
Glazed porcelain	10	38.333	27.734	8.770	769.194	72.351
Polished porcelain	8	10.185	18.740	6.626	351.199	183.999
Human tooth	10	13.090	8.915	2.819	79.469	68.102

(Courtesy of Tietge JD, Dixon DL, Breeding LC: *Int J Prosthodont* 5:523–526, 1992.)

TABLE 2.—Duncan's Multiple Range Test for Wear Variations
in the Combined Contacting Surface I-Bar Groups

Group	Mean (μm)	Duncan grouping*
Glazed porcelain/ I-bar	45.024	A
Human tooth/ I-bar	38.333	A
Polished porcelain/ I-bar	10.185	B

* Means with the same letter are not significantly different at α < .05.
(Courtesy of Tietge JD, Dixon DL, Breeding LC: Int J Prosthodont 5:523–526, 1992.)

Methods.—Eight extracted teeth with cemented partial-coverage porcelain-laminate restorations were studied. After recontouring and polishing, placement and removal movements of the corresponding I-bar clasps were made using a simulated function machine. The simulated 2 years of wear assumed that the RPD would be placed and removed an average of 4 times a day. Wear was quantitated by means of scannning electron photomicrographs and computer imaging and compared to previous wear data on I-bar tips moved against human enamel and glazed, luted porcelain-laminate restorations.

Results.—The laminate specimens showed no measurable wear. For the I-bar groups, wear was greatest against glazed porcelain and least against polished porcelain (Table 1). The combined wear of the human tooth/I-bar combination and the glazed porcelain/I-bar combination was significantly greater than the mean wear of the polished porcelain/I-bar combination, according to Duncan's multiple range test (Table 2).

Conclusion.—There was no significant difference between the mean wear of I-bar clasps tested against polished porcelain vs. human enamel, but there was significantly greater wear of I-bar clasps tested against glazed porcelain vs. polished porcelain or human enamel. The mean wear of the I-bar/polished porcelain combination is significantly less than that of the other 2 combinations. Porcelain-laminate restorations placed for retention of I-bar retainers should be polished rather than glazed.

▶ The porcelain laminate veneer offers a good means of altering an abutment tooth to achieve the necessary contours and undercuts to provide the needed retention for a removable partial denture. The veneer also provides a very pleasing appearance. All of this can be achieved with a minimal amount of tooth removal. The porcelain can present a problem for the partial denture clasps, however. The potential abrasive quality of porcelain can cause significant wear of the clasps if the porcelain is not well polished. The dentist

Moving?

I'd like to receive my *Year Book of Dentistry* without interruption.
Please note the following change of address, effective:

Name: _____

New Address: _____

_____

City: _____ State: _____ Zip: _____

Old Address: _____

_____

City: _____ State: _____ Zip: _____

Reservation Card

Yes, I would like my own copy of *Year Book of Dentistry*. Please begin my subscription with the current edition according to the terms described below.* I understand that I will have 30 days to examine each annual edition. If satisfied, I will pay just $64.95 plus sales tax, postage and handling (price subject to change without notice).

Name: _____

Address: _____

City: _____ State: _____ Zip: _____

Method of Payment
○ Visa   ○ Mastercard   ○ AmEx   ○ Bill me   ○ Check (in US dollars, payable to Mosby, Inc.)

Card number: _____ Exp date: _____

Signature: _____

LS-0909

*Your *Year Book* Service Guarantee:

When you subscribe to the *Year Book*, we'll send you an advance notice of future volumes about two months before they publish. This automatic notice system is designed to take up as little of your time as possible. If you do not want the *Year Book*, the advance notice makes it quick and easy for you to let us know your decision, and you will always have at least 20 days to decide. If we don't hear from you, we'll send you the new volume as soon as it's available. And, of course, the *Year Book* is yours to examine free of charge for 30 days (postage, handling and applicable sales tax are added to each shipment.).

BUSINESS REPLY MAIL

FIRST CLASS MAIL   PERMIT No. 762   CHICAGO, IL

POSTAGE WILL BE PAID BY ADDRESSEE

Chris Hughes
Mosby-Year Book, Inc.
200 N. LaSalle Street
Suite 2600
Chicago, IL 60601-9981

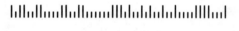

BUSINESS REPLY MAIL

FIRST CLASS MAIL   PERMIT No. 762   CHICAGO, IL

POSTAGE WILL BE PAID BY ADDRESSEE

Chris Hughes
Mosby-Year Book, Inc.
200 N. LaSalle Street
Suite 2600
Chicago, IL 60601-9981

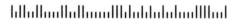

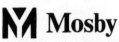 **Mosby**

Dedicated to publishing excellence

needs to assess exactly where the clasps meet the porcelain and then polish the porcelain very well. Contrary to what was traditionally taught, the glazed porcelain is more abrasive than the polished porcelain. Leaving the porcelain glazed can lead to premature wear and, subsequently, loss of retention or the need to replace the clasps.—T.G. Berry, D.D.S., M.A.

Amalgam

A Concept of Restorative Treatment During Orthodontic Therapy

Baumann MA, Ruppenthal T (Johannes-Gutenberg-Univ of Mainz, Germany)
Quintessence Int 23:695–700, 1992   105-94-12–17

Background.—Fixed orthodontic appliances make efficient oral hygiene difficult, and they are associated with a high risk of plaque accumulation, leading to demineralization and new carious lesions. A treatment concept based on interdisciplinary teamwork between restorative dentists and orthodontists has been developed that allows comprehensive dental treatment during orthodontic therapy with fixed appliances.

Discussion.—Occlusal defects in fissures and pits requiring class I and II restorations are easily handled. Larger lesions up to the proximal boxes, however, require the use of wedges and matrices to achieve adequate restoration. In some cases, the pre-existing band may be used as the matrix. The arch wire may also be retained; whereas in other circum-

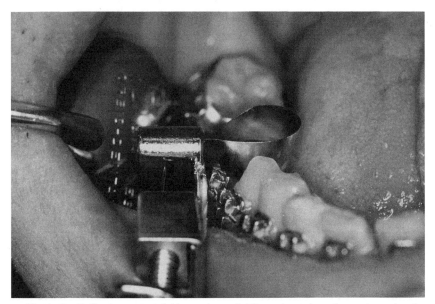

Fig 12–25.—Tofflemire matrix is held over the tooth. The position where the matrix touches the arch wire has been marked with a blue lithographic pencil. (Courtesy of Baumann MA, Ruppenthal T: *Quintessence Int* 23:695–700, 1992.)

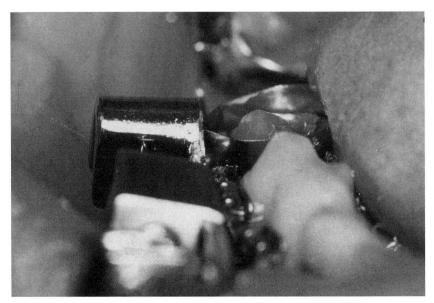

Fig 12–26.—The Tofflemire matrix fits well after 2 notches are made. (Courtesy of Baumann MA, Ruppenthal T: *Quintessence Int* 23:695–700, 1992.)

stances, partial or complete removal will be required. Tofflemire matrices can be fitted for these restorations by placing the matrix in the required position and marking the points of contact between the matrix and arch wire (Fig 12-25). A gap is then made at the indicated areas with crown scissors, and the matrix is fitted and secured with proximal wedges (Fig 12-26). Class III and IV restorations may be treated in a fairly normal fashion with acetate matrices. An adequate dry working area may be achieved with cotton balls, a rubber dam, or both. Good adaption is achieved by slitting the matrix around the arch wire.

Conclusion.—A prognostic evaluation of all teeth should be made before beginning orthodontic treatment. A close partnership between the dental practitioner and the orthodontist will allow a quick resolution of any difficulties that do arise.

▶ This article addresses a well-known problem facing the dentist: how to restore teeth after the orthodontic bands and arch wires are in place. Orthodontic procedures are performed on young patients at a time during which their oral hygiene may not be good and they may be particularly susceptible to carious activity. Additionally, the bands and wires interfere with the normal hygiene procedures. It is therefore especially important to institute preventive measures before and then during the orthodontic treatment. Topical fluoride application, restoration of all active carious lesions, and placement of pit and sealants should be done before orthodontic appliances are placed. Use of oral antimicrobial agents, such as chlorhexidine, while the orthodontic treatment is ongoing will help to prevent new carious lesions. If treatment is needed, however, the techniques offered by the authors allow the means of successfully accomplishing that treatment.—T.G. Berry, D.D.S., M.A.

Finishing Techniques for Amalgam Restorations: Clinical Assessment at Three Years

Bryant RW, Collins CJ (Univ of Sydney, Westmead, Australia)
Aust Dent J 37:333–339, 1992   105-94-12–18

Background.—Optimally finishing an amalgam restoration may enhance the marginal integrity of the restoration and discourage unnecessary replacement. Amalgam restorations finished in 1 of 3 ways were evaluated clinically.

Methods.—Fifty-six patients were included in the study. A total of 228 high copper amalgam restorations were assessed by clinical criteria up to 3 years after placement. Each patient had had at least 1 carved-only amalgam, at least 1 immediately finished restoration, and at least 1 amalgam that was polished at a subsequent visit.

Findings.—Regardless of the finishing method, the restorations showed similar marginal integrity up to 3 years after placement. Polished restorations had markedly better surface texture and were less likely to show surface discoloration. The findings did not support the use of immediate finishing techniques.

Conclusion.—Restorations polished at least 24 hours after placement have superior surface texture and somewhat less surface discoloration than carved-only or immediately finished restorations. One to 3 years after placement, the integrity of the 3 restorations studied was similar, regardless of the finishing technique. No long-term advantages are gained from the use of immediate finishing methods, compared with the use of carved-only or delayed polishing methods. Carefully placed, carved high copper amalgam restorations may have a longevity similar to that of polished restorations.

▶ The study supports past findings that polishing the restoration does not increase the life span of the restoration. This contradicts what has been taught in the past. Article 105-94-12–24 demonstrates that burnishing after the carving is finished actually is detrimental to the margins. If the restoration is not to be polished, it is critical that (1) the margins are well carved; (2) all contours are established; (3) the occlusal and proximal contacts are satisfactory; and (4) the surfaces are smoothed to compensate for no polishing at a later date. If the dentist does wish to polish the amalgam restoration, it must be recognized that the procedure is only to provide a very shiny appearance rather than to improve the performance. Polishing releases mercury, albeit a small amount, so high-speed suction and a water spray should be used.—T.G. Berry, D.D.S., M.A.

Initial Preparations for Amalgam Restorations: Extending the Longevity of the Tooth-Restoration Unit

Summitt JB, Osborne JW (Univ of Texas Health Science Ctr, San Antonio; Univ of Colorado, Denver)
J Am Dent Assoc 123(11):67–73, 1992   105-94-12–19

Background.—A number of factors affect the longevity and serviceability of cavity restorations. Despite advances in instrumentation and amalgam technology, dentists continue to prepare teeth the way they did 2 decades ago. Some of the alternative materials and techniques that can extend the longevity of restorations were discussed.

Amalgam Preparations.—For the purposes of discussion, a groove was defined as the depression formed by the junction of 2 lobes of a tooth. Lobes that have fused may show coalesced enamel at the base of a groove. Those with an imperfect junction may show a fissure, which may extend past the dentoenamel junction or terminate within the enamel. The junction of 2 or more fissures is the usual location of pits.

Many of the traditional principles of cavity preparation no longer apply, such as extending class II amalgam restorations through the grooves across the occlusal surfaces of posterior teeth without occlusal caries or making faciolingually wide preparations in occlusal surfaces, even if they are caries-free. Over the years, a number of laboratory and clinical studies have clearly demonstrated that making a smaller amalgam restoration will extend the life of the tooth-restoration unit.

Recommendations.—Specific recommendations for conservative class I and class II amalgam restorations include the following: class I preparations should be made only in areas where caries has been diagnosed, not just where fissures are present. If a single tooth shows multiple carious areas, make a separate preparation for each. Preparations should be kept as narrow as possible, especially if they extend through a noncarious fissure. Only if diagnosed caries is present should a class II preparation be extended into occlusal grooves. Resin sealant should be used to seal occlusal fissures. Adequate retention locks should be used in the approximal slot preparation. If an occlusal extension is less than about 1.2 mm in width, retention to the approximal segment should be augmented with retention points. Finally, a dentinal bonding agent should be used to line preparations using combined amalgam and resin fissure sealant restorations. Copal varnish should not be used with combined preparations.

Summary.—The size of the amalgam restoration is a vital consideration. It should be no larger than necessary for removal of the carious process and to provide adequate resistance and retention.

▶ This article states a very important principle of conservation of tooth structure when preparing a tooth for restorative treatment. Despite studies showing an increased longevity for the restoration and greater strength of the tooth when the preparations are very conservative, dentists continue to cut traditional preparations. Current methods of preventing carious activity in pits and fissure adjacent to the carious area, such as preventive resin restorations or pit and fissure sealants, can be used when they seem to be indicated. The preparations and restorations proposed by the authors depart radically from the "extension for prevention" philosophy of previous years, but new materials and techniques allow the successful use of a very conservative restorative treatment.—T.G. Berry, D.D.S., M.A.

In Vitro Marginal Leakage in Varnished and Lined Amalgam Restorations

Grossman ES, Matejka JM (Univ of the Witwatersrand, South Africa)
J Prosthet Dent 69:469–474, 1993   105-94-12-20

Background.—Until the margins of silver amalgam restorations are sealed over time, the restoration remains vulnerable to attack by bacteria. A logical combination of restorative materials that quickly promotes a demonstrable seal is needed.

Methods.—Two types of silver amalgam and 5 different bases, with or without cavity varnish, were compared for their resistance to marginal leakage in 440 extracted, intact human premolars (Table 1). Twenty different combinations were used to restore Black's class I classic cavity preparations. The teeth were stored for 1 year in 1% sodium chloride solution and assessed for percentage of marginal leakage by a standard fluorescent dye test.

Findings.—As time passed, sealing improved. In the initial months, sealing was better without varnish, but this difference was not significant after 1 year. Sealing was better with low-copper amalgam than with high-copper amalgam. Sealing was enhanced by the use of a calcium hydroxide base, and the next-best results were achieved in base-free cavities. Teeth in which Dycal base was used had decreased sealing at 1 year. Zinc-containing bases were associated with poor sealing, even if they also contained tin (Table 2).

Conclusion.—Sealing is quick with unvarnished calcium hydroxide-based cavities, regardless of whether a high- or low-copper amalgam is used. Sealing is slow with varnished high-copper amalgam, regardless of the base used. Leakage will occur after 1 year in restorations lined with zinc-containing bases.

▶ It is well known that an amalgam corrodes at the margins. This results in an elevated level of tin, which is associated with decreased leakage. This, in turn, decreases problems associated with leakage, such as pulpal sensitivity and recurrent caries; therefore, methods for preventing leakage are of real interest. In the past, the use of cavity varnish under the restoration was advocated. This study challenges the use of cavity varnish because the high-cop-

TABLE 1.—Abbreviations and Details of the Dental Materials

Abbrev.	Material	Manufacturer	Batch
P	Polyvar	Lorvic Corp St Louis, Mo.	B032
C	E Merck	Darmstadt, Germany	431A895847
F	Poly-F Plus	De Trey, Zurich, Switzerland	FB61 86/02
K	Kalzinol	De Trey, Zurich, Switzerland/ E. R. Bernard Johannesburg, South Africa	DC1
Z	Zinc oxide	Kalzinol powder as above	
Y	Dycal	L. D. Caulk Division, Dentsply International Inc. Milford, Del.	102488
D	Dispersalloy	Johnson & Johnson Dental Products East Windsor, New York, USA	8C816
N	New True Dentalloy	S.S. White Dental Products Int. Philadelphia, Pa.	033081 # 6798101 and 102684 # 0428410
X	The base/varnish is absent		

(Courtesy of Grossman ES, Matejka JM: J Prosthet Dent 69:469–474, 1993.)

TABLE 2.—Percentage Seal in Tooth Specimens

Restoration combination	Percentage seal		
	7 day	3 month	1 year
Varnish + KALZ + Cu(low)	8	6	18
Varnish + KALZ + Cu(high)	0	0	0
Varnish + ZO + Cu(low)	0	6	12
Varnish + POLYF+ + Cu(low)	0	18	31
Varnish + POLYF+ + Cu(high)	0	6	0
Varnish + Ca(OH)$_2$ + Cu(low)	33	62	68
Varnish + Ca(OH)$_2$ + Cu(high)	25	18	56
Varnish + DYCAL + Cu(low)	91	31	12
Varnish + Cu(low)	16	6	31
Varnish + Cu(high)	16	6	56
KALZ + Cu(low)	0	12	37
KALZ + Cu(high)	8	6	0
ZO + Cu(low)	8	43	6
POLYF+ +Cu(low)	0	0	25
Poly + + Cu(high)	0	6	0
Ca(OH)$_2$ + Cu(low)	66	87	100
Ca(OH)$_2$ + Cu(high)	58	43	68
DYCAL + Cu(low)	58	18	25
Cu(low)	33	31	43
Cu(high)	41	25	37

Abbreviations: Varnish, Polyvar; *KALZ,* Kalzinol; *ZO,* zinc oxide mixed with distilled water; *POLYF +,* Poly-F Plus; *Ca(OH)$_2$,* calcium hydroxide mixed with distilled water; *DYCAL,* Dycal; *Cu(low),* New True Dentalloy; *Cu(high),* Dispersalloy.
(Courtesy of Grossman ES, Matejka JM: *J Prosthet Dent* 69:469–474, 1993.)

per amalgam gained a seal more slowly when varnish was used. The varnish does offer some early protection before the corrosion products start to form, so the elimination of varnish from the procedures would forgo this early benefit. It has recently been suggested that a resin/resin varnish cured over the margins can provide an early seal more effectively. More investigation is needed.—T.G. Berry, D.D.S., M.A.

Intraoral Galvanic Corrosion: Literature Review and Case Report

Meyer RD, Meyer J, Taloumis LJ (North Rivera Ridge Dental Clinic, Fort Drum, NY; Cave Junction, Ore; Fort Meade, Md)
J Prosthet Dent 69:141–143, 1993   105-94-12-21

Introduction.—Galvanic corrosion is an electrochemical reaction between dissimilar metals that can produce unpleasant and even painful intraoral effects. One patient had a persistent complaint of a burning, tingling sensation in several teeth and a metallic taste after placement of a gold crown.

Case Report.—A dentist in general practice for 30 years had a complete gold crown (FGC, type III alloy) placed on the maxillary left permanent first molar, opposing a similar restoration on the mandibular left first molar. A mesial occlusal lingual silver amalgam alloy was present in the mandibular second molar. There were no centric occlusal stops between these teeth. After about 2 months the patient noted a metallic taste resembling tinfoil, which became more pronounced over time, as well as vague discomfort in the left mandible that radiated to the left side of the face. Symptoms persisted after the contact between the new FGC and the amalgam alloy was removed, and they were noted primarily during chewing on the left side. Placing dental floss between the mandibular first and second molars relieved the symptoms; a rubber band also was effective. A more permanent solution was provided by placing class II posterior composite resin within the existing amalgam restoration to remove the contact point.

Discussion.—Oral galvanism occurs most often when cast type III gold and silver amalgam restorations are present. Pain caused by galvanic current usually is relieved by physically separating the teeth. The best management is to precipitate silver nitrate on the surface of the new restoration or to coat the entire surface of the restoration with unfilled composite resin, which then is cured.

▶ It has long been known that the contact of dissimilar metals can create a galvanic current that leads to problems. Dissimilar metals in opposing teeth can give a galvanic shock every time they contact. Constant contact of dissimilar metals that are side by side in the arch creates a more subtle problem because the signs and symptoms are much more difficult to recognize. Once suspected, however, a simple diagnostic test may reveal the problem. A separator to break the contact is easy to place without real discomfort to the patient. If the symptoms are relieved, any one of several procedures can be taken to eliminate future galvanic response problems. It is important to recognize the patient's often vague symptoms and determine the cause to apply the relatively simple solution. The increased use of composite resins and ceramic materials on posterior teeth would predict that fewer of these problems will occur in the future.—T.G. Berry, D.D.S., M.A.

Oral Amalgam Tattoos: A Diagnostic Study
Owens BM, Schuman NJ, Johnson WW (Univ of Tennessee, Memphis)
Compend Contin Educ Dent 14:210–215, 1993   105-94-12-22

Background.—Oral amalgam tattoos resulting from accidental dental amalgam placement into intraoral soft tissue may occur in both the maxillary and mandibular arches. Amalgam tattoos occur most often in the

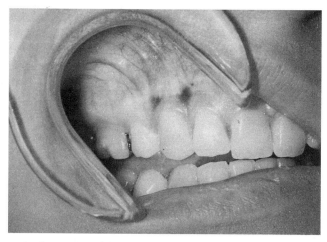

Fig 12–27.—Amalgam tattoos of the maxillary gingiva. (Courtesy of Owens BM, Schuman NJ, Johnson WW: *Compend Contin Educ Dent* 14:210–215, 1993.)

buccal mucosa, gingiva, and alveolar mucosa (Fig 12–27), but they have also been found in the lip, palate, tongue, and retromolar mucosa (Fig 12–28). Data on oral amalgam tattoo lesions submitted to the oral pathology department of one university were examined.

Results.—During a 10-year period, 74 dentists submitted 168 pathology reports of oral amalgam tattoos for histologic verification; 148 reports contained a preliminary clinical diagnosis by the attending dentist (table). Amalgam tattoo lesion was included in the diagnosis in 122 of the 148 case reports. Almost 42% of the dentists submitting pathology

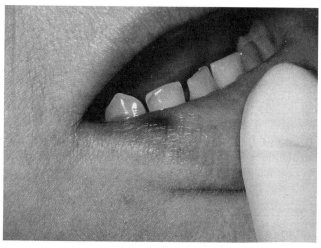

Fig 12–28.—Amalgam tattoo of the lower lip. (Courtesy of Owens BM, Schuman NJ, Johnson WW: *Compend Contin Educ Dent* 14:210–215, 1993.)

	Lesion Diagnoses	
Lesion/Dx	Total Cases Dx*	% Cases Final Dx (N = 168)
Amalgam tattoo	122	72.6
Nevus	28	16.7
Melanoma	28	16.7
Pigmented lesion	12	7.1
Vascular lesion	10	6.0
Other lesions	10	6.0

* The total number of cases was greater than 168, because total cases includes sole and secondary diagnoses.
(Courtesy of Owens BM, Schuman NJ, Johnson WW: *Compend Contin Educ Dent* 14:210–215, 1993.)

reports for verification were general dentists and 58% were dental specialists. Melanoma was suspected in 28 case reports submitted by 20 attending dentists, of which 7 were general practitioners. Oral surgeons and periodontists comprised 60% of the sample.

Conclusion.—Oral amalgam tattoos are usually clinically diagnosed by the attending dentist. When a suspicious lesion is identified, a biopsy specimen should be obtained and submitted for histologic verification.

▶ Amalgam tattoos are relatively common in adult patients who have received several amalgam restorations. Although they are harmless, they may create patient concern, and they must be differentiated from other pigmented lesions, such as melanoma, that have potentially serious consequences. The authors have outlined well the clinical features of an amalgam tattoo and have listed the most likely areas of occurrence. It is important that the dentist carefully examine every pigmented area to determine whether it is an amalgam tattoo or a lesion. Biopsies should be performed whenever there is a real question about the diagnosis.—T.G. Berry, D.D.S., M.A.

Clinical Study of Oral Galvanism: No Evidence of Toxic Mercury Exposure but Anxiety Disorder an Important Background Factor
Herrström P, Högstedt B (Primary Care Ctr Hertig Knut, Halmstad, Sweden; Central Hosp, Halmstad, Sweden)
Scand J Dent Res 101:232–237, 1993   105-94-12–23

Background.—The public has become concerned that dental amalgams may be detrimental to their health because of oral galvanism and mercury release. However, epidemiologic studies have failed to show that these amalgams pose a major health hazard. Two hundred eighteen patients with self-diagnosed oral galvanism were examined in a prospective study.

Patients and Methods.—Self-diagnosed patients were referred from medical and dental professionals. General medical (including the main organ systems) and psychological status were evaluated. Whole blood mercury concentration tests (B-Hg) were performed on 172 patients. Normal concentration was defined as less than 50 nmol/L. The patients were subdivided based on amalgam load. Twenty percent of the patients had 0 to 5, 37% had 6 to 10, and 43% had 11 or more amalgam fillings.

Results.—The mean B-Hg was 17.3 nmol/L, with no values exceeding 50 nmol/L. No correlation was found between amalgam burden and B-Hg, or the presence of oral, somatic, or psychological main symptoms. No incidents of mercury intoxication were found. The majority of the patients (62%) reported symptom durations in excess of 5 years. Mental disorders comprised the main diagnosis in 43% of the cases, including 41 patients with general anxiety disorder. Amalgam removal was recommended for 65 patients, mainly because of psychological implications, although in 22 patients removal was recommended because of oral conditions.

Conclusion.—Although some patients with oral galvanism do have allergies to dental materials or other oral conditions, the most frequent main diagnosis in these patients is generalized anxiety or other mental disorders. No generalized toxic effects of amalgam fillings were noted.

▶ The use of dental amalgam continues to stir controversy among health-care providers and the public, despite the absence of any research proving amalgam harmful to patients or dental personnel. This study, which showed no connection between patient's symptoms and the number of restorations, adds to the body of evidence debunking theories of mercury hazards to patients. A conference held by the Food and Drug Administration in March 1991 noted that no evidence supports the contention that the mercury in dental amalgam presents a danger to the patient. Furthermore, epidemiologic studies have shown that although allergic responses to mercury can occur, they are very rare.—T.G. Berry, D.D.S., M.A.

Determining Amalgam Marginal Quality: Effect of Occlusal Surface Condition

Woods PW, Marker VA, McKinney TW, Miller BH, Okabe T (Baylor College of Dentistry, Dallas)
J Am Dent Assoc 124(5):60–65, 1993   105-94-12-24

Background.—There have been no standard criteria for determining when replacement of amalgam restorations is needed. In addition, there are no standard finishing and polishing procedures for these restora-

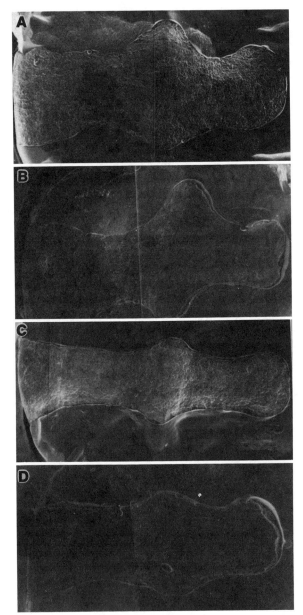

Fig 12–29.—Twelve-week micrographs. **A,** CO, Tytin; **B,** CB, Tytin; **C,** BC, Dispersalloy; **D,** CB, Dispersalloy. Original magnification, ×20. (Courtesy of Woods PW, Marker VA, McKinney TW, et al: *J Am Dent Assoc* 124(5):60–65, 1993.)

tions. The effect of 4 different finishing techniques on the durability of dental amalgam restorations as determined by marginal breakdown was investigated.

Patients and Methods. —Thirty-two class II restorations were placed in the first and second molars of removable, partial dentures. Two high-copper alloys, Tytin and Dispersalloy, were used, and the 4 finishing procedures were carve-only (CO), burnish-carve (BC), carve-burnish (CB), and burnish-carve-burnish (BCB). The finishing times were constant for all 4 procedures. After 12 weeks, the restorations were switched. Each patient received 4 restorations of each type of alloy. At the 12th week, scanning electron micrographs were obtained of the occlusal surfaces and the marginal ridge, illustrating each of the 4 finishing procedures and the Tytin and Dispersalloy copper alloys used in the restorations (Fig 12–29).

Results. —There was no overall correlation between the amount of breakdown and the location on the restoration. The amount of wear occurring in denture teeth was only slightly accelerated compared with that of natural teeth. The micrographs showed that Tytin restorations finished with the CO and the BC procedures had the least amount of marginal breakdown. The CB and the BCB procedures seemed to have a damaging effect on the Tytin restorations. The CO and the BC treatment were ranked superior to the BCB procedure. The Dispersalloy restorations showed similar results.

Conclusion. —Both the CO and the BC techniques showed similar postive effects on marginal breakdown; therefore, a subjective variable, ease of handling, was applied to assist in recommending the standard finishing technique. Burnishing immediately before carving or as part of the condensation process seemed to improve the carving characteristics of the amalgam. The BC procedure is recommended as the standard finishing technique.

▶ The finish of the surface of an amalgam restoration has been considered important to the longevity of the restoration's performance. However, research has not shown any real advantage to polishing the restoration, although other finishing procedures and sequences do affect the long-term success of the restoration. This article demonstrates that disturbing the amalgam surface after carving (e.g., burnishing) has a detrimental effect on the performance of the material. Because the burnishing after carving creates a relatively shiny surface, it is tempting to perform the step. It would seem that burnishing after carving shortens the life span of the restoration, and there is no real benefit to polishing the surface at a later appointment.—T.G. Berry, D.D.S., M.A.

Prosthodontics

Retention Properties of a Split-Shaft Threaded Post: Cut at Different Apical Lengths

Cohen BI, Condos S, Musikant BL, Deutsch AS (Essential Dental Labs, South Hackensack, NJ)

J Prosthet Dent 68:894–898, 1992   105-94-12-25

Introduction.—Successful restoration requires retention of the post to the root of an endodontically treated tooth. Post length is often modified to accommodate a specific clinical situation. The retentions of apically shortened and full-length no. 1 and no. 2 Flexi-Post dowels were compared.

Methods.—No. 1 and no. 2 Flexi-Post restorations were shortened apically from 1 to 5 mm (Fig 12-30). Ten groups of experimental material with 10 samples in each group were studied.

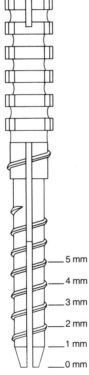

— 5 mm
— 4 mm
— 3 mm
— 2 mm
— 1 mm
— 0 mm

Fig 12–30.—Illustration of Flexi-Post No. 2 dowel with positions for apical cutting (1 to 5 mm). (Courtesy of Cohen BI, Condos S, Musikant BL, et al: *J Prosthet Dent* 68:894–898, 1992.)

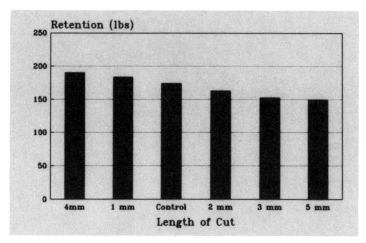

Fig 12–31.—Retention vs. apical cutting of No. 1 Flexi-Post dowel. (Courtesy of Cohen BI, Condos S, Musikant BL, et al: *J Prosthet Dent* 68:894–898, 1992.)

Findings.—According to analysis of variance with a Tukey-Student range (multiple-comparison test), there were no significant differences among retentions of no. 1 dowels shortened by 1, 2, 3, and 5 mm and full-length dowels. However, 4 mm of apical shortening produced significantly greater retention. There were no significant differences with apical reductions of 1 to 4 mm or full-length control Flexi-Post no. 2 dowels. However, 5 mm of apical shortened was associated with significantly less retention (Figs 12–31, 12–32, and 12–33).

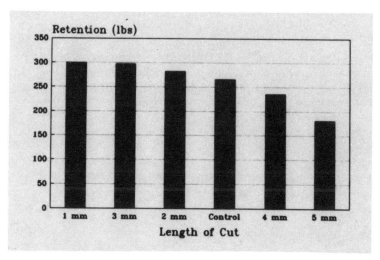

Fig 12–32.—Retention vs. apical cutting of No. 2 Flexi-Post dowel. (Courtesy of Cohen BI, Condos S, Musikant BL, et al: *J Prosthet Dent* 68:894–898, 1992.)

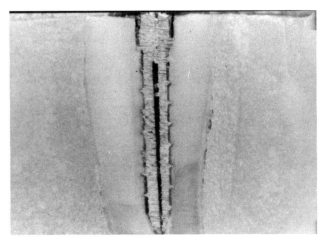

Fig 12–33.—Longitudinal section of cemented Flexi-Post dowel in root. Note apical three threads are barely engaged in dentin. (Courtesy of Cohen BI, Condos S, Musikant BL, et al: *J Prosthet Dent* 68:894–898, 1992.)

Conclusion.—When endodontic posts are shortened, fewer flexible threads are present at the apex than with the original, unaltered Flexi-Post dowel. The apical threads of the post then invade the dentin more deeply, and almost all threads fully engage dentin from the apex to the coronal surface of the root instead of the 3 or 4 levels of threads not engaging dentin near the apex in the unaltered post.

▶ The post and core restoration offers a very crucial means of restoring the badly broken-down tooth, but it is not without its problems. It is not always easy to achieve a post that is adapted to the canal along its entire length well enough to offer excellent retention without creating a wedging force.

The Flexi-Post system offers a post that can create retention without undue internal pressures. Many of the posts (29%) must be shortened, so it is reassuring that shortening the post actually adapts it better to the canal walls. The remaining threads do cut into the dentin to gain excellent retention. For many situations, the Flexi-Post has proved to be an excellent choice for restoring the tooth.—T.G. Berry, D.D.S., M.A.

The Resistance to Tensile, Compression, and Torsional Forces Provided by Four Post Systems
Burgess JO, Summitt JB, Robbins JW (Univ of Texas Health Science Ctr, San Antonio)
J Prosthet Dent 68:899–903, 1992   105-94-12–26

Background.—Past experience shows that threaded endodontic posts are most retentive, followed by parallel posts, and tapered posts are least

| | Post Systems Tested | |
Post	Luting agent	Canal treatment
Experimental post	Experimental resin	1. Dry—paper point 2. Polyacrylic acid—20 sec (Dentin prep) 3. Drying agent—10 sec (Methyl ethyl ketone) 4. Cement Bis-GMA
Experimental post with over-sized preparation	Experimental resin	1. Same as above
Para-Post	Flexi-Flow	1. Dry—paper point 2. Cement
V Lock	Flexi-Flow	1. Dry—paper point 2. Cement
Flexi-Post	Flexi-Flow	1. Dry—paper point 2. Cement

(Courtesy of Burgess JO, Summitt JB, Robbins JW: *J Prosthet Dent* 68:899–903, 1992.)

retentive. A longer post is more retentive, but an increased post diameter increases retention only minimally. A number of methods of preparing the post space have been described; their effects on apical seal are variable. Studies of luting agents have failed to show that one is better than the others. Whether a post strengthens an intact anterior tooth remains uncertain.

Objective.—Four endodontic posts (table) were assessed under conditions of tensile, torsion, and compressive force application. A total of 120 extracted mandibular premolars were used in the study.

Methods.—The teeth were decoronated at the cementoenamel junction, pulp tissue was removed, and the canals were enlarged, cleaned, and filled with gutta percha. Posts then were cut and cemented into prepared spaces with resin cement. Pins were placed into the coronal dentin paralleling the post, and composite resin cores were made around the coronal part of the post and pins.

Results.—The tensile load needed to pull the post and resin was significantly less than that required to remove the threaded posts. Flexi-Posts provided the most resistance to tensile and torsional loading (Figs 12–34 and 12–35). The compressive load needed to fracture the core

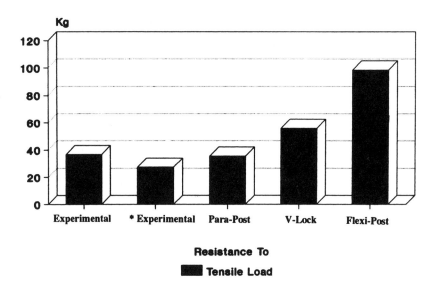

Experimental Post- Oversized Canal

Fig 12–34.—Resistance to tensile loading provided by 4 post systems. (Courtesy of Burgess JO, Summitt JB, Robbins JW: *J Prosthet Dent* 68:899–903, 1992.)

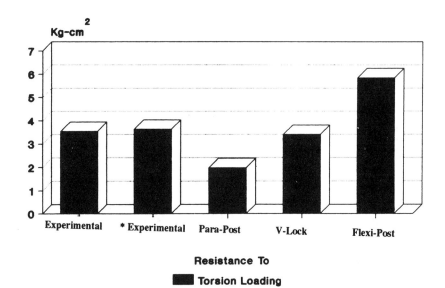

• Experimental Post- Oversized Canal

Fig 12–35.—Resistance to clockwise torsion loading provided by 4 post systems. (Courtesy of Burgess JO, Summitt JB, Robbins JW: *J Prosthet Dent* 68:899–903, 1992.)

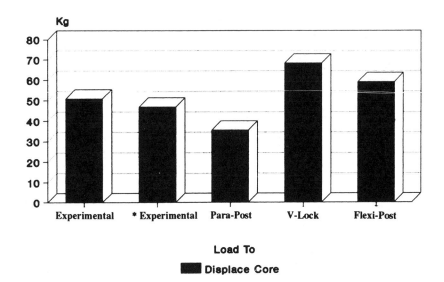

Load To

■ **Displace Core**

• **Experimental Post- Overslzed Canal**

Fig 12–36.—Resistance to compressive loading provided by 4 post systems. (Courtesy of Burgess JO, Summitt JB, Robbins JW: *J Prosthet Dent* 68:899–903, 1992.)

over the V Lock post was significantly greater than with the other post systems (Fig 12–36).

Conclusion.—The experimental post system failed to improve significantly on posts cemented with a conventional nonadhesive resin cement in this trial. Failures were primarily adhesive at the dentinal surface. Threaded post systems provide higher tensile resistance than do cemented post systems.

▶ Much research and discussion has been conducted regarding which is the best post system for use with endodontically treated teeth. Threaded, parallel, and tapered posts all offer some distinct advantages. The threaded post appears the most advantageous, even though the possibility of root fracture is a concern. A truly adhesive luting agent, such as a resin adhesive, could give the tensile resistance of a nonthreaded post equal to or greater than for a threaded post. The failure of the experimental system in this study to achieve better results may not be because of the experimental parallel-sided post design, but because of the failure of the resin cement system. Other adhesive systems are proving more promising. The design of the post may soon be of less consequence than the nature of the bonding system used to bond the metal to the canal wall.—T.G. Berry, D.D.S., M.A.

Effect of Post Design on Resistance to Fracture of Endodontically Treated Teeth With Complete Crowns
Assif D, Bitenski A, Pilo R, Oren E (Tel Aviv Univ, Israel)
J Prosthet Dent 69:36–40, 1993   105-94-12–27

TABLE 1.—Failure Loads (in kg) in Various Groups in Increasing Order

Sample No.	C1 Cast dowel-core	C2 Cylindrical post cast dowel-core	C3 Tapered-end post cast dowel-core	C4 Control
1	92.5	170	137.5	125
2	140	185	175	162.5
3	187.5	232.5	195	185
4	210	242.5	202.5	210
5	245	260	205	220
6	250	275	207.5	230
7	250	310	210	245
8	270	315	255	250
9	320	342.5	260	300
10	395	435	435	325
11	440	—	—	—

(Courtesy of Assif D, Bitenski A, Pilo R, et al: *J Prosthet Dent* 69:36–40, 1993.)

TABLE 2.—Mean, Median, and Standard Deviation for Each Group

	C1	C2	C3	C4
		Group No.		
Mean	254.2	276.7	228.2	225.2
Median	250.0	267.5	206.2	225.0
SD	102.3	78.3	80.7	60.1

(Courtesy of Assif D, Bitenski A, Pilo R, et al: *J Prosthet Dent* 69:36–40, 1993.)

Background.—Usually a post-core system is inserted to restore damaged teeth after endodontic treatment. The best dowel design for these teeth remains uncertain. Strong metal posts concentrate stress in the less rigid root, increasing the risk of root fracture. A tooth with a post is commonly restored with an artificial crown having its finish line on healthy tooth structure. The effects of post design on the fracture resistance of endodontically treated teeth subjected to simulated occlusal loads was examined.

Methods.—A post-core system was restored with a complete cast crown, leaving 2-mm margins on healthy tooth structure apical to the border of the core. In the experimental groups, endodontically treated teeth were restored with a conventional cast dowel-core (C1), a cast cylindrical dowel and core (C-2), or a cast cylindrical tapered-end dowel and core (C3). Teeth in group C4 were controls. The cast dowel-cores were cemented with zinc phosphate cement. In control teeth, gutta-percha was removed from the canal to a depth of 9 mm, and the access cavity was closed with glass ionomer cement.

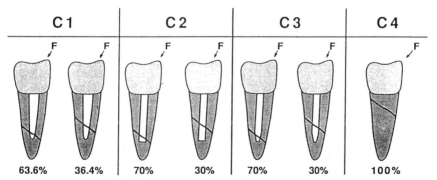

Fig 12–37.—Fracture patterns in the various groups. (Courtesy of Assif D, Bitenski A, Pilo R, et al: *J Prosthet Dent* 69:36–40, 1993.)

Results.—When the dowel and core had identical rigidity, the dowel design did not influence the fracture resistance of the teeth. Tables 1 and 2 list the forces that caused failure in the various groups. There were no statistically significant differences between the groups. All teeth failed by oblique root fracture. There were no vertical or longitudinal fractures paralleling the long axis of the teeth and no cohesive or adhesive cement failures. The fracture lines in teeth containing a dowel-core usually passed through the apex, but in some instances the fracture line passed through the apical third of the post (Fig 12–37). One dowel fracture occurred in group C2. In 3 instances, the post tip was bent.

Conclusion.—When a dowel-core system is used to restore endodontically treated teeth, a dowel that preserves the most tooth structure and provides suitable retention of the core should be chosen. No dowel is needed if the anatomical crown is adequately preserved and core retention is achievable from within the natural crown or if it is not necessary to complete the coronal surface.

▶ This study, which tested the resistance to fracture as related to the design of the post-core system, addresses some of the areas of controversy that exist. Various materials, designs, and lengths have been touted as the best to protect the tooth and to provide for retention of the restoration. Studies have shown that different post designs result in different stress concentrations. This study brings a different factor into discussion. If the crown margins are established on 2 mm or more of sound tooth structure when cemented to the abutment, the apical and cementoenamel junction stress concentrations are reduced. This margin location is not always possible, but it should be considered when there are not contraindications. If this can be accomplished, the most important factors in choosing a post system are preservation of tooth structure and retention of the post.—T.G. Berry, D.D.S., M.A.

Fracture Resistance of Amalgam and Composite Resin Cores Retained by Various Intradentinal Retentive Features
Tjan AHL, Dunn JR, Lee JK-Y (Loma Linda Univ, Calif)
Quintessence Int 24:211–217, 1993   105-94-12-28

Introduction.—Problems exist with the use of a self-threading pin system for tooth restoration or core construction. An alternative for retention of complex amalgam restorations may be the use of intradentinal retentive features.

Methods.—The fracture resistive strength of amalgam and composite resin cores retained by 3 types of intradentinal retentive features—(4 cylindrical channels, 2 U-form slots, or a post with a countersink)—was compared with that of cores retained by 4 self-threaded retentive pins (Figs 12–38 and 12–39). The cores were prepared with only facial and lingual inclined planes (Fig 12–40). Fracture resistance was assessed by an Instron testing machine (Fig 12–41).

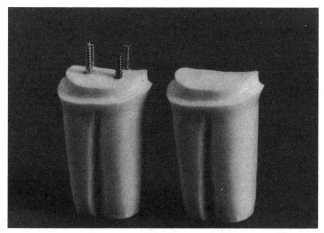

Fig 12–38.—Ivorine molar analogues: (**left**) with self-threaded retentive pins installed and (**right**) before the placement of the intradentinal retentive features. (Courtesy of Tjan AHL, Dunn JR, Lee JK-Y: *Quintessence Int* 24:211–217, 1993.)

Results.—Fracture resistance was significantly greater for composite resin cores with any of the retentive features tested. In the amalgam cores, fracture resistance was significantly greater with pins than with channels or slots. The fracture resistance of pins and post-countersink was comparable. In composite resin cores, fracture resistance was higher with pins than with any of the intradentinal retentive features (table).

Conclusion.—Fracture resistance is greater in amalgam and composite resin cores retained by self-threaded retentive pins than by various intradentinal retentive features. The exception is the fracture strength of post-countersink in amalgam cores, which is comparable to that of pins. There are no differences in fracture resistance among the intradentinal retentive features tested. Composite resin cores have significantly greater

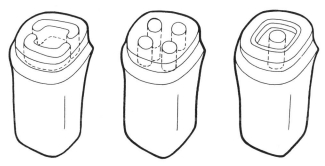

Fig 12–39.—Three types of intradentinal retentive features: (**left to right**) facial and lingual U-form slots, 4 cylindrical channels, and a post and countersink. (Courtesy of Tjan AHL, Dunn JR, Lee JK-Y: *Quintessence Int* 24:211–217, 1993.)

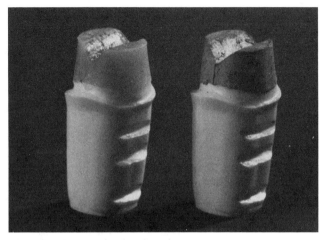

Fig 12–40.—Finished cores: (**left**) composite resin and (**right**) amalgam. (Courtesy of Tjan AHL, Dunn JR, Lee JK-Y: *Quintessence Int* 24:211–217, 1993.)

resistance to fracture than do amalgam cores with any of the retentive features.

▶ Many means are available to retain core materials in the tooth. Self-threading pins work quite well to retain either amalgam or resin cores, but the pins

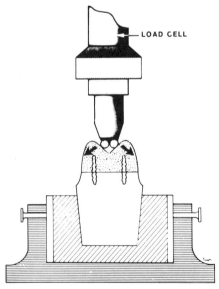

Fig 12–41.—Schematic setup used for fracture testing. The load is applied by means of 2 small cylinders, which yield combined stresses in axial and nonaxial directions, but predominantly nonaxial. (Courtesy of Tjan AHL, Dunn JR, Lee JK-Y: *Quintessence Int* 24:211–217, 1993.)

Summary of Results of Duncan's Tests		
Core material	Retentive feature	Mean (SD)
Amalgam*	Pins	84.3 (12.6)
	Post and countersink	74.6 (10.5)
	Channels	64.6 (9.8)
	Slots	62.7 (8.1)
Composite resin	Pins	149.8 (26.6)
	Post and countersink	121.6 (24.7)
	Channels	112.8 (22.7)
	Slots	127.2 (31.5)

Note: Vertical lines connect means that are not significantly different.
* Analysis of variance indicated a highly significant difference between amalgam and composite resin ($P < .0001$).
(Courtesy of Tjan AHL, Dunn JR, Lee JK-Y: *Quintessence Int* 24:211–217, 1993.)

can fracture the tooth or penetrate into the pulp, and pins do weaken the core material. These disadvantages make it important to have other available means of retaining a core. Composite resin can be easily placed and finished in one appointment, so it offers some advantage. This study indicates that a composite resin core requires greater force for fracture than does an amalgam core. Intradentinal retentive features produce adequate strength, but they do not offer the retention and resistance of the self-threading pins. If intradentinal retentive features are selected for retention of an amalgam core instead of pins, it would be good to select a post-countersink that offers strength comparable to self-threading pins.—T.G. Berry, D.D.S., M.A.

A Seven-and-a-Half-Year Survival Study of Resin-Bonded Bridges
Creugers NHJ, Käyser AF, Van't Hof MA (Univ of Nijmegen, The Netherlands)
J Dent Res 71:1822–1825, 1992   105-94-12-29

Purpose.—Studies of the efficacy of resin-bonded bridges (RBB) have shown great variability in survival, although 1 recent meta-analysis calculated an overall 4-year survival of 74%. Prospective clinical studies are still needed for evaluation of this restorative technique. In a 7.5-year follow-up study, the survival of RBBs placed under controlled clinical conditions was assessed, and the possible relationships between survival and retention type, cementation material, and patient-related variables were assessed.

Methods.—The study included 203 RBBs placed in 183 patients. There were 92 perforated bridges (P-bridges) and 111 electrolytically

TABLE 1.—Survival Rates, Conditional Relative Risk Values, Confidence
Intervals, and P Values of the Compared Resin-Bonded Bridges

Comparison[*]	7.5-year Survivals(%)	CRR Value	95% C.I	p-Value
Ant. - Post.	75 - 44	2.8	1.6 - 4.8	0.0002
P/Si - P/Cl	61 - 60	1.3	0.6 - 2.9	0.50
E/Cl - P/Cl	89 - 60	2.9	1.4 - 6.0	0.004
E/Cl - E/Pa	89 - 70	1.4	0.5 - 4.1	0.50
E/Cl - E/Co	89 - 60	3.1	1.3 - 7.2	0.01
E/Pa - E/Co	70 - 60	2.2	0.8 - 6.3	0.15

[*] *Abbreviations: Ant.,* anterior; *Post.,* posterior; *P,* perforated resin-bonded bridge; *E,* etched
resin-bonded bridge; *Cl,* Clearfil F; *Si,* Silar; *Pa,* Panavia EX; *Co,* Conclude.
(Courtesy of Creugers NHJ, Käyser AF, Van't Hof MA: *J Dent Res* 71:1822–1825, 1992.)

TABLE 2.—List of Co-Variables and Significance of Tested
Effects on Survival Rates

Co-variable	Significance
Etiology of open space	N.S.
Number of teeth replaced	N.S.
Occlusion on pontic	N.S.
Maxilla/mandible	interaction [*]
Mobility	N.S.
Initial occlusion	N.S.
Occlusion on retention wings	N.S.
Restorations in abument teeth	N.S.
Anterior spatial relation	0.03 [†]

[*] Interaction with anterior/posterior location.
[†] 'Deep bite' vs. 'normal'.
(Courtesy of Creugers NHJ, Käyser AF, Van't Hof MA: *J Dent Res* 71:1822–1825,
1992.)

etched NP2 alloy bridges (E-bridges). The bridges were cemented with Clearfil F, Panavia Ex, Silar, or Conclude. Two abutment teeth were used in all cases. Ninety-two percent of patients were examined at the 7.5-year recall.

Results.—Survival was 75% for anterior RBBs and 44% for posterior RBBs. E-bridges had a survival rate of 78%, significantly better than the 63% rate for P-bridges. The most retentive combination was an E-bridge cemented with Clearfil F, which had an anterior and posterior survival of 89% (Table 1). Significant interactions were seen between the variables of anterior spatial relation and maxilla mandible, with maxillary anterior RBBs being significantly less retentive than mandibular RBBs (Table 2).

Conclusion.—Significant relationships between certain variables and the survival of RBBs were documented. Survival is much better for anterior vs. posterior location of the RBB, and a conservative approach using minimal tooth preparation can be successful in anterior bridges. Other than location, however, no clear clinical criteria were found by which to identify the "high-risk" patient or to clarify the role of patient selection.

▶ The RBB is a conservative means of replacing teeth, but there exists the question of how well it will function over time. There have been numerous reports of bridges becoming debonded from the abutment teeth. This study reports that the survival rates depend on several factors, including the area of the mouth and the material used to lute it to the abutment. Anterior RBBs last longer than do posterior ones, and mandibular RBBs last longer than do the maxillary ones. This is likely the result of not only the amount of force, but also the direction the occluding force is directed. The overall success rate is good enough, however, that the RBB provides long-term successful replacement and restoration of teeth if the patient, location of area in the mouth, and luting agent are carefully selected.—T.G. Berry, D.D.S., M.A.

Masticatory Function in Patients With Extensive Fixed Cantilever Prostheses

Carlson BR, Carlsson GE, Helkimo E, Yontchev E (Univ of Göteborg, Sweden)
J Prosthet Dent 68:918–923, 1992   105-94-12–30

Background.—The use of extensive fixed partial dentures (FPDs), especially those with cantilevered extensions, has been controversial, and the detailed function of these prostheses needed to be studied. Oral function was monitored by using established methods in a group of patients treated with extensive cantilevered FPDs that included only 2 abutments.

Methods.—Eleven patients with complete maxillary dentures and 12-unit fixed partial dentures including the mandibular canines were evaluated before and during prosthodontic treatment. The last evaluation was 30 months after treatment.

Findings.—All patients said their masticatory function had been improved substantially. There were no symptoms of dysfunction in the masticatory system. Masticatory efficiency improved after prosthodontic treatment, which reduced both the number of cycles before the initial swallow and the total number of strokes, including time for completed mastication. Prosthodontic treatment was also associated with increased occlusal force. Individual variations were high for all occasions and force levels, but the forces recorded on the extensions of the cantilever were comparable to those on the canine regions.

Conclusion.—Patient reports of improved mastication after treatment were verified by functional tests. The increase in occlusal force after treatment was minimal. The functional improvements resulting from this prosthodontic treatment were consistent with previous findings.

▶ The choice of treatment for patients requiring extensive replacement and restoration of teeth with distal extension always raises questions. The treatment could include leaving the distal area edentulous; placing a distal extension removable partial denture, a fixed partial denture with a cantilevered extension(s); or placing implants to serve as abutments. Although implants are establishing an excellent record of success as their use becomes routine, not every situation allows placement of an implant and not all patients tolerate a removable partial denture. This study is reassuring because it demonstrates that the cantilevered fixed partial denture improves the patient's chewing efficiency without destruction of periodontal support. The cantilevered extension can be of real benefit to patients if carefully prescribed and then carefully fabricated and placed. It is important to distribute the occlusal forces over several teeth to avoid overtaxing the supporting mechanism of a few teeth.—T.G. Berry, D.D.S., M.A.

"The Gingiva Is Red Around My Crowns": A Differential Diagnosis
Kois J (Tacoma, Wash)
Dent Economics 83:101–105, 1993   105-94-12-31

Objective.—There are widespread myths about the gingival response to restorative dentistry and the determination of cervical limitations of intracrevicular tooth preparation. Rather than attempting to follow unrealistic doctrines, the practitioner will be better served by developing a differential diagnosis of bacterial plaque accumulation, marginal integrity, contour, alloy sensitivity, and marginal location.

Bacterial Plaque.—Plaque can accumulate on crowns of various materials, increasing with surface roughness. Yet, in some patients, the initial tissue response of the provisional restoration is better than the long-term response of the final crowns (Fig 12–42). The answer to this question cannot be simply oral hygiene.

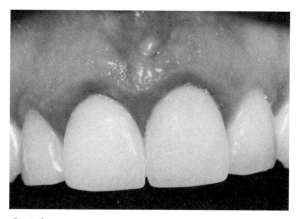

Fig 12–42.—Gingival response to plaque accumulation on maxillary central incisor crowns. (Courtesy of Kois J: *Dent Economics* 83:101–105, 1993.)

Marginal Integrity.—There is no clear relationship between the degree of marginal opening and periodontal disease. Patient-resistance factors appear to play a more important role than the mechanical aspects of margin design (Fig 12–43).

Contour.—The relationship between coronal contour and gingival form is confusing because of the difficulty in distinguishing the effect of margin location commensurate with coronal alteration. The environment and relationships between the proximal surfaces of the teeth appear to be more important to gingival health than the emergence profile. The only unacceptable contour is one that interferes with oral hygiene procedures or places pressure on the gingiva.

Alloy Sensitivity.—Although alloy sensitivity can occur, it is very rare. In most cases, alloy has nothing to do with gingival response problems.

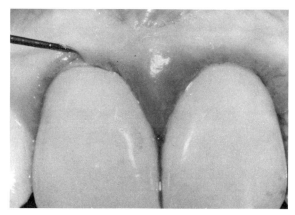

Fig 12–43.—Crowns with acceptable contours. (Courtesy of Kois J: *Dent Economics* 83:101–105, 1993.)

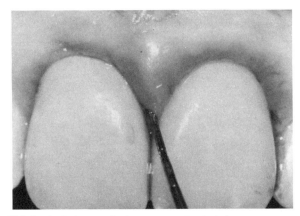

Fig 12–44.—Violation in the interproximal area creates the gingival response seen on the facial aspect of the crowns. (Courtesy of Kois J: *Dent Economics* 83:101-105, 1993.)

Margin Location.—Crown margin has important effects on plaque and periodontal health, especially the relation between the gingival attachment and margin location. In restorations, the dentist can easily go past the base of the sulcus without recognizing the cervical limitations of intracrevicular tooth preparation. A gingival response on the facial aspect of a crown results from violation of the zone of biological width in the interproximal area (Figs 12-44 and 12-45). The restoration must not encroach on the attachment, approximately 2.5 mm from the bone (Fig 12-46). When this problem is addressed, the gingival reaction resolves (Figs 12-47 and 12-48).

Clinical Application.—The osseous scallop, which follows the cementoenamel junction, is greatest for the anterior teeth and flattens toward the posterior (Fig 12-49). Biological width follows the scallop as well

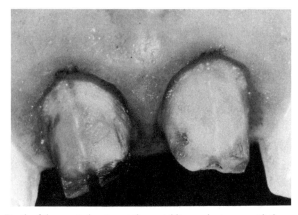

Fig 12–45.—Depth of the margin location at the mesial line angles is seen with the crowns removed. (Courtesy of Kois J: *Dent Economics* 83:101-105, 1993.)

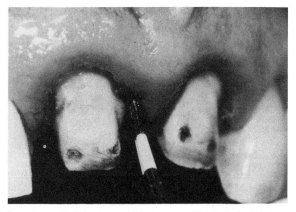

Fig 12–46.—Surgery was needed to reestablish the zone of biological width interproximally only. Restoration must not encroach on the attachment approximately 2.5 mm from the bone. (Courtesy of Kois J: *Dent Economics* 83:101–105, 1993.)

(Fig 12-50). Packed retraction cord can play an important role in preventing inadvertent excessive apical preparation (Fig 12-51). Generally, in the restoration of anterior teeth, margins should be developed at the base of the sulcus, then follow the normal scallop of the sulcus base (Fig 12-52). A horizontal margin can be avoided by the use of a round- rather than a flat-ended diamond bur, even for shoulder-type preparations (Fig 12-53).

Discussion.—Margin location relative to the attachment fibers is the most important biological factor in the differential diagnosis of a gingival response to restorative dentistry. Encroachment on these fibers should be checked for feeling the tooth structure beyond the margins without resulting discomfort for the patient. The cervical interproximal aspect,

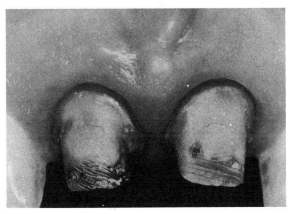

Fig 12–47.—Tissue returns to health after surgery. (Courtesy of Kois J: *Dent Economics* 83:101–105, 1993.)

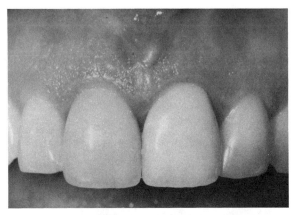

Fig 12–48.—Final crowns 2 years later. (Courtesy of Kois J: *Dent Economics* 83:101–105, 1993.)

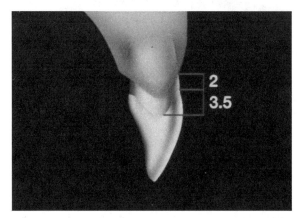

Fig 12–49.—The osseous scallop, which is greatest for the anterior teeth and flattens toward the posterior. (Courtesy of Kois J: *Dent Economics* 83:101–105, 1993.)

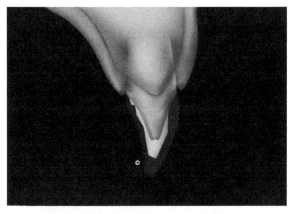

Fig 12–50.—The biological width follows the scallop. (Courtesy of Kois J: *Dent Economics* 83:101–105, 1993.)

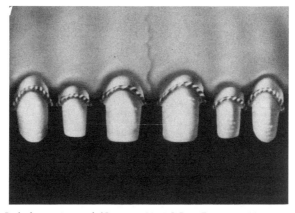

Fig 12-51.—Packed retraction cord. (Courtesy of Kois J: *Dent Economics* 83:101-105, 1993.)

the most difficult to control, accounts for most of the gingival response problems.

▶ No restoration, whether placed primarily for patient comfort, function, or esthetic reasons, can be considered successful if the soft tissue and underlying bony tissue are not healthy. Certainly, the beauty of any anterior restoration is marred by an inflamed gingiva. The author lists several factors that must be controlled to achieve the desired results. The most important factor is the placement of the restoration margins. If the zone of biological width is not well protected by placement of the finish lines in a position definitely incisal/occlusal to the zone, then inflammation will persist. Careful planning of the preparation design is critical to ensure good tissue health. The desire to achieve maximum esthetic results by locating the margins subgingivally can actually create esthetic problems as a result of chronic gingival inflammation.

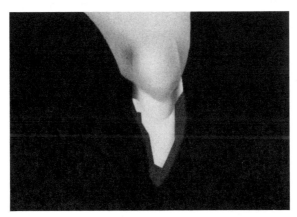

Fig 12-52.—Illustration of restoration of anterior teeth showing margins developed at the base of the sulcus, after which the normal scallop of the base of the sulcus is followed. (Courtesy of Kois J: *Dent Economics* 83:101-105, 1993.)

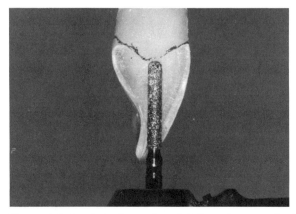

Fig 12–53.—Change of the bur design from a flat-ended diamond to a round-ended diamond is recommended, even for shoulder-type preparations. (Courtesy of Kois J: *Dent Economics* 83:101–105, 1993.)

When the situation dictates location of the preparation finish lines near or in the zone, some relatively minor surgery may prevent long-term periodontal problems.—T.G. Berry, D.D.S., M.A.

Influence of Finish-Line Geometry on the Fit of Crowns
Syu J-Z, Byrne G, Laub LW, Land MF (Natl Taiwan Univ Hosp, Taipei; Loyola Univ, Maywood, Ill)
Int J Prosthodont 6:25–30, 1993   105-94-12–32

Objective.—Many studies have examined factors that influence the seating and fit of full cast crown preparations, including the influence of cementation variables. However, the internal adaptation of the castings before cementation has not previously been examined. The potential influence of 3 commonly used margin designs on internal casting adaptation was investigated.

Methods.—By using standard procedures, 3 Ivorine maxillary central incisors were prepared for metallic ceramic crowns and given different labial finish lines: a shoulder, a shoulder-bevel, and a chamfer. Each tooth preparation was duplicated, and 10 dies for each finish line were obtained. The crowns were seated on their corresponding dies, embedded in epoxy without cementation, and sectioned. Axial and marginal gap widths of the castings were measured at predetermined sites. Two faciolingual sections were made 1 mm on either side of the midline (Fig 12-54).

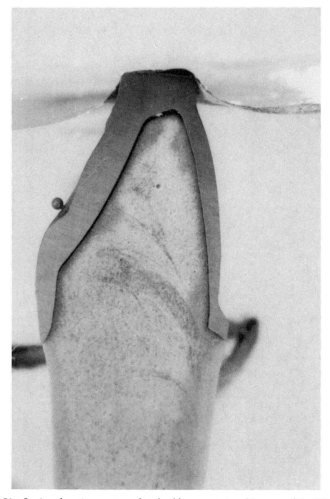

Fig 12–54.—Sectioned casting on stone die: shoulder preparation. (Courtesy of Syu J-Z, Byrne G, Laub LW, et al: *Int J Prosthodont* 6:25–30, 1993.)

Results.—There were no significant differences for marginal and axial gaps among the 3 types of finish lines. Castings with well-fitting margins showed axial wall spaces of between 15 and 33 μm but negligible horizontal marginal metal overhangs (Fig 12–55).

Conclusion.—The use of different finish-line designs does not influence casting accuracy.

▶ Despite the long-waged arguments and much research, there still exists controversy as to the preparation finish line configuration that provides the best marginal adaptation and, less directly, the best adaptation to the axial

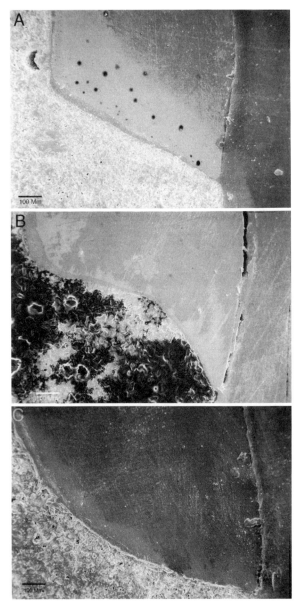

Fig 12–55.—Facial sites for castings on their respective dies. Scanning electron micrographs. Original magnification, ×100. **A,** shoulder; **B,** shoulder-bevel; **C,** chamfer. (Courtesy of Syu J-Z, Byrne G, Laub LW, et al: *Int J Prosthodont* 6:25–30, 1993.)

walls of the preparation. Apparently, it does not make much difference as to which type of finish line is chosen. All of the factors other than variation in the finish-line type in this in vitro study were well controlled, which is not so easy to do in vivo. Clinically, it is more difficult to ensure that adaptation of the walls is close, without fitting so tightly in some area(s) that complete seating of the crown cannot be accomplished. In this study, no die spacer was used, so the fit of the castings was controlled entirely by the waxing process and by careful investment and burnout procedures. It is possible to conclude that the close attention and precise control of each step was more important to the fit of the casting than was the marginal finish line chosen.—T.G. Berry, D.D.S., M.A.

Effect of Adhesive Luting Agents on the Marginal Seating of Cast Restorations
White SN, Kipnis V (Univ of Southern California, Los Angeles)
J Prosthet Dent 69:28–31, 1993   105-94-12–33

Background.—Zinc phosphate cement has traditionally been the luting agent of choice for cementing castings. Several new classes of adhesive luting agents (ALA) have been introduced, and some have markedly better properties than zinc phosphate cement. The effect of the new adhesive luting agents on the marginal seating of cast restorations was investigated.

Methods.—Standardized preparations were performed on newly extracted human premolars. Impressions were made, and complete metal veneer crowns were cast using a base metal alloy. The castings were then placed on their respective teeth and the degree of marginal opening was noted. The samples were then assigned to 1 of 5 groups: glass ionomer cement (GI), polycarboxylate cement (PC), microfilled BIS-GMA composite resin with NPG-GMA/PMDM dentinal bonding agent (GMA + NPG), microfilled BIS-GMA/phosphate ester composite resin (GMA/PE), or zinc phosphate cement (ZP). Marginal openings were measured again after castings were cemented.

Findings.—Table 1 and Fig 12–56 display the means and standard deviations of the marginal openings for each ALA group before and after cementation. Tukey's multiple comparisons test (Table 2) showed that the least marginal openings were recorded in groups with GI, ZP, and PC luting agents. The differences between these 3 groups were not significant. The greatest marginal openings were observed with GMA/PE and GMA + NPG luting agents.

Conclusion.—Significant differences in marginal seating resulted from various luting agents used to cement routine castings to human teeth.

TABLE 1.—Marginal Openings Before and After Cementation

Group	Precementation			Postcementation		
	Mean	SE	RCV	Mean	SE	RCV
GI	57.2	6.0	10.4	82.8	12.6	15.2
ZP	58.0	12.8	22.0	111.0	17.2	15.5
PC	69.5	11.6	16.6	141.6	24.2	17.1
GMA/PE	35.1	7.2	20.6	263.0	52.4	19.9
GMA + NPG	66.5	12.0	17.9	333.1	45.9	13.8

Note: Means and standard errors (SE) in micrometers and relative coefficients of variation (RCV) in percent.
(Courtesy of White SN, Kipnis V: J Prosthet Dent 69:28–31, 1993.)

The resin cements tested resulted in greater marginal openings than did the other luting agents.

▶ The introduction of adhesive luting agents offers some major advantages over the commonly used zinc phosphate cement. Zinc phosphate cement is

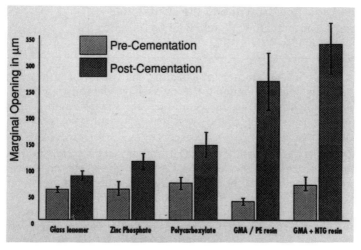

Fig 12–56.—Effect of adhesive luting agents on marginal seating of cast restorations. (Courtesy of White SN, Kipnis V: *J Prosthet Dent* 69:28–31, 1993.)

not adhesive and it is soluble, whereas the adhesive luting agents do not present a real problem with solubility. The adhesive luting agents are a bit more technique-sensitive. Although the use of the adhesive agents did result in a greater marginal opening in this study, other investigators have not noted as great a marginal discrepancy with the use of the resin luting agents. Manufacturers are decreasing the film thickness of these agents, so there is real promise of a superior material in the near future. At the present time, use of these materials requires adherence to manufacturer's directions and the use of die spacers and, perhaps, venting of the crown to accommodate the film thickness of this material.—T.G. Berry, D.D.S., M.A.

TABLE 2.—Multiple Comparisons Test of
ALA Groups

ALA group	Mean marginal opening (μm)
GI	82.8
ZP	111.0
PC	141.6
GMA/PE	263.0
GMA + NPG	333.1

Note: ALA groups connected by vertical lines are not statistically different.
(Courtesy of White SN, Kipnis V: *J Prosthet Dent* 69:28–31, 1993.)

Microleakage: Full Crowns and the Dental Pulp
Goldman M, Laosonthorn P, White RR (Tufts Univ, Boston)
J Endodont 18:473–475, 1992   105-94-12–34

Objective.—Several studies investigating the causes of pulp inflammation and pulp necrosis under full crowns have demonstrated the presence of microleakage. Certain techniques of crown margin preparation were investigated to determine whether they contribute to the occurrence of microleakage.

Methods.—Thirty freshly extracted molar teeth were mounted in acrylic resin blocks and divided into 3 groups of 10. The crown margins were prepared with a full shoulder in 10 teeth, with a chamfer in another 10 teeth, and with a shoulder and bevel in the remaining 10 teeth. The height of the preparations, measured from gingival shoulder to occlusal plane, was standardized at 4.5 mm. All crowns were cemented with zinc

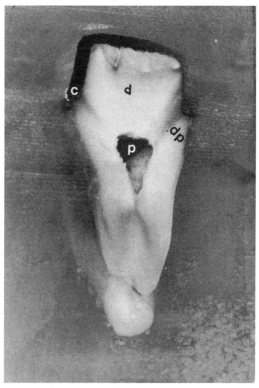

Fig 12–57.—*Abbreviations: c,* crown; *d,* dentin; *p,* pulp; *dp,* dye penetration. Typical section examined under dissecting microscope. Note the penetration of the dye along the path of the dentinal tubules directly into the pulp (original magnification, ×10). (Courtesy of Goldman M, Laosonthorn P, White RR: *J Endodont* 18:473–475, 1992.)

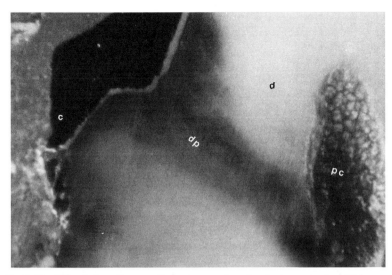

Fig 12–58.—*Abbreviations:* C, crown; D, dentin; *pc,* pulp cavity; *dp,* dye penetration. Higher magnification of another specimen. Note the penetration of the dye into the pulp cavity (original magnification, ×40). (Courtesy of Goldman M, Laosonthorn P, White RR: *J Endodont* 18:473–475, 1992.)

phosphate cement. After storage for 7 days in 100% humidity, the teeth were thermocycled in a water bath containing crystal violet dye, encased in clear acrylic resin, and sliced into 3 sections to test for microleakage.

Results.—All crowns showed microleakage that followed the dentinal tubules directly into the pulp chamber (Figs 12-57 and 12-58). The use of different crown margin preparations did not prevent the microleakage.

Conclusion.—Microleakage around the margins of full crowns can be an important cause of pulp inflammation and pulp necrosis.

▶ In the past, pulpitis and necrosis after cementation were thought to be the result of preparation trauma, dehydration, or a reaction to the initial low pH of zinc phosphate cement. Research has shown that the real culprit is often microleakage. This study indicates that no matter what type of finish lines were prepared, the crowns cemented with zinc phosphate cement still exhibited significant microleakage. This would seem to offer strong support for the use of a glass-ionomer or resin luting agent because of its adherence to the tooth, structure, and relative insolubility in oral fluids. The long-term marginal seal is likely to be better than that of zinc phosphate cement. Allowances for the greater film thickness of resin luting agents need to be made, however.—T.G. Berry, D.D.S., M.A.

Adhesive Cements and Cementation

White SN (Univ of Southern California, Los Angeles)
J Calif Dent Assoc 21(6):30–37, 1993   105-94-12–35

Introduction.—In patients with fixed prostheses, luting cements may be the weak link between the prosthesis and the supporting tooth structures. The physical properties of luting cements are poor compared with bulk restorative filling materials, but they must meet additional requirements such as low film thickness. The wide range of applications for luting cements prohibits recommendations of a single material in all clinical situations. The necessary qualities of luting agents and the available agents and cementation procedures were reviewed.

Properties.—Luting cements need compressive and tensile strength, an elastic modulus matching that of the tooth structure, resistance to plastic deformation, solubility and stability in water, low film thickness, and adequate working time. Obviously, no one material can meet all of these properties ideally. Other important considerations include marginal integrity, seating, and tilting; avoidance of microleakage; proper mixing and application to avoid problems with pH and sensitivity; translucency; adhesion and retention; and fluoride release.

Available Materials.—Available luting agents include zinc phosphate cements, polycarboxylate cements, glass ionomer cements, composite resin, composite resin-glass ionomer hybrid, and hydroxyapatite. The specific properties of the various materials make them best for different situations (table).

Conclusion.—Significant clinical improvements are possible using modern adhesive cements, glass ionomer-composite resin hybrids, and adhesive composite resins or composite resins with dentinal bonding agents. However, these materials are technically more difficult to use than zinc phosphate cements.

▶ Dentistry has long sought the ideal luting agent, which would be easy to use, insoluble, flow easily with a favorable film thickness, and have true adhesion to the tooth and restoration. Zinc phosphate cement has long been the most popular luting agent, although it is soluble, nonadhesive, and highly acidic in its early stages. Recent advances in resin and glass-ionomer cements have made them much more promising. They possess excellent strength, are relatively insoluble, and have the great advantage of adhering to both the restoration and to the tooth. The only definite disadvantages are that they are more technique-sensitive, making them more difficult to use with multiple units, and they do not have a long history of clinical use to allow a prediction of long-term success. The film thickness for the resin cements is now somewhat greater than desirable.

Because of the adhesive qualities, strength, and lower solubility they offer, adhesive luting agents are likely to be the agent of choice in most situations in the near future.—T.G. Berry, D.D.S., M.A.

	Suggested Materials
Type III Gold	Glass ionomer
Porcelain Fused to Metal	Glass ionomer. Glass ionomer composite resin hybrid. Glass ionomer composite resin hybrid with a dentin-bonding agent.
Porcelain Labial Margin	Glass ionomer. Glass ionomer composite resin hybrid. Glass ionomer composite resin hybrid with a dentin-bonding agent.
Long Span/Mobile Abutments	Glass ionomer composite resin hybrid with a dentin-bonding agent. Adhesive filled composite resin. Filled Composite resin with a dentin-bonding agent.
Post Cores	Glass ionomer. Glass ionomer composite resin hybrid. Glass ionomer composite resin hybrid with a dentin-bonding agent. Adhesive filled composite resin. Filled composite resin with a dentin-bonding agent.

(continued)

Table (*continued*)

All Ceramic	Adhesive filled composite resin.
	Filled composite resin with a dentin-bonding agent.
	Dual-cured composite resin, with a dentin-bonding agent.
Maryland Bridge	Adhesive filled composite resin.
Poor Environmental Control	Zinc phosphate.
Poor Retention or Resistance Form	Glass ionomer composite resin hybrid with a dentin-bonding agent.
	Adhesive filled composite resin.
	Filled composite resin with a dentin-bonding agent.

(Courtesy of White SN: *Can Dent Assoc J* 21:30–37, 1993.)

Comparisons of Tactile Thresholds Between Implant-Supported Fixed Partial Dentures and Removable Partial Dentures

Garrett NR, Hasse AL, Kapur KK (West Los Angeles Med Ctr, Calif; Dept of Veteran Affairs Med Ctr, Palo Alto, Calif; Univ of California, Los Angeles)
Int J Prosthodont 5:515–522, 1992   105-94-12–36

Background.—Oral sensations play an important role in efficient masticatory function. In patients with Kennedy class I or II edentulous conditions, placement of a removable or fixed partial denture (RPD or FPD) supported by a blade implant only partially restores masticatory efficiency. There is a lack of information on how tactile sensitivity, masticatory performance, and oral perception are affected by splinting teeth and placing RPDs and FPDs.

Methods.—The tactile sensitivity of splinted abutment and denture teeth of 32 patients with Kennedy class I or II edentulous conditions were examined. Tactile thresholds were ascertained by the application of nylon fibers of various diameters, which exerted forces of .07 to 215.0 g.

Results.—Neither group showed any appreciable differences between the tactile thresholds of the natural abutment teeth and artificial teeth. Stimulus detection by the splinted abutment teeth required an occlusal load up to 5.8 times higher than that needed for the comparable nonsplinted teeth. Thresholds increased an additional 54% with the FPD and by more than 100% with the RPD. On a patient questionnaire, both groups were largely satisfied with the masticatory function of their den-

TABLE 1.—Comparison (%) of RPD and FPD With Most Favorable Response to Patient Satisfaction Questionnaire

Item	RPD (%)	FPD (%)	Chi-square comparison P value
1. Eat with denture mostly	81.3	100.0	0.19
2. Experience no discomfort	100.0	87.5	0.14
3. Can chew everything	93.8	100.0	0.31
4. Enjoy eating very much	75.0	100.0	0.10
5. Does not restrict food choices	100.0	100.0	1.00
6. Food particles never or sometimes get under dentures	75.0	100.0	0.03*
7. No difference in food taste	81.3	100.0	0.07
8. Very satisfied with speech	87.5	100.0	0.14
9. Experience no odor	100.0	100.0	1.00
10. Easy to clean	100.0	68.8	0.02*
11. Very satisfied with cleanliness	100.0	93.8	0.31
12. Feel very secure	93.8	100.0	0.31
13. Marked improvement in social life	6.3	25.0	0.31
14. Completely satisfied	93.8	100.0	0.31
15. Would select the same treatment	81.3	100.0	0.19

* $P < .05$.

(Courtesy of Garrett NR, Hasse AL, Kapur KK: *Int J Prothodont* 5:515–522, 1992.)

TABLE 2.—Correlation Between Tactile Thresholds and Masticatory Performance Scores With Peanuts and Carrots When Chewing on the Side of the Tactile Tests

Comparison	Total sample		RPD		FPD	
	r	P	r	P	r	P
Abutment occlusal threshold						
vs Masticatory performance—Peanuts	0.43	0.02*	0.39	0.15	0.46	0.08
vs Masticatory performance—Carrots	0.46	0.01**	0.41	0.13	0.50	0.05
Abutment facial threshold						
vs Masticatory performance—Peanuts	0.15	0.43	0.17	0.52	0.10	0.72
vs Masticatory performance—Carrots	0.23	0.21	0.20	0.45	0.15	0.57
Artificial molar occlusal threshold						
vs Masticatory performance—Peanuts	0.37	0.04*	0.35	0.18	0.40	0.12
vs Masticatory performance—Carrots	0.42	0.02*	0.33	0.22	0.51	0.04*
Artificial molar facial threshold						
vs Masticatory performance—Peanuts	0.25	0.17	0.42	0.10	0.06	0.83
vs Masticatory Performance—Carrots	0.23	0.20	0.32	0.23	−0.02	0.95

* $P < .05$.
** $P < .01$.
(Courtesy of Garrett NR, Hasse AL, Kapur KK: *Int J Prothodont* 5:515–522, 1992.)

tures (Table 1). Tactile thresholds showed a moderately positive correlation with masticatory performance (Table 2).

Conclusion.—Splinting of teeth appears to increase their tactile thresholds, increasing the load needed to perceive the stimulus by at least 5 times. Because of cross-arch splinting and mucosal support, load distribution is better with the RPD. The observed reduction in tactile perception does not appear to cause the incomplete restoration of masticatory function in patients with RPDs or FPDs.

▶ The old debate over whether a fixed or a removable partial denture will best serve a patient must now include the effect that an implant or several implant teeth will have on the function of either partial denture. This study showed there was an increased tactile threshold on the implants. This would be expected because there is distribution of the occlusal load over the remaining teeth or basal seat area of the denture. It is good that the implant abutments apparently have about the same tactile sensitivity and load receiving capacity as do the other teeth that are splinted together. This allows the patient to more effectively control the biting strokes. Although there is some reduction in tactile sensitivity because of the distribution of the load over a wider areas (as seen with a removable partial denture with cross-arch splinting), this does not really affect the patient's ability to masticate.—T.G. Berry, D.D.S., M.A.

Phenytoin Hyperplasia Occurring Under Complete Dentures: A Clinical Report

McCord JF, Sloan P, Quayle AA, Hussey DJ (Univ Dental Hosp, Manchester, England; The Queens Univ, Belfast, Northern Ireland)

J Prosthet Dent 68:569–572, 1992   105-94-12–37

Background.—Phenytoin is an antiepileptic drug that has been widely used since the 1930s. Its adverse effects include gingival hyperplasia. The following cases illustrate phenytoin-induced hyperplasia in edentulous patients.

Case 1.—Man, 73, had been edentulous for 20 years. On presentation, the maxillary alveolar ridge was flabby anteriorly. In 1985, the patient had been prescribed phenytoin, 300 mg daily, for "blackouts." In 1989, he had sought dental care for denture replacement, and during that visit, multiple nodular hyperplasia was noted on the palate. Histologic sections of the biopsy specimen suggested phenytoin-induced hyperplasia. Few candidal hyphae were evident in and on the mucosa. Treatment was nonsurgical because of the patient's age. After tissue conditioning, replacement complete dentures were provided through selective impression techniques.

Case 2.—Man, 45, was referred for replacement dentures. He had been edentulous for 5 years. In 1988, he had a cerebrovascular incident and was prescribed phenytoin, 150 mg daily. His maxillary ridges and palate were beefy red, and the tuberosities were covered with hyperplastic tissue. No hyperplasia had been present when the initial dentures were provided. Treatment consisted of leaving the dentures out for 1 week before a tissue conditioner was applied to the denture, then surgically removing the hyperplasia. Histologic study of the biopsy specimen suggested phenytoin-related hyperplasia. Replacement dentures were provided after healing was complete.

Conclusion.—Varying degrees of gingival hyperplasia reportedly occur in about 66% of patients receiving phenytoin. Bacterial plaque is thought to be an essential etiologic factor in this condition. In the cases described, the dentures were ill-fitting and plaque was noted, suggesting that plaque was a stimulus in these patients.

▶ It is well documented that dentulous patients medicated with phenytoin (Dilantin) have gingival hyperplasia develop. The effects are not as well known for patients who wear dentures. These case histories demonstrate that the effect is very similar. Hyperplasia is definitely provoked by phenytoin. This hyperplasia is recognized as a problem for the denture wearer, but its cause my not be so readily determined. A thorough health history and, when indicated, a biopsy will greatly aid in the diagnosis of the precipitating agent. The patient must be educated to recognize that ill-fitting dentures and the accumulation of plaque inside the dentures appear to be contributing factors. The patient population for most dental offices consists of an ever-increasing percentage of people who are taking some medication. Recognition of the relationship of these drugs to tissue health is critical to the dentist to provide the best care for the patients.—T.G. Berry, D.D.S., M.A.

The Effect of Reducing the Number of Clasps on Removable Partial Denture Retention
Ahmad I, Sherriff M, Waters NE (UMDS-Guy's Campus, London)
J Prosthet Dent 68:928–933, 1992   105-94-12-38

Background.—Many disadvantages are associated with the use of clasps for removable partial denture (RPD) retention. Clasps can abrade tooth surfaces and collect plaque, and they may fail because of breakage or distortion. Furthermore, clasps exert lateral force on abutment teeth, which can cause periodontium damage. The use of guide planes could provide added frictional resistance, thereby contributing to RPD retention. The retention of an RPD was examined when the number of clasps was reduced, and it was determined what frictional resistance, if any, was provided by guide planes. In addition, the direction and position of the dislodging force was assessed.

Methods.—Ten nominally identical chrome-cobalt RPD castings, with standardized bilateral molar and premolar casts engaging .25 mm undercuts, and 10 castings, with clasps engaging .50 mm undercuts were constructed to evaluate retention to a master model (Fig 12–59). Retention was measured using an Instron universal testing machine. Two frameworks groups were created. Each comprised 5 frameworks with .25 undercuts and 5 with .50 undercuts. Five vertical pull tests were conducted, with the position and direction of the dislodging force kept constant in the framework's center. Retention measurements were recorded with all 4 clasps in place and repeated after removing each clasp. Each group

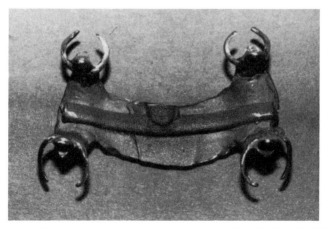

Fig 12–59.—Test framework with all clasps present. (Courtesy of Ahmad I, Sherriff M, Waters NE: *J Prosthet Dent* 68:928–933, 1992.)

Centre

Left

Right

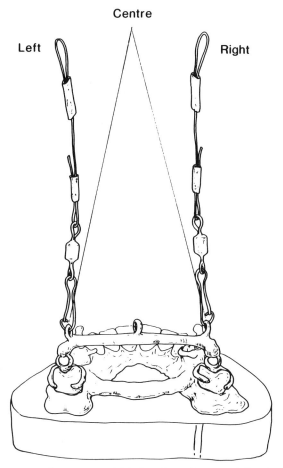

Fig 12–60.—Diagram to show position of dislodging force. (Courtesy of Ahmad I, Sherriff M, Waters NE: *J Prosthet Dent* 68:928–933, 1992.)

was assigned a different order for clasp removal. Five additional RPD frameworks with casts engaging .25 undercuts were tested. In this series, the dislodging force was first in the center, then vertically above the right edentulous area, and, finally, vertically above the left edentulous area (Fig 12–60).

Results.—Significant differences between frameworks, number of clasps, and undercut depth were noted, although the order in which the clasps were removed was not statistically significant. The position of the dislodging force was also found to be statistically significant.

Conclusion.—The dislodging force was dependent on framework fit, undercut depth, number of clasps, and point of application.

▶ This study had a predictable result. One would expect that reducing the number of clasps on a partial denture would reduce the retention. It is interesting to note that some retention was achieved just from the guide planes. Even more retention is possible, perhaps, if a design using more guide planes per abutment were used. The secret of the retention of the framework depends directly on how well it fits. The fit depends on the finishing procedures that remove some metal from contacting surfaces. Increasing the undercuts to .5 mm would increase retention, but it could overtax the supporting structures of the abutment teeth. Increasing retention may be easiest to accomplish by improving the fit of the framework, especially the guiding planes.—T.G. Berry, D.D.S., M.A.

The Tooth-Removable Partial Denture Interface
Brudvik JS, Reimers D (Univ of Washington, Seattle)
J Prosthet Dent 68:924–927, 1992   105-94-12–39

Background.—Several factors can compromise the fit of chrome-based alloys used for removable partial dentures (RPDs). Loss of metal in the finishing of the framework has received the least attention in the literature. Because dentists seldom finish and polish a metal framework, they are generally unaware of the potential for uncontrolled loss of metal during the procedures. Therefore, the procedures and resultant metal loss were reviewed.

Methods and Findings—Four teeth were prepared, and the model was blocked out to keep wax below the height of contour during blockout. The model was duplicated in hydrocolloid, resulting in 5 refractory casts to which an analog RPD form was waxed. The forms were invested and cast in a partial denture alloy. The analogue form provided a long- and short-span edentulous region for assessment, with a total of 10 posterior spaces. Castings were related with individual resin forms to permit exact replacement for repeated measures; they were then calibrated. The castings were finished by standard methods and returned to their vernier caliper for measurement after each of 3 finishing stages: electropolishing, stoning, and rubber wheeling and final polishing. The mean values of metal lost in finishing for the 10 edentulous spaces were .041 mm after electropolishing, .024 mm after stoning, and .062 mm after rubber wheeling and polishing.

Conclusion.—A contact between the guiding plane surface of a prepared abutment tooth and the minor connector of the RPD casting may help in partial denture retention. Controlling laboratory procedures is essential to obtain this level of contact. There are many advantages to precision at the tooth-RPD interface.

▶ As Article 105-94-12–38 indicates, some limited retention of the removable partial denture framework can be obtained from the relationship of the framework to the guiding plane surfaces of the abutments. An even greater amount would be obtained if the framework were designed to fit additional guiding planes. If, however, the finishing process removes metal from the framework of more than .1 mm, the resistance to placement offered by the fit of the framework to the guiding planes and other surfaces is compromised. Good communication with the laboratory about control of the finishing procedures must occur if a truly precise fit is to occur.—T.G. Berry, D.D.S., M.A.

Reinforcement of Complete Denture Bases With Continuous High Performance Polyethylene Fibers

Ladizesky NH, Ho CF, Chow TW (Univ of Hong Kong)
J Prosthet Dent 68:934–939, 1992   105-94-12–40

Background.—Highly drawn linear polyethylene (HDLPE) fibers posses high tensile stiffness and strength. When oriented longitudinally, they provide composite resins with high tensile and compressive moduli. Flexural strength significantly exceeds that of unreinforced resin. During bending and impact, HDLPE fiber-reinforced composite resins do not

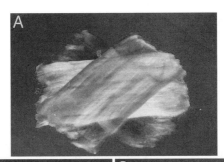
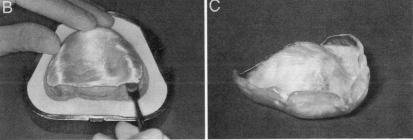

Fig 12–61.—**A**, set of "pre-pregs" ready for adaptation on duplicate cast. **B**, adaptation of pre-pregs to maxillary mold after being cut to correct shape. **C**, maxillary denture base reinforced with 4 layers of parallel fibers. Fiber content 26% by volume. (Courtesy of Ladizesky NH, Ho CF, Chow TW: *J Prosthet Dent* 68:934–939, 1992.)

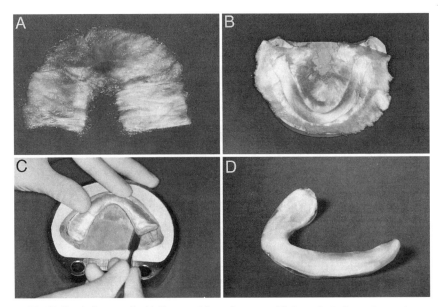

Fig 12–62.—A, "pre-preg" with fibers at right angles to mandibular arch. **B,** first and second pre-pregs adapted to duplicate cast, ready to receive third pre-preg. **C,** adaptation of pre-preg to mold after cutting to correct shape. **D,** mandibular base reinforced with pre-preg parallel fibers. Fiber content 39% by volume. (Courtesy of Ladizesky NH, Ho CF, Chow TW: *J Prosthet Dent* 68:934–939, 1992.)

exhibit propagation of cracks, and they maintain their coherence over many test cycles. Their fatigue performance, however, is uncertain.

Objective.—A protocol was developed for making HDLPE fiber-reinforced maxillary and mandibular bases. A high-fiber content was used without increasing prosthetic thickness. Both PMMA syrup and Trevalon C resin were used.

Techniques.—Maxillary bases are reinforced with 4 layers of parallel fibers by using a form of the preimpregnated "pre-preg" technique (Fig 12–61). For mandibular bases, 2 bundles of fibers are prepared and cut into 5 bundles. Adaptation of the pre-pregs to the duplicate cast and the mold is illustrated in Figure 12–62. A cross section of a mandibular base with fibers following the arch, sandwiched between fibers at right angles to the ridge, is shown in Figure 12–63.

Results.—These reinforced bases (Fig 12–64) should provide significantly improved clinical performance.

▶ The breakage of a denture represents a major functional and esthetic loss to a patient. Although the fractured denture can usually be repaired satisfactorily, the patient is without her or his denture for some time. Sometimes, alterations in the fit or the occlusion cause discomfort and additional trips to the dentist. The incorporation of fibers into the denture base for reinforcement offers a marked improvement in the strength of the base. These fibers

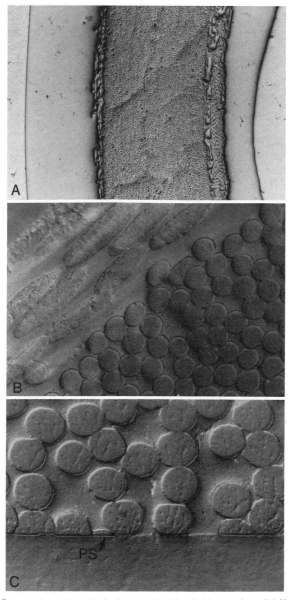

Fig 12–63.—Cross section of mandibular base reinforced with 3 layers of parallel fibers. **A,** 3 layers of fibers (original magnification, ×35). **B,** boundary betwen 2 layers of fibers (original magnification, ×400). **C,** cross section of mandibular base at region where fibers reach polished surface (PS) (original magnification, ×800). (Courtesy of Ladizesky NH, Ho CF, Chow TW: *J Prosthet Dent* 68:934-939, 1992.)

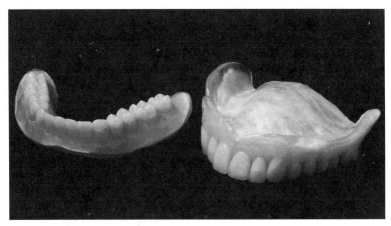

Fig 12–64.—Complete dentures with fiber-reinforced bases. (Courtesy of Ladizesky NH, Ho CF, Chow TW: *J Prosthet Dent* 68:934–939, 1992.)

do not affect the thickness of the base or simulation of oral tissues. This system offers a real advantage to denture wearers.—T.G. Berry, D.D.S., M.A.

Cephalometric Evaluation of the Changes in Patients Wearing Complete Dentures: A 20-Year Study

Douglass JB, Meader L, Kaplan A, Ellinger CW (Univ of Kentucky, Lexington)
J Prosthet Dent 69:270–275, 1993   105-94-12–41

Objective.—The findings at 20 years are now available from an ongoing longitudinal study of 64 complete denture wearers that was designed to monitor changes in the craniofacial complex. Initially, patients had a mean age of 53 years and had been edentulous for at least 1 year and for a mean time of 13.5 years. Twenty-four patients were evaluable after 20 years.

Methods.—Lateral cephalometric radiographs were acquired immediately after denture placement, annually for the first 5 years, and after 7, 10, 15, and 20 years. The same cephalostat was used throughout, and all films were exposed with the dentures in place and with the teeth in centric occlusion. Metallic implants had been placed in the denture acrylic resin to aid in the cephalometric analysis.

Observations.—The bony maxilla and alveolus remained relatively stable throughout the study period. The mandible rotated counterclockwise (when viewed in the right profile), and the chin moved anteriorly and superiorly. Resorption of the mandibular alveolus was documented. The anterior part of the maxillary denture moved slightly forward and upward, whereas the posterior portion remained relatively stable in the vertical dimension of occlusion. No significant differences were seen between patients with standard dentures and those whose dentures were made by a complex technique. There were no substantial gender-related differences.

▶ This rather unique study followed patients for 20 years after insertion to measure changes in the jaws and their relationships. The results were not particularly surprising as to bone loss and shifts in jaw relationships. Clinical observations would predict to some degree these results. The maxillary alveolus, with its much larger load-bearing area, showed much less resorption than did the mandibular ridge, which also shifted in an anterior and clockwise direction. It is interesting that there was no difference in the group wearing dentures made using more complex jaw relationship records and the group wearing dentures made without those records. Despite the concern of osteoporosis among female patients, there appeared to be no real difference between men and women.—T.G. Berry, D.D.S, M.A.

Attitudes to Identification of Dentures: The Patients' Perspective
Cunningham M, Hoad-Reddick G (Turner Dental School, Manchester, England)
Quintessence Int 24:267–270, 1993   105-94-12–42

Introduction.—Dental practitioners are increasingly accepting the value of adding identification to dentures, a practice that is frequent in nursing homes and on geriatric and psychiatric wards. Some have proposed that identifying marks be added to all dentures when they are manufactured, so they can readily be retrieved if mislaid. In addition, there are instances where it may be possible to identify the patient from the denture.

A Survey.—Only 2 of 63 denture wearers questioned (3.2%) had had their dentures marked, and more than 90% of the respondents had not heard about the possibility of this being done. After the marking process was explained, 85% of the group thought it would be useful for their dentures to bear an identifying mark.

Discussion.—It appears that dentists are not often making denture identification available to their patients. Cost is likely the chief objection. Most patients probably would be willing to bear the cost, but it would be best if this were included in the basic fee to allow laboratories to routinely place names on the dentures they make.

▶ Despite the obvious advantages of the patient being able to identify his or her own denture or of being able to identify an unconscious or dead person by marking the denture with identification, most dentures are not so marked. Such identification would be especially important in hospitals, nursing homes, and the military. This article lists several relatively easy means of identifying the denture that can be performed in the laboratory without undue costs. The survey, conducted in England, indicates that many patients are not informed by their dentists that such identification is possible. Such an easy procedure should be routinely done. The "graying" of our population will likely result in a greater number (though not necessarily a larger percentage of the population) of denture wearers, so such marking could be even more important in the future.—T.G. Berry, D.D.S., M.A.

Prevention, Infection Control, Biocompatibility

Effects of Chlorhexidine-Containing Gel and Varnish on Abutment Teeth in Patients With Overdentures
Keltjens HMAM, Creugers TJ, Schaeken MJM, Van Der Hoeven JS (Univ of Nijmegen, The Netherlands)
J Dent Res 71:1582–1586, 1992   105-94-12-43

Introduction.—Previous studies have shown that daily application of a 1% chlorhexidine gel to the notches of overdentures almost completely prevents caries formation in the abutment teeth. A single application of a 40% chlorhexidine varnish was compared to daily 1% chlorhexidine gel application as a means of preventing caries formation in abutment teeth.

Patients.—Thirty-one patients with a mean age of 62 years were randomly allocated to receive chlorhexidine varnish, placebo varnish, chlorhexidine gel, or placebo gel. All had been wearing overdentures for about 3 years. A single dose of 40% chlorhexidine varnish was applied to the abutment teeth by the investigator; a 1% chlorhexidine gel was applied daily for 7 days by the patients at home. Plaque samples from the abutment teeth were cultured at baseline and at regular intervals during an 8-week follow-up period.

Results.—A single application of 40% chlorhexidine varnish and daily application of a 1% chlorhexidine gel both significantly suppressed mutans streptococci (table). However, the beneficial effect of chlorhexidine on plaque formation was not long-lasting.

Conclusion.—Both methods of chlorhexidine application appear to be useful in preventing caries formation in overdenture abutments.

▶ Chlorhexidine has proved to be quite effective against organisms that are involved in the carious process, especially mutans streptococci. Because chlorhexidine demonstrates a strong affinity for hard structures of the mouth, it remains on the surface of those structures for some period of time no matter which form of application is used. By interrupting the metabolism of the organisms, it quickly decreases the colonies present. It is logical to apply the solution to abutment teeth to prevent caries. The denture itself should also be treated to prevent it from serving as a reservoir of organisms that would reinfect the abutment teeth.—T.G. Berry, D.D.S., M.A.

Number of Abutments Without Detectable Mutans Streptococci

Treatment	Total number of sampled surfaces	B	Time after treatment				
			1 day	1 wk	2 wks	4 wks	8 wks
Placebo varnish	16	5	-	7	5	4	4
CHX. varnish	14	5	-	9	9	6	5
Placebo gel	16	6	6	6	4	3	3
CHX. gel	16	7	14	14	11	12	8

Note: Plaque samples were taken after treatment with either varnish or gel.
(Courtesy of Keltjens HMAM, Creugers TJ, Schaeken MJM, et al: *J Dent Res* 71:1582–1586, 1992.)

Disinfection of Irreversible Hydrocolloid Impressions: A Comparative Study

McNeill MRJ, Coulter WA, Hussey DL (Queen's Univ, Belfast, Northern Ireland)

Int J Prosthodont 5:563–567, 1992   105-94-12-44

Introduction.—Cross-contamination of the dental technician by the dental patient can potentially occur via contaminated impressions and prostheses. Guidelines for the handling of impressions for patients without a history of exposure to hepatitis B virus or HIV vary. Potential for bacterial and viral cross-contamination from impression materials was assessed as well as the effectiveness of various methods of disinfection.

Methods.—An acrylic resin template contaminated with *Streptococcus sanguis* or poliovirus was used to make irreversible hydrocolloid impressions. The impressions were then disinfected by 1 of 4 methods: washing under running water for 15 seconds, soaking in 2% glutaraldehyde, soaking in hypochlorite solution, and using the Hygojet disinfection system, which uses aldehydes, quaternaryamines, surfactants, etc. Microorganisms remaining on the impressions were harvested by sonication, cultured, and counted.

Results.—Simply washing the impressions reduced the number of *S. sanguis* organisms from 60×10^3 cfu to 7×10^3 cfu/mL. The 3 chemical methods of disinfection each removed all organisms (Table 1). Likewise, washing greatly removed poliovirus carriage and chemical disinfection virtually eliminated it (Table 2). On inoculation of the templates with a virus suspension but without serum, more virus remained after

TABLE 1.—Efficacy of Four Disinfection Regimens
on Impressions Contaminated With
Streptococcus sanguis

Disinfection method	Bacterial counts (mean cfu/mL x 10^3)
Unwashed	60.00
Washed	7.25
2% Glutaraldehyde	0.00
10% Hypochlorite	0.00
Hygojet cycle	0.00

TABLE 2.—Assessment of Four Disinfection Regimens on
Impressions Contaminated with Poliovirus

Disinfection method	Suspension media (virus titre)	
	Eagles MEM (mean pfu/mL)	HIFCS (mean pfu/mL)
Unwashed		390
Washed	230	10
2% Glutaraldehyde	0	0
10% Hypochlorite	0	0
Hygojet cycle	0	0

(Courtesy of McNeill MRJ, Coulter WA, Hussey DL: *Int J Prosthodont* 5:563–567, 1992.)

washing and disinfection with the Hygojet system. Breakup and blending of the impression material resulted in a rise of viral titers from 15 to 182 pfu/mL.

Conclusion.—Impression material can serve as a vehicle for bacterial and viral transfer. Virus is present in the body of the impression itself and may thereby evade decontamination measures. Cross-contamination can be avoided by washing, followed by disinfection of impressions.

▶ Impressions are undeniably a potential source of infection transmission, presenting a possible danger to dental personnel in the office and to technicians in the laboratory. This study emphasizes the concern for disease transmission. Because the chemical agents used are known to be effective against bacteria and viruses, it is not surprising that they were effective against *S. sanguis* and poliovirus. These 2 organisms are reasonably representative of the bacteria and viruses likely to be encountered in the mouth. Each impression should be treated as if it came from an infectious patient, so disinfecting each impression is required. It is interesting that a 15-second rinse with running water does remove significant numbers of bacteria and even viruses. The rinse also seems to allow the chemical agents to be more effective when they are applied. However, as noted in another study, a disinfectant spray does not eliminate all organisms, especially the viruses that have already penetrated into the material.—T.G. Berry, D.D.S., M.A.

Effects of Disinfecting Irreversible Hydrocolloid Impressions on the Resultant Gypsum Casts: Part I. Surface Quality

Tan H-K, Wolfaardt JF, Hooper PM, Busby B (Univ of Alberta, Edmonton)
J Prosthet Dent 69:250–257, 1993   105-94-12-45

Objective.—Controlling infection in dental practice is of critical importance. The effects of disinfection time on the surface quality of gypsum casts poured against irreversible hydrocolloid impression material were evaluated.

Methods.—The casts were poured against disinfected alginate impressions. Four disinfectants meeting the criterion of tuberculocidal activity in 10 minutes were studied, including Sporicidin spray, sodium hypochlorite, iodophor spray, and Sporicidin cold sterilization solution for immersion. In addition, Cidexplus glutaraldehyde solution for immersion was included because past studies of glutaraldehyde solutions have yielded confusing results. Disinfection times of 10, 30, and 60 minutes were compared. The cast surfaces were examined stereomicroscopically by 3 experienced raters who scored the surfaces for smoothness and reproduction of detail.

Results.—Both immersion disinfectants were unacceptable. Disinfection time significantly influenced the quality of the cast surface for Sporicidin spray and sodium hypochlorite, but not for the iodophor spray. Disinfection with the sodium hypochlorite for 10 or 30 minutes yielded casts with low scores, but treatment for 1 hour had adverse effects on the cast surface. Similar results were obtained with Sporicidin spray.

Conclusion.—Immersion disinfectants are unsuitable for use with alginate impressions made of Jeltrate. Iodophor spray, but not sodium hypochlorite or Sporicidin sprays, is safe to use for 1 hour on alginate impressions.

▶ It is well known that certain chemical agents are effective against infectious organisms. The conditions under which the agents are effective against organisms that contaminate dental impressions but do not harm the surface characteristics or dimensional stability of the impression are not well known. Different impression materials may call for different agents or modes of application to be most effective. The use of the immersion, disinfectants, Sporicidin, and Cidexplus had a deleterious effect on the surfaces of casts made from alginate impression. The effect was noticed even when the disinfectants were used for a short time. Spray disinfectants did not cause surface deterioration, but they are not as effective against microorganisms. There does not seem to be a single disinfectant regimen that works well for every combination of impression material and dental stone. More investigation is needed to provide a true disinfectant that does not decrease the accuracy of the casts.—T.G. Berry, D.D.S., M.A.

The Use of Sterile Versus Nonsterile Gloves During Out-Patient Exodontia

Giglio JA, Roland RW, Laskin DM, Grenevicki L (Med College of Virginia/Virginia Commonwealth Univ, Richmond)
Quintessence Int 24:543–545 1993   105-94-12-46

Introduction.—Sterile surgical gloves were not routinely used during outpatient exodontia before the required use of barrier techniques. Nevertheless, postoperative infections did not appear to be a serious problem. Whether nonsterile, but clean, gloves might be used without increasing the risk of postoperative infection was assessed.

Methods.—Patients without evidence of acute infection, who were not taking antibiotics, and who were scheduled for removal of erupted teeth were alternately assigned to surgeons wearing sterile gloves (control group) or nonsterile but clean gloves (experimental group). Before each of the first 50 procedures (24 control and 26 experimental), a sterile swab was passed over the palm of the surgeon's gloved hand to obtain a specimen for culture. Surgery proceeded in the usual manner and no postoperative antibiotics were prescribed. The patients returned in 7 days for examination and suture removal.

Results.—Ninety-one teeth were removed in the sterile glove group and 92 teeth in the nonsterile glove group. The mean surgical times were comparable for patients in the 2 groups. No patient in either group was found to be infected at the 7-day recall. There were 7 cases of localized alveolar osteitis—4 in the control and 3 in the experimental group. Specimens tested positive for bacterial growth in 50% of the sterile gloves and 85% of the nonsterile gloves.

Conclusion.—Dental extractions are performed in a surgically clean, but nonsterile, environment. The use of nonsterile, but clean, gloves would appear to be appropriate for routine exodontic procedures. The high rate of positive cultures obtained from the sterile gloves suggests contamination during the gloving process. If sterile gloves are desired, the practitioner must be careful during gloving to maintain a sterile field.

▶ The AIDS epidemic has raised great concern with the public and with health-care workers. The result has been better control of infection to protect the patient and the health-care worker, but there has been an overreaction that has added significant time and considerable cost to health care. This study offers evidence that the patient undergoing routine dental care, including surgery, is not jeopardized by the use of nonsterile gloves as opposed to the more expensive sterile gloves. This supports the contention that clean but nonsterile gloves can be routinely used if a careful patient history is taken to rule out situations requiring extra precautions. A second message of this study is that bacterial growth can occur even when sterile gloves are used if the techniques and procedures are not sterile.—T.G. Berry, D.D.S., M.A.

An In Vitro Evaluation of Simplified Quantitative Diagnostic Aids for Detection of *Candida albicans*
Nikawa H, Iwanaga H, Hamada T (Hiroshima Univ, Japan)
J Prosthet Dent 68:629–633, 1992   105-94-12-47

Background.—Denture stomatitis, the pathologic reaction of denture-bearing mucosa, is one of the most common pathogenic states of chronic candidosis. However, this condition is not a specific disease entity caused by *Candida* species; thus, some mycologic assessments must be done to establish or increase the validity of the diagnosis. Many simplified methods to detect *Candida* species from dentures or oral mucosa have been developed to facilitate the diagnostic procedure. The sensitivity and ability for quantitative detection of C. *albicans* of 5 simplified diagnostic aids are compared to detect denture stomatitis.

Methods and Findings.—The 5 aids tested in vitro were Microstix-Candida, Stomastat medium, Mizuno-Takada medium, CA-TG medium, and the "milk test" (Table 1). After 30 hours of incubation, Microstix-Candida and Stomastat media reacted with 10^2 cells ml^{-1} yeast suspension. After 48 hours of incubation, some colonies or color change were noted in 10^2 cells inoculated samples of CA-TG medium or milk test (Table 2). Within 48 hours, some differences were found among each of 0, 10^2, 10^3, and 10^4 cells ml^{-1} yeast suspension inoculated samples of the 4 commerical systems. However, among these 4, Stomastat's action could not be detected, whereas it was difficult to differentiate the color changes of each sample of the milk test. There were good correlations

TABLE 1.—Simplified Diagnostic Methods for
Denture Stomatitis

Method	Manufacturer or author	Colonies or color change
Microstix-Candida	Miles-Sankyo Co. Ltd. Tokyo, Japan	Colonies Brown to black
Stomastat	Sankin Industry Co. Ltd. Osaka, Japan	Color change Red → yellow
Mizuno-Takada medium	Fujisawa Pharmaceutical Co. Ltd. Osaka, Japan	Colonies Black
CA-TG medium	Hokuiken Co. Ltd. Sapporo, Japan	Colonies Green to brown
Milk test	Cardash & Rosenberg[15]	Color change Blue → white

(Courtesy of Nikawa H, Iwanaga H, Hamada T: *J Prosthet Dent* 68:629-633, 1992.)

TABLE 2.—Sensitivity and Ability for Quantitative Detection
for *Candida albicans* of Simplified Diagnostic Methods

Method	Sensitivity*	Ability for quantitative detection*
Microstix-Candida	HS	HQ
Stomastat	HS	Q
Mizuno-Takada medium	PS	HQ
CA-TG medium	S	HQ
Milk test	S	PQ

* Sensitivity and ability for quantitative detection for C. *albicans* were determined according to the criteria described in the Materials and Methods section of the original article.
(Courtesy of Nikawa H, Iwanaga H, Hamada T: *J Prosthet Dent* 68:629–633, 1992.)

between the results of Microstix-*Candida*, CA-TG, or Mizuno-Takada mediums, corroborating their quantitative abilities.

▶ For debilitated patients or those who are taking long-term medication, *C. albicans* is a distressing pathogen that often proves difficult to treat effectively. It is especially difficult if the treatment protocol is not based on correct diagnosis of the organism. This listing of diagnostic tests and their mechanisms should be valuable to the dentist treating a patient suspected to have *C. albicans.* The varying complexities of the tests and the differences in their sensitivities give the dentist a choice in diagnostic aids. Whatever the aid chosen, it should help in determining the cause of the stomatitis and in the selection of the therapeutic agent.—T.G. Berry, D.D.S., M.A.

Cytotoxicity of Impression Materials
Sydiskis RJ, Gerhardt DE (Univ of Maryland, Baltimore)
J Prosthet Dent 69:431–435, 1993   105-94-12-48

Objective.—A previous in vitro study showed that certain impression materials are potentially cytotoxic. The cytotoxicity of impression materials was further evaluated.

Methods.—Six commercially available impression materials, including Surgident, Permlastic, Jeltrate Regular Set, Jeltrate Fast Set, Impregum, and Reprosil were used in 3 different cell culture assays to measure their effect on cell viability. Individual components of the impression materials were similarly tested.

Results.—After 3 days of incubation with Vero cell cultures, all tested impression materials showed varying degrees of cytotoxicity (Fig 12–65). Some of the components also were cytotoxic. The effect that each of the

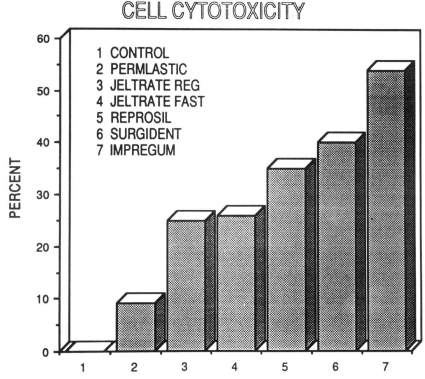

Fig 12–65.—Average percent of cell cytotoxicity of various impression materials in Vero cells after 3 days of incubation. Effect was scored with 0 to 4+ cytotoxicity (CTE) scale for each dilution of test materials. Scores from each dilution series were averaged for 3 experiments and presented as total percent CTE values. (Courtesy of Sydiskis RJ, Gerhardt DE: *J Prosthet Dent* 69:431–435, 1993.)

materials had on cell viability after 3 days of incubation on dividing Vero cells is shown in Figure 12–66.

Conclusion.—Impression materials show varying degrees of cytotoxicity in in vitro assessment. However, the probability of allergic or toxic reactions from the use of impression materials in clinical practice is small.

▶ Various impression materials are routinely used in general and prosthodontic practices without any thought as to the relative biocompatibility of the materials. Because most patients seem to tolerate the relatively short period of contact with the impression material without significant allergic or toxic reactions, it may be assumed that these materials are innocuous. This study, involving the commonly used categories of materials, indicated all categories demonstrated cytotoxicity. Earlier reports have stated that patients have experienced toxic or allergic reactions to zinc oxide-eugenol and polyether impression materials. This report confirms their cytotoxicity and further

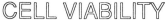

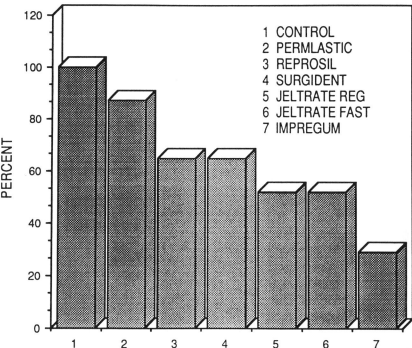

Fig 12–66.—Average percent of viable cells after exposure to various dilutions of impression materials in Vero cells after 3 days of incubation. The cell viability scores from each dilution series were averaged and presented as total percent cell viability values. (Courtesy of Sydiskis RJ, Gerhardt DE: *J Prosthet Dent* 69:431–435, 1993.)

declares that zinc oxide-eugenol and polyether are more damaging to cells than are the vinyl polysiloxane and the irreversible hydrocolloid materials. Although this evidence is not enough to recommend cessation of their use, it is important that dentists carefully observe their patients for any sign of a reaction and carefully remove any piece of the impression left after removal of the impression tray.—T.G. Berry, D.D.S., M.A.

Occlusal Adjustment Therapy for Craniomandibular Disorders: A Clinical Assessment by a Double-Blind Method
Tsolka P, Morris RW, Preiskel HW (United Med and Dental Schools, London)
J Prosthet Dent 68:957–964, 1992   105-94-12-49

Background.—Occlusal disharmony may be an important causative factor of craniomandibular disorders (CMDs). Despite the extensive use of occlusal adjustment as a treatment modality, there has been only a limited number of controlled studies of its efficacy. The effects of elimi-

TABLE 1.—Prevalence of Symptoms in Placebo and Real Treatment Group Before Treatment and After First Session Treatment

| | A Session | | | | B Session | | | |
| | Placebo | | Real | | Placebo | | Real | |
Symptoms	n	%	n	%	n	%	n	%
Jaw pain	17	74	16	57	14	61	11	39.2
Face pain	9	39	8	28.5	7	30.4	7	25
Headache*	22	95.6	17	61	19	82.6	15	53.5
Click	17	74	19	68	13	56.5	18	64.2
Lock	6	26	12	43	1	4.3	3	11

Note: **A,** before treatment; **B,** 10 days after first treatment session, real or mock occlusal adjustment.
* Significant difference ($P < .05$) between placebo and real treatment group in both sessions.
(Courtesy of Tsolka P, Morris RW, Preiskel HW: J Prosthet Dent 68:957–964, 1992.)

nating occlusal disorders on the signs and symptoms of CMDs were evaluated in a placebo-controlled study.

Patients and Methods.—A total of 51 patients with CMD aged 15 to 52 years underwent pretreatment examinations and were then randomly

TABLE 2.—Prevalence of Anamnestic Dysfunction Index by Helkimo in 2 Groups Before Treatment and After First Session Treatment

Helkimo index	A Session*				B Session*			
	Placebo		Real		Placebo		Real	
	n	%	n	%	n	%	n	%
AiII (severe)	23	100	22	78.6	19	82.6	15	53.6
AiI (mild)	0		3	10.7	2	8.6	9	32.1
AiO (absence)	0		3	10.7	2	8.6	4	14.2

Note: **A,** before any treatment; **B,** 10 days after first treatment session, real or mock occlusal adjustment.
* Significant differences (P < .05) between placebo and real treatment in both sessions.
(Courtesy of Tsolka P, Morris RW, Preiskel HW: J Prosthet Dent 68:957–964, 1992.)

divided into 2 groups. Group 1 comprised 23 patients treated with mock occlusal adjustments and group 2 included 28 patients treated with real chairside adjustments to remove significant slides and nonworking side interferences. Each patient was also questioned regarding TMJ sounds,

TABLE 3.—Changes in Symptoms in Both Groups Between A and B Session

Symptoms	Placebo group						Real treatment group					
	1 Unchanged		2 Better		3 Worse		1 Unchanged		2 Better		3 Worse	
	n	%	n	%	n	%	n	%	n	%	n	%
Overall symptoms	13	56.5	10	43.5	0		12	42.8	15	53.6	1	3.6
Headache	10	43.5	9	39.1	3	13	9	32.1	8	28.5	0	
Clicking	12	52.1	5	21.7	0		13	46.4	6	21.4	0	
Locking	1	4.3	5	21.7	0		3	10.7	9	32.1	0	
Pain jaw	9	39.1	8	34.7	0		5	17.8	10	35.7	1	3.5
Pain face	5	21.7	4	17.3	0		3	10.7	4	14.2	1	3.5

(Courtesy of Tsolka P, Morris RW, Preiskel HW: J Prosthet Dent 68:957–964, 1992.)

TABLE 4.—Prevalence of Clinical Dysfunction Index by Helkimo Between 2 Groups Before Treatment and After First Session Treatment

Helkimo index	A session* Placebo		A session* Real		B session* Placebo		B session* Real	
	n	%	n	%	n	%	n	%
DiIII (severe)	6	26	5	17.8	1	4.4	2	7.2
DiII (moderate)	14	61	15	53.6	14	60.8	15	53.6
DiI (mild)	3	13	7	25	8	34.8	10	35.6
DiO (absent)	0	0	1	3.6	0	0	1	3.6
Painful muscle sites (mean)	6		5.5		4.3		4.3	
Total No.	137		154		99		120	

Note: **A,** before treatment; **B,** 10 days after first treatment session, real or mock occlusal adjustment.
* None of the differences between groups were significant.
(Courtesy of Tsolka P, Morris RW, Preiskel HW: J Prosthet Dent 68:957–964, 1992.)

TMJ luxation and locking, oral habits, chewing ability, and face, jaw, and head pain before and after treatment. The Helkimo anamnestic dysfunction index was completed according to patients' responses. Follow-up sessions were conducted 10 days after treatment.

Results.—The initial pretreatment examination revealed that the groups differed significantly in terms of headache prevalence and anamnestic dysfunction index (Tables 1 and 2). When all symptoms were considered together, no significant between-group differences were noted from pretreatment to follow-up sessions (Table 3). The Helkimo clinical dysfunction index did not appear to be affected by either treatment mode (Table 4).

Conclusion.—No significant differences in improvement in CMDs were noted after the first treatment by either mock or real occlusal adjustment.

▶ Starting in the 1960s and continuing for the next 2 decades, occlusal adjustments were highly touted as the solution to a variety of patient problems, such as muscle tenderness, trismus, headaches, tooth mobility, and lessened masticatory function. Unfortunately, much of what was taught was not based on solid research with which to support the sometimes dramatic claims. More recently, good research has shown that occlusal adjustment and selective grinding as common treatment procedures have little value and should not be routinely performed. This study adds to a growing body of clinical research refuting the extravagant claims made in the past.—T.G. Berry, D.D.S., M.A.

Effect of a Full-Arch Maxillary Occlusal Splint on Parafunctional Activity During Sleep in Patients With Nocturnal Bruxism and Signs and Symptoms of Craniomandibular Disorders
Holmgren K, Sheikholeslam A, Riise C (Karolinska Inst, Stockholm)
J Prosthet Dent 69:293–297, 1993   105-94-12-50

Introduction.—In patients with nocturnal bruxism and subsequent craniomandibular disorders (CMD), a full-arch maxillary occlusal splint or bite plate can reduce the level of cumulative nightly electromyographic activity of the masseter muscle. There are no data on the long-term effects of the occlusal splint in these patients and insufficient data on parafunctional activity of nocturnal bruxism.

Patients and Methods.—Thirty-one patients with nocturnal bruxism and signs and symptoms of CMD were studied to explore the long-term effects of occlusal splinting on the kinesiology of their parafunctional oral motor behavior, i.e., grinding and clenching, during sleep. There were 26 women and 5 men (median age, 27 years). All wore a full-arch maxillary occlusal splint in heat-cured acrylic resin during sleep. Every 2 weeks, up to 6 months or until signs and symptoms were eliminated, the

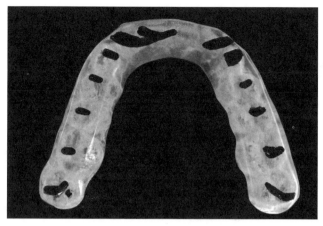

Fig 12–67.—Pattern of wear facets on occlusal splint of a patient with bilateral mandibular movements. (Courtesy of Holmgren K, Sheikholeslam A, Riise C: *J Prosthet Dent* 69:293-297, 1993.)

wear facets and retruded contact position on the splint were recorded. At each visit, the splint was reexamined for stability and, if necessary, readjusted. The signs and symptoms of CMD were also recorded.

Results.—Sixty-one percent of patients showed active, shiny wear facets at each visit, which appeared in the same location and with a similar pattern and direction. The rest showed wear facets only from time to time. Seventy-one percent had facets caused by bilateral mandibular clenching excursions (Fig 12–67). In 13%, the facets were caused by unilateral excursions (Fig 12–68). The facets were caused by protrusive movements in 1 patient and by isometric clenching of the elevator muscles with small lateral movement in the remaining 13% (Fig 12–69). Signs

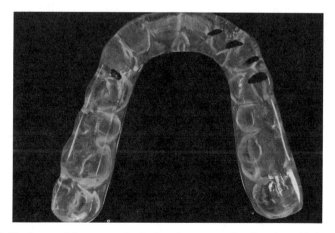

Fig 12–68.—Pattern of facets on occlusal splint of a patient with unilateral mandibular movements. (Courtesy of Holmgren K, Sheikholeslam A, Riise C: *J Prosthet Dent* 69:293-297, 1993.)

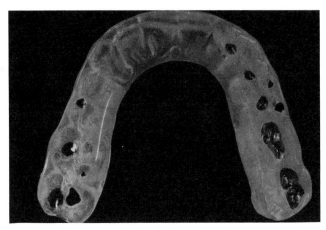

Fig 12–69.—Pattern of facets on occlusal splint of a patient with isometric contraction of the elevator muscles with small lateral movements. (Courtesy of Holmgren K, Sheikholeslam A, Riise C: *J Prosthet Dent* 69:293-297, 1993.)

and symptoms fluctuated and gradually improved or went away (Figs 12-70 and 12-71).

Conclusion.—The full-arch maxillary occlusal splint does not stop the habit of nocturnal bruxism. Wear facets on the splint occur in the same location and in the same pattern, mainly as the result of grinding. In patients with eccentric bruxism, lateral movement of the mandible is far past the edge-to-edge contact relationship of the canines.

▶ Patients with parafunctional grinding or clenching of their teeth, especially during their sleep, are often prescribed occlusal splints. The common result reported by the patients is relief of muscle tenderness and other symptoms. Despite theories indicating that the splints provide new stimuli that disrupt the destructive old habits, the question remains as to whether the splint cures the problem or merely alleviates the symptoms. This study strongly suggests that a splint decreases the stress on the teeth, the bony support, and the jaws, so that the symptoms are greatly abated. However, the splint does not eliminate the habit. It is interesting that the wear facets detected on the splint are in the same pattern even when the splint is adjusted and that patients re-experience the signs and symptoms that provoked them to seek treatment originally. The dentist needs to inform the patient that splint therapy is not truly curative. It is prescribed primarily for relief of symptoms.—T.G. Berry, D.D.S., M.A.

Percentage of patients

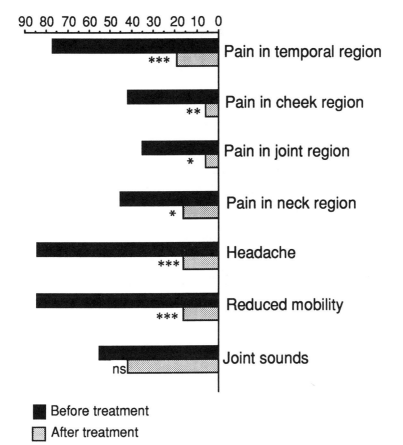

Fig 12–70.—Symptoms of craniomandibular disorders in 31 patients with nocturnal bruxism before and after occlusal splint therapy. Levels of significance: ns = not significant, $P > .05$; $*$ = $.01 < P < .05$; $**$ = $.001 < P < .01$; $***$ = $P < .001$. (Courtesy of Holmgren K, Sheikholeslam A, Riise C: *J Prosthet Dent* 69:293–297, 1993.)

Percentage of patients

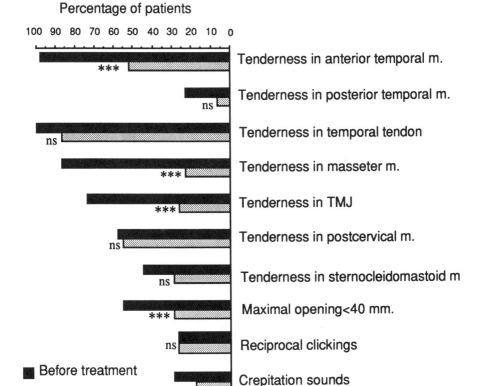

Fig 12–71.—Signs of craniomandibular disorders in 31 patients with nocturnal bruxism before and after occlusal splint therapy. Levels of significance: *ns* = not significant, $P > .05$; * = $.01 < P < .05$; ** = $.001 < P < .01$; *** = $P < .001$. (Courtesy of Holmgren K, Sheikholeslam A, Riise C: *J Prosthet Dent* 69:293-297, 1993.)

Tooth Sensitivity: Mechanisms and Management
Markowitz K (Columbia Univ, New York)
Compend Contin Educ Dent 14:1032–1046, 1993   105-94-12–51

Introduction.—Tooth sensitivity is a common complaint encountered in clinical dental practice. The phenomenon of sensitivity in superficial dentin with no nerve endings has long puzzled researchers. Dentin has numerous thin tubules that extend from the dentinoenamel or dentinocementum junction to the pulp. Some research has indicated that 3 types of sensory nerves exist in the pulp: A-delta fibers, unmyelinated C-fibers, and A-beta fibers. The A-beta fibers respond to similar stimuli as the A-delta and the C-fibers, but they are more sensitive to the electric stimulation.

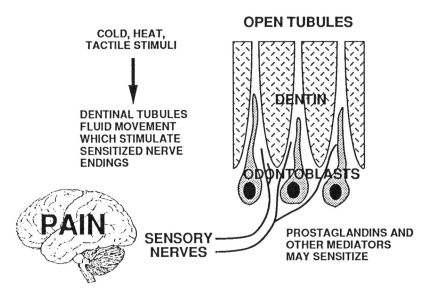

Fig 12–72.—The mechanism of dentin sensitivity involves movements of fluid through the dentinal tubules when stimuli are applied to the dentin surface. This movement of fluid in turn leads to activation of the intradental nerves. Inflammatory mediators in the pulp can modulate the responses of the nerve fibers to dentinal stimulation. (From Markowitz K: *Compend Contin Educ Dent* 14:1032-1046, 1993. Courtesy of Markowitz K, Kim S: *Dent Clin North Am* 34:491-501, 1990.)

Discussion.—Tooth pain can be caused by stimuli such as air blasts, probing dentin surfaces, and fluid movements, which in turn can activate the intradental nerves (Fig 12–72). Some structural factors can actually contribute to lessened hypersensitivity, including mineral precipitates and the age-related reduction in size and subsequent obstruction of the dentinal tubules. Several clinical practice treatments for sensitivity, including resins and bonding agents, are based on tubule obstruction. Early tests with these materials yielded good results in the laboratory, but they have not held up in clinical practice.

Teeth that have exposed dentin and healthy pulp can be sensitive, but the degree of sensitivity can be influenced by the internal environment of the pulp. Caries and faulty restorations can lead to prolonged and extreme sensitivity to temperature changes and sweets in these affected teeth. Healthy teeth respond only briefly to temperature and little, if any, to sweets. In addition, microorganisms on exposed dentin, especially those with caries and/or defective restorations, can make teeth more sensitive.

Therapeutic approaches to reducing sensitivity in teeth have involved either occlusion of the dentinal tubules or attempts to decrease activation on the intradental nerves. A desensitizing agent could effectively reduce the excitability of the intradental nerves. A number of compounds were tested and found to be effective, some of which were potassium-based. It was found that the potassium was responsible for the reduction in sensitivity. The potassium solutions caused a drop in pupal flow, which may be the factor that inhibits the nerve activity. Strontium solutions also proved effective in nerve activity reduction. The type of treatment a dentist uses depends on the severity of the problem, the physical findings, and prior interventions. Some interventions include desensitizing dentifrices, topical treatments, and composites.

Conclusion.—Tooth sensitivity treatment should be based on the etiology of the patient's problem, the extent of dentinal damage, and the use of the appropriate therapy.

▶ Dentists very often deal with patients who complain of a sensitive tooth. The incidence of patients with this complaint may increase as the population ages while retaining its teeth. Exposure of the root surface, which frequently occurs with older patients, often results in sensitivity. This article offers a good explanation of why the pain is often disproportional to the apparent pathology of trauma present. A better understanding of the mechanisms involved will help dentists to better explain the problems to their patients and to aid in selection of a more efficacious treatment to solve the problem. Many modalities, such as placement of dentin bonding agents, have offered promise, but they have not proven consistently effective. It appears that older methods using stannous or sodium fluoride or the recently developed fluoride in a resin base are providing relief to sensitive teeth. A better seal at the cavosurface margins to reduce microleakage, often a cause of sensitivity, is now possible.—T.G. Berry, D.D.S., M.A.

Enamel Roughness After Air-Powder Polishing
Gerbo LR, Lacefield WR, Barnes CM, Russell CM (Univ of Alabama, Birmingham)
Am J Dent 6:96–98, 1993   105-94-12–52

Objectives.—An attempt was made to quantify differences in enamel surface roughness after treatment with an air abrasive system, when compared with the use of a rubber cup and pumice. In addition, whether sodium bicarbonate remains on or in the enamel surface after treatment was investigated.

Methods.—Forty extracted anterior bovine teeth were used in the study. Half the teeth were cleansed with a rubber cup and pumice, and half were treated with an air-powder polisher. All teeth were exposed for a period equivalent to a 15-year recall program. A surface profilometer was used to assess surface changes, and representative samples were examined by scanning electron microscopy.

Results.—There were no marked differences between the 2 groups. Scanning electron microscopy demonstrated surface irregularities in both groups, but no substantial differences in the degree of surface roughness. There was no evidence that sodium bicarbonate particles remained embedded in the enamel surface.

Conclusion.—The use of the air-powder polisher does not alter the enamel surface of a tooth to an important degree. No enamel roughness or ditching was noted in this study, even after an exposure equivalent to that of a 15-year recall program.

▶ Various means of removing stain and plaque from the tooth surface have been tried. The efficacy of the method has always been tempered by the effect that method has on the tooth surface itself. No method that significantly abrades the tooth can be tolerated even if it proves very effective in removing stain and plaque. The air-powder polisher seems to be a means of plaque and stain removal that must be used with caution. It is a more effective agent than a rubber cup and pumice or a hand instrument, but it must be confined to enamel only. The much softer cementum is removed by the air-powder polisher. However, this precaution also applies to most rotary polishing agents and to use of hand instruments. Cementum is a relatively soft surface that must be protected during dental procedures.—T.G. Berry, D.D.S., M.A.

13 Restorative Dental Materials: Direct Systems

Introduction

The field of restorative dental materials continues to be one of the major areas of interest for the private practitioner. Advances in both restorative systems and associated techniques have been modified so extensively that it is virtually impossible for the busy clinician to keep abreast of new developments. This is particularly true for the area of composite resins and dentin adhesive systems. Present day composite resins are far superior to those that were on the market only 4 and 5 years ago. Many of the materials available to the practitioner today exhibit such good color matching ability that it is virtually impossible in many cases to distinguish between the restoration and the adjacent tooth structure. In addition, the wear resistance of many of the new materials has been improved so dramatically that many of them are nearly as wear resistant as amalgam. Unfortunately, however, the material remains technique-sensitive. Consequently, the clinician still remains challenged by the potential problems for marginal adaptation, proximal contour, contact, and secondary caries.

The most recent trend in modifying or improving composite resins has been to reduce the size of the filler particle. Until recently, the most popular materials contained filler particles ranging from 3 to 5 μ. Unfortunately, however, although these materials were fairly wear-resistant, they were not highly polishable. In an effort to develop composite resins that could be used as a restorative system both in anterior as well as posterior teeth, the particle size has been reduced even further. Many of the materials on the market today now contain mean filler particle sizes ranging from approximately .6 to .9 μ. Particle sizes this small are necessary if the material is to exhibit a surface smoothness resembling that of enamel. Although these new universal materials perform extremely well in anterior situations, they do not necessarily function at the same level in posterior teeth. Although there are a number of exceptions, there is a tendency for many of the universal materials to exhibit minor ditching or crevicing along the margins.

Undoubtedly, the greatest advance in restorative systems has been that of dentin adhesives. During the past 25 years, the adhesive bond strength of these systems has increased from approximately 2 MPa (300 psi) to nearly 20 MPa (3,000 psi) or even higher. The mechanism by which these dentin adhesives work is different from their predecessors. Specifically, after removing the hydroxyapatite from the dentinal surface, the resultant vacancies are filled with a polymer as a hybrid layer. The dentinal tubules and the dentin become impervious to the infiltration of microorganisms. Furthermore, such a process has been shown to eliminate or substantially reduce postoperative sensitivity.

Although amalgam has been and continues to be the material of choice for the direct filling of posterior teeth, its safety is being challenged by a number of different groups. Although some argue about the biological compatibility of mercury in the body, much of the pressure has come from environmental agencies and academic institutions that are concerned about mercury as a pollutant in the environment. Consequently, there is a major effort by dental researchers to find a suitable substitute for the amalgam restoration. Such an objective will be difficult to attain, particularly when considering amalgam's ease of manipulation, low cost, and relative independence from manipulative variables. In spite of potential problems with amalgam, however, the dental profession continues to use this material as a posterior restorative system and will probably do so for the next several years.

Karl F. Leinfelder, D.D.S., M.S.

Composite Resins

The Influence of Lining Techniques on the Marginal Seal of Class II Composite Resin Restorations

Blixt M, Coli P (Karolinska Inst, Huddinge, Sweden)
Quintessence Int 24:203–210, 1993   105-94-13–1

Objective.—An important problem in Class II resin restorations is the cervical contraction gap that may occur, particularly when the cervical margin of the cavity is at the cementoenamel junction. Many cross-cut dentinal tubules at this site increase the risk of pulp irritation, inflammation, and necrosis. Whether a bonding agent, Scotchbond 2, improves sealing and prevents the occurrence of gaps was studied.

Study Design.—Scotchbond 2 was used with 1 of 5 thin liners in treating 203 class II cavities prepared in premolar teeth. A light-curing resin-bonded ceramic, P-50, was used in conjunction with Scotchbond 2. In 1 group, use of a liner was combined with renin impregnation of the gap after the composite had set. A fluorescent resin-penetrating technique was used to study the number of gaps and their width.

Results.—Scotchbond 2 and a light-curing glass-ionomer lining frequently failed to prevent gap formation at the cervical wall (table). Gaps usually occurred between the liner and dentin, with penetration of dye into the dentin. Liners containing polytrifluorethylene sodium fluoride

Number of Cervical Gaps Revealed With the Dye Technique

Group	Lining	Total No. of restorations	No. of restorations with cervical gaps	No. of restorations with penetration to dentin	Restorations with gaps nearest dentin (%)[†]
IIb	VB	20	18	12	60.0
III	TH[‡]	24	24	24	100.0
IV	HL	20	20	20	100.0
V	BR	20	20	20	100.0
VI	TP/L[§]	35[II]	29	4	11.4
VII	TP/L plus Resin impregnation	19[¶]	2	0	0.0

Note: All cavities cleaned with tubulicid red label.
† Revealed by dye penetration into the dentin.
‡ Four restorations with Scotchbond 2 placed only on the enamel.
§ Nineteen restorations with Scotchbond 2 placed only on the enamel.
II Three additional restorations were excluded.
¶ One additional restoration was excluded.
(Courtesy of Blixt M, Coli P: *Quintessence Int* 24:203–210, 1993.)

and calcium fluoride, polyamide resin, and calcium hydroxide did not prevent dye penetration into dentin, but good protection was achieved by treating cavities with a hydrophilic shellac film before placing a polystyrene liner. The best results were achieved when this treatment was followed by resin impregnation of the contraction gap after the composite resin had set.

▶ Although the current posterior composite resins are considerably more wear-resistant than their predecessors, they are still characterized with less than perfect marginal adaptation or seal. It is speculated that the problem can be ultimately resolved either by using a composite resin that does not undergo polymerization shrinkage or by using a bonding agent that provides sufficient adhesion to the surface of the dentin and enamel. Although non-contracting types of polymers have not been developed satisfactorily for dental purposes, the adhesive agents are being improved constantly. There has recently been an interest in developing agents that would penetrate into the interfacial gap between the restoration and the tooth structure after the restoration has been completed. A number of companies are now interested in producing a surface penetrating sealant that would effectively fill in any interfacial gap that may be present.—K.F. Leinfelder, D.D.S., M.S.

Three-Year Follow-Up of Five Posterior Composites: In Vivo Wear
Willems G, Lambrechts P, Braem M, Vanherle G (Katholieke Universiteit te Leuven, Belgium; Universitair Centrum Antwerpen, Belgium)
J Dent 21:74–78, 1993   105-94-13–2

Introduction.—Because of increasing interest in natural-appearing posterior restorations, the wear of 5 posterior composites was examined in class II cavities during a 3-year period.

Methods.—Fifty-two class II restorations were placed in mandibular and maxillary first and second permanent molars. The materials tested were an ultrafine midway-filled composite (Exp.LF), 3 ultrafine compact-filled composites (P-30, P-30 APC, P-50 APC), and a fine compact-filled composite (Marathon). Dental students aged 20–25 years with normal occlusions and complete dentitions served as subjects. Four dental practitioners familiar with the acid-etch technique inserted the fillings. Wear at occlusal contact area (OCA) and contact-free occlusal areas was estimated using a 3-dimensional measuring technique.

Results.—The ultrafine compact-filled composites had acceptable OCA-wear rates, ranging from 110 to 149 μm after 3 years, similar to the OCA-wear rate of human enamel on molars. The fine compact-filled composite had an unacceptable OCA-wear value of 242 μm at 3 years. The ultrafine midway-filled composite had a very high contact-free occlusal area wear value of 151 μm. Seventy percent of restorations made with this material exhibited excellent color match after 3 years. Most compact-filled composite restorations appeared at least slightly opaque, and many were clearly opaque. Nearly all restorations were ranked as dull, but Exp.LF restorations had mostly smooth surfaces at 3 years.

Conclusion.—With respect to wear resistance, ultrafine compact-filled composites are the best alternatives to amalgam for posterior restorations.

▶ Unfortunately, it is very difficult to predict the wear resistance of posterior composite resins. No laboratory test or mechanical characteristic is presently capable of indicating how much material will wear over time. It is necessary to conduct well-controlled clinical studies to measure this important property.—K.F. Leinfelder, D.D.S., M.S.

A 3-Year Clinical Study of a Hybrid Composite Resin as Fissure Sealant and as Restorative Material for Class I Restorations

Städtler P (Karl-Franzens-Univ, Graz, Austria)
Quintessence Int 23:759–762, 1992   105-94-13–3

Introduction.—The preventive resin restoration (PRR) uses composite materials as well as glass-ionomer cements to restore minimal occlusal caries while preventing future caries through the acid-etch technique. A type I PRR is used when a pit and fissure lesion is minimal, and a type II restoration is used when caries extend into dentin but remain confined to a small area. In a type III PRR, only filled resin is used to restore a cavity preparation, and pit and fissure sealant is applied to adjacent fissures.

Objective.—In a prospective 3-year study, whether Luxafill, a radiopaque hybrid composite resin, is suitable for fissure restorations and minor class I restorations was determined. A total of 104 teeth in 50 patients were treated.

Results.—Thirty-seven fissure restorations and 27 PRRs were evaluated at 3 years. Seventy-eight percent of these restorations were clinically acceptable or excellent. Six percent had fractured, whereas 16% were no longer acceptable for other reasons. More than 80% of type II and III PRRs received A ratings for color, anatomical form, and surface, but only 75% received A ratings for marginal discoloration and 67% for marginal seal. None of the restorations was lost. Twenty-seven percent of fissure sealants and type I PRRs and 15% of type II and III PRRs had to be replaced.

Conclusion.—The acid-etch composite resin technique may be used to treat small occlusal defects, although some repairs and replacements will be required. Proper dental hygiene and regular dental examinations will permit needed corrections or repairs to be made in a timely manner.

▶ During the past several years, a considerable number of investigators have tried to determine the best method for treating occlusal surfaces with minimal caries involvement. Before the advent of composite resins, it had been suggested that ultra-small amalgam restorations would suffice. More recently, it has been recommended that small restorations of composite be inserted, followed by surfacing with a pit and fissure sealant. The sealant then is extended over the adjacent fissures, thereby inhibiting the potential for future caries development.—K.F. Leinfelder, D.D.S., M.S.

Esthetic Alternatives for Posterior Teeth: Porcelain and Laboratory-Processed Composite Resins
Walton JN (Univ of British Columbia, Vancouver, Canada)
J Can Dent Assoc 58:820–823, 1992   105-94-13–4

Introduction.—Concern over esthetics and toxicity from mercury have encouraged a search for alternative restorative materials. Etched porcelain and laboratory-processed composite inlays and onlays are increasingly being used, but these restorations continue to pose a variety of problems.

The Problems.—The high cost of indirect procedures can be a strong deterrent to their use, but it is much easier to work on a laboratory bench than in the mouth. Lab processing permits better control over the physical properties of composite materials. It has been difficult to obtain consistent results in studies of microleakage. Some posterior esthetic restorations have produced encouraging initial results; however, long-term assessments are lacking. Finishing and polishing of composites have been fairly well accepted, but this is not the case for the intraoral finishing of porcelain. The abrasiveness of porcelain, including that which has been properly glazed or polished, compared with other restorative materials or to natural teeth is recognized. Wear resistance is the other side of this effect, although the wear resistance of posterior composites has been improving.

Outlook.—In addition to research on dentin bonding and resins that expand rather than contract on polymerization, computer-assisted design and machining of ceramic restorations represents an exciting initiative. Although the use of computers to design and produce dental restorations could lead to significant savings of both time and labor, the search continues for the ideal restorative material.

▶ Because of the complexities associated with the placement of a posterior composite resin, many clinicians have had difficulty in obtaining satisfactory results. These include improper proximal contour and contact, leakage, secondary caries, and postoperative sensitivity. The composite resin inlay and the ceramic restoration were designed to offset the undesirable properties associated with the composite resin. Because the inlay restorations are commonly generated outside the oral cavity, many of these problems, particularly marginal adaptation, have been resolved.—K.F. Leinfelder, D.D.S., M.S.

Effects of Cements and Eugenol on Properties of a Visible Light-Cured Composite
Powell TL, Huget EF (Univ of Tennessee, Memphis)
Pediatr Dent 15:104–107, 1993   105-94-13-5

Objective.—Because it is diffcult in the clinical setting to determine whether a visible light-cured (VLC) restoration is adequately polymerized, the effects of barrier materials on the mechanical properties of a VLC composite restorative material, Silus Plus Universal, were determined in an in vitro study.

Methods.—The composite material was cured and aged over Dycal, a widely used cavity liner, as well as a variety of cements (Fleck's, Durelon, Vitrabond, ZOE B&T), and free eugenol. Testing was performed after 1 week and 4 weeks to determine tensile stress at rupture, compressive strain, and the stress-strain ratio at rupture.

Results.—The barrier materials neither aided nor impeded the ability of the restorative material to withstand compressive strain and tensile stress. Tensile strength was highest for 28-day specimens that were cured and aged over eugenol; it was lowest for 1-week specimens cured and aged in contact with calcium hydroxide or eugenol. Strain at tensile rupture was highest for the eugenol 4-week group. One-week specimens cured and aged over zinc polycarboxylate cement (Durelon) exhibited the highest mean stress-strain ratio.

Conclusion.—These in vitro studies failed to show that various barrier materials significantly affect the tensile and compressive properties of a VLC-microfilled composite restorative material.

► One of the problems associated with composite resin restorations is that the use of various liners or bases is contraindicated. It has been demonstrated by some investigators that zinc oxide and eugenol may retard polymerization of the overlying composite resin. In this particular study, the authors demonstrated that the presence of eugenol had no effect on either the tensile or compressive strength of a visible light-cured microfilled composite resin.—K.F. Leinfelder, D.D.S., M.S.

Megafill: A New Posterior Composite Technique
Freedman G (Case Western Reserve Univ, Cleveland, Ohio)
Am J Dent 6:55–56, 1993   105-94-13-6

Introduction.—Restorative dentistry benefits from the rapid pace of research and the improvements in dental material technology. Dentists appear to favor tooth-colored materials for dental amalgam. The information available to date for the megafill insert was reviewed.

Methods.—Review of the dental literature provided information about the new posterior composite technique using the megafill insert, a stabilized, stuffed lithium aluminosilicate glass used in combination with modifier oxides.

Results.—The megafills increase the filler-to-resin ratio of a restoration via bulk-replacement of the hybrid composite material. Glass-ceramic inserts have several advantages over other materials, including lowering the polymerization shrinkage, reducing microleakage, raising restoration strength and dimensional stability, and promoting insert functions. Enough experience has accumulated with the glass-ceramic inserts to determine a standard procedure for megafill restorations. The typical treatment protocol comprises conservative preparation, using the largest insert to fit the cavity, etching and preparing the insert, placing the composite into the cavity, treating it with a monomer bonding agent, removing excess materials, light curing of the restoration, and finishing the restoration with a diamond bur and disk.

Conclusion.—Dentists can achieve better restoration results with glass-ceramic inserts, an innovative alternative to direct composites. The glass-ceramic inserts perform especially well for posterior restorations.

▶ Because composite resins undergo a polymerization shrinkage during the curing process, there is a tendency for the material to pull away from the margins, leaving an interfacial gap. To try to minimize the polymerization shrinkage of the composite resin, the beta quartz insert was developed. After filling the preparation with the composite resin and before curing with light, the insert is forced downward through the composite until it contacts the pulpal floor. After polymerizing, the surfaces are contoured to normal anatomical form. Theoretically, the glass insert should not only decrease polymerization shrinkage, but it should also reduce the coefficient of thermal expansion. It should also serve to increase the wear resistance of the composite resin restoration.—K.F. Leinfelder, D.D.S., M.S.

Effects of the Removal of Composite Resin Restorations on Class II Cavities
Millar BJ, Robinson PB, Davies BR (King's College School of Medicine and Dentistry, London)
Br Dent J 173:210–212, 1992   105-94-13-7

Background.—The esthetic qualities of composite resin are so good that it can be difficult to identify the tooth-restoration interface. However, it is important that it be identifiable if the material must be removed completely. The effects of removing composite resin on cavity size and shape were studied.

Methods and Results.—Direct and indirect composite resin restorations were removed from class II cavities, and significant changes in cavity size and shape were documented. Thirty-eight cavities were assessed from the occlusal and proximal aspects. When final cavity sizes were compared with the originals, cavity size had increased significantly, with a mean increase of 37% for direct composite cavities and 35% for indirect cavities; the range of values was wide. After the removal of restorations, occlusal surfaces were found to increase in 71% of teeth and proximal surfaces in 75% of teeth. The results for direct and indirect composite restorations did not differ significantly. Occlusal dovetails and cavity undercuts were produced in cavities that did not initially contain these features.

Conclusion.—There were significant changes in the size and shape of cavities after the removal of composite resin restorations. Dentists should use repair methods, when applicable, instead of trying to remove an entire composite resin restoration.

▶ One of the disadvantages of posterior composite resins is that they are rather difficult to remove from the preparation without increasing the size of the preparation itself. Under most circumstances, not only is the composite resin of the same color, translucency, and opacity as the adjacent enamel, but it is actually bonded to it.—K.F. Leinfelder, D.D.S., M.S.

Clinical Evaluation of a Highly Wear Resistant Composite
Dickinson GL, Gerbo LR, Leinfelder KF (Med College of Georgia, Augusta; Univ of Alabama, Birmingham)
Am J Dent 6:85–87, 1993   105-94-13–8

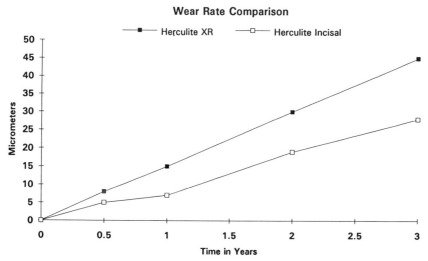

Fig 13–1.—Wear rate comparison of Herculite XR and Herculite Modified. (Courtesy of Dickinson GL, Gerbo LR, Leinfelder KF: *Am J Dent* 6:85-87, 1993.)

Introduction.—The use of posterior resin composites has grown considerably in recent years, despite the fact that such composites are less wear-resistant than are amalgam or cast restorative materials. A slightly modified formulation of the Herculite XR resin composite appears to perform more reliably as a posterior restorative material. Sixty-two restorations of Herculite Incisal formulation were evaluated.

Methods.—The test material was inserted into 13 class I and 49 class II cavity preparations. The restorations were complex in nature in that each class II included replacement of at least 1 cusp. The occlusal component generally involved at least one third of the intercuspal distance. In a control group of class I and II cavity preparations the conventional Herculite formulation was used. Each restoration was independently evaluated at baseline, 6 months, 1, 2, and 3 years by 2 clinicians.

Results.—The color-matching ability of Herculite Incisal never fell below 96%; the percent of restorations exhibiting a surface texture similar to that of the adjacent enamel never decreased below 90% alfa. During follow-up, the wear rate for the incisal form was nearly one half that of the conventional formulation (Fig 13–1). The total average loss of material at the end of 3 years was 45 μm for Herculite XR, but only 28 μm for the incisal formulation. Marginal integrity values were similar for the 2 formulations at 3 years.

Conclusion.—The increased wear resistance of modified Herculite can probably be attributed to the lack of pigmentation, allowing for a more efficient penetration of the curing light during polymerization. There may be some advantage for this formulation in areas of high occlusal stress and in extensive restorations, but marginal crevicing remains a problem.

▶ Herculite XRV has been shown to be a clinically acceptable material for the restoration of anterior and posterior teeth. Much of its acceptance has been based on its excellent color-matching ability. This study demonstrated that the wear resistance of Herculite XRV could be improved substantially by using the incisal component as a restorative material. Because the material is translucent, it lacks the appropriate color-matching abilities. However, it is suggested that if the incisal component is used to veneer the body form of Herculite XRV, the wear resistance of the restoration could be improved substantially.—K.F. Leinfelder, D.D.S., M.S.

Three-Year Follow-Up of Five Posterior Composites: SEM Study of Differential Wear

Willems G, Lambrechts P, Lesaffre E, Braem M, Vanherle G (Katholieke Universiteit te Leuven, Belgium; Universitair Centrum Antwerpen, Belgium)
J Dent 21:79–86, 1993   105-94-13–9

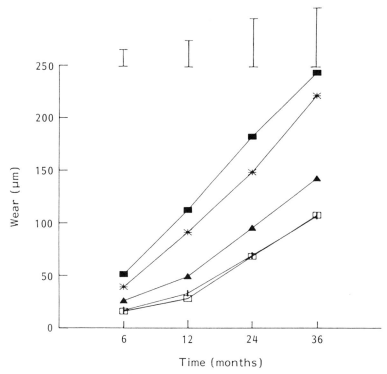

Fig 13–2.—Wear results of all materials tested together with an overall mean standard deviation. *Solid box*, Marathon; *star*, Exp.LF; *solid triangle*, P-30; *vertical rule*, P-30 APC; *open box*, P-50, APC. (Courtesy of Willems G, Lambrechts P, Lesaffre E, et al: *J Dent* 21:79–86, 1993.)

Background.—Evaluating the wear of enamel and composite at a shared occlusal contact area allows study of the differential wear between enamel and composite on 1 tooth. The differential wear of 5 posterior composite restorations was investigated.

Methods and Findings.—An accurate 3-dimensional measuring method was used to assess differential wear. The materials studied were 1 ultrafine midway-filled composite, 3 ultrafine compact-filled composites, and 1 fine compact-filled composite. Scanning electron photomicrographs were used to visualize the distinct wear step between enamel and composite. Both ultrafine midway-filled and fine compact-filled composites had a much higher differential wear value and were less suitable for rehabilitating posterior teeth. The ultrafine compact-filled composites had a very satisfactory differential wear rate, appeared to be highly wear resistant and, thus, are suitable for stress-bearing regions (Fig 13–2).

Conclusion.—The dental wear process of resin composites is determined by many factors. Both the ultrafine midway-filled and fine compact-filled composites had a high differential wear value and, therefore, are not suitable for rehabilitation of posterior teeth. However, the ultra-fine compact-filled composites would be suitable for use in posterior teeth.

▶ The rate of wear and the general overall clinical performance of posterior composite resins is greatly influenced by the presence of an occlusal contact from an antagonistic cusp. In general, strong occlusal contact on the surface of the composite resin may accelerate both localized and general wear and may also result in bulk fracture. It is therefore recommended that the clinician try to minimize contact of the antagonistic cusp on the surface of the finished composite resin. In fact, it is suggested that if the contact area of the cusp could be moved up the incline plane onto the surface of the enamel and off the surface of the composite resin without interfering with functional occlusion, such a technique would substantially enhance the wear resistance of the composite resin.—K.F. Leinfelder, D.D.S., M.S.

Effect of Matrix Systems and Polymerization Techniques on Microleakage of Class II Resin Composite Restorations

Cvitko E, Denehy GE, Boyer DB (Federal Univ of Rio Grande do Sul, Porto Alegre, Brazil; Univ of Iowa, Iowa City)
Am J Dent 5:321–323, 1992   105-94-13-10

Background.—Microleakage can result in marginal staining, marginal breakdown of restorations, secondary caries, and postoperative sensitivity, including pulp pathosis. The effects of different-sized light-curing tips on microleakage of posterior composite materials placed with Mylar or metal matrix systems and their associated polymerization methods were investigated.

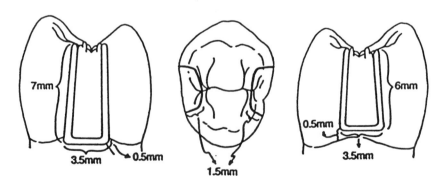

Mesial View   **Occlusal View**   **Distal View**

Fig 13–3.—Slot cavity preparations. (Courtesy of Cvitko E, Denehy GE, Boyer DB: *Am J Dent* 5:321–323, 1992.)

Methods and Findings.—Curing tips of 2 mm and 11 mm were used. Eighty class II mesial and distal slot preparations were divided randomly into 4 groups; metal matrix, large tip; Mylar matrix, light-emitting wedge, large tip; Mylar matrix, light-emitting wedge, small tip; and metal matrix, small tip. No significant differences were found among groups using small and large curing tips. Significantly more leakage occurred in the dentin gingival cavosurface margin groups than in the enamel cavosurface margin groups. Significantly greater leakage was also found in the polymerization procedures associated with the metal matrix groups compared with polymerization procedures associated with the Mylar matrix groups (Fig 13-3).

Conclusion.—The cervical margins in dentin leaked more than those in enamel. Microleakage occurred at most cervical margins ending on dentin, regardless of the matrix system or diameter of curing tip used. Only a few specimens showed no leakage or less leakage than in enamel.

▶ One of the major problems associated with composite resins, particularly in posterior teeth, is inadequate polymerization of the resin matrix. Failure either to have access from the light or inadequate intensity will substantially retard the potential for polymerization. Under such conditions, the material is considerably weakened and has a substantial reduction in wear resistance.—K.F. Leinfelder, D.D.S., M.S.

Interfacial Morphology of Resin Composite and Shiny Erosion Lesions
Gwinnett AJ, Kanca J III (State Univ of New York, Stony Brook; Middlebury, Conn)
Am J Dent 5:315–317, 1992   105-94-13–11

Background.—As the population ages and the number of surviving teeth increases, abrasion and erosion lesions requiring treatment may be expected to increase. Previous studies have found that occlusal wear may be associated with the presence of a burnished, shiny appearance of the lesion. Although acid conditioning removes the tubular plugs in the tubules of eroded dentin, allowing some superficial resin penetrations, there is little information on the extent of such changes after phosphoric acid treatment.

Methods and Findings.—Ten shiny erosion lesions were divided in vivo horizontally so that the gingival half could be prepared and the incisal half could serve as an untreated control. Both halves were simultaneously etched with 32% phosphoric acid for 20 seconds and rinsed. They were then restored using the All Bond wet technique and P50 composite. The teeth were extracted as part of the patients' treatment plan and were sectioned vertically midway through the restorations. Polyvinyl siloxane impressions were obtained and examined for gaps. The teeth were then demineralized, and the restoration fitting surfaces were assessed for resin penetration into the dentin. There were no gaps in any

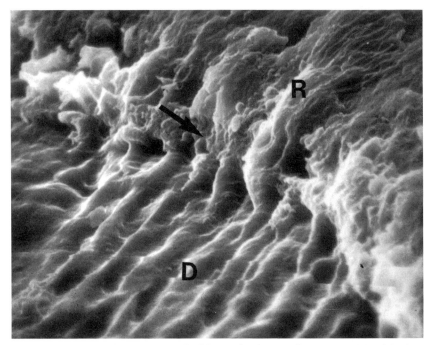

Fig 13–4.—Scanning electron micrograph of the interface between the restoration (R) and the dentin (D) in the uncut portion, showing a discontinuous zone of the hybridization (*arrow*); original magnification, ×4,000. (Courtesy of Gwinnett AJ, Kanca J III: *Am J Dent* 5:315–317, 1992.)

of the interfaces. The most proliferative, deep serin penetration was noted in the halves that were prepared and etched (Figs 13-4 and 13-5).

Conclusion.—The absence of gaps suggests significant interfacial bonding. The presence of a continuous zone of hybridization and uniform resin penetration deep into the tubules suggests that cutting the surface of shiny erosion or abrasion lesions may be beneficial in the long-term clinical retention of a restoration.

▶ Because of the development of the most recent dentin adhesive agents, it is now possible to bond composite resins to cervical lesions without the aid of mechanical undercuts. Such a process is possible by substituting a resin for the hydroxyapatite component of the dentin itself. As a result, it can be anticipated that when used under the appropriate conditions, little or no gap formation will occur between the dentin and the composite resin restoration.—K.F. Leinfelder, D.D.S., M.S.

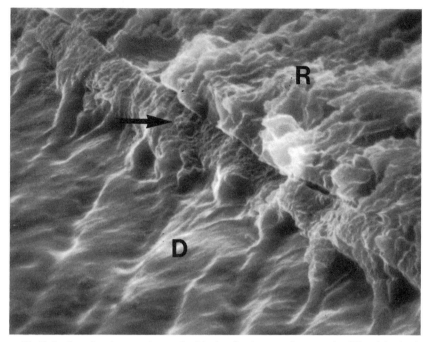

Fig 13–5.—Scanning electron micrograph of the interface between the restoration (R) and the dentinal (D) that was cut, showing a continuous zone of the hybridization (*arrow*); original magnification, ×4,000. (Courtesy of Gwinnett AJ, Kanca J III: *Am J Dent* 5:315–317, 1992.)

Reliability of Three Dental Radiometers

Hansen EK, Asmussen E (Univ of Copenhagen)
Scand J Dent Res 101:115–119, 1993   105-94-13-12

Introduction.—The curing unit is an important factor in obtaining good clinical results with light-activated resin. The difficulty of determining the intensity of curing and of distinguishing between a properly and an inferiorly cured resin has prompted the use of light intensity testers, or radiometers.

Objective.—Three dental radiometers were used to record light intensity from 80 different curing units. The devices tested included the CL-tester, the Demetron Curing Radiometer Model 100, and the Sure Cure Tester. Depth of cure with 20 light sources was examined in cavities prepared in extracted human third molars.

Results.—Readings made with the 3 testers correlated at a fairly high level, but some units were rated as good by 1 radiometer and poor by another. In some instances, there were marked differences in output within the same type of unit. When cavities were filled with microfilled resin and irradiated for 40 seconds, the radiometers were not able to rank the units according to depth of cure (table).

Depth of Cure (Mean ± SD) in Extracted Third Molars vs. Average Recording on
CL-Tester (CL), Demetron Radiometer (DM), and Sure Cure Tester (SC).

| Curing unit | | | | Mean radiometer recordings | | |
No.	Type	Depth of cure (mm)		CL	DM	SC
1	‡ Heliomat	2.25±0.10		1.5	50	2
2	‡ Visilux 2	2.71±0.17		1	40	6
3	‡ Command II	2.81±0.03		3	120	12
4	*Servolite	3.04±0.13		3	170	16
5	‡ Visilux 2	3.21±0.19		2.5	140	5
6	†LC-80 (barrel)	3.71±0.34		7	300	47
7	†Luxor	3.76±0.25		7	460	34
8	*LC-80	3.86±0.13		8	300	62
9	‡ Visilux 2	3.91±0.22		6.4	420	44
10	*LC-80	3.92±0.23		9	360	72
11	*LC-80	4.01±0.19		7	295	62
12	†Visilux 2	4.13±0.27		6.6	380	37
13	*Servolite	4.14±0.19		6.5	350	43
14	*Elipar, new tip	4.15±0.21		7.8	400	50
15	†Visilux 2	4.26±0.09		7.4	390	40
16	*Translux EC	4.39±0.09		6	380	33
17	*Translux CL	4.58±0.26		10	750	84
18	†Visilux 2	4.59±0.24		9.5	550	54
19	*Translux EC, no tip	4.65±0.22		10	550	99
20	*Translux CL	4.82±0.08		10	680	72

Vertical bars connect means with no statistically significant difference (P > .05)
* = New units.
† = Used/worn out units.
‡ = Mishandled/damaged units.
(Courtesy of Hansen EK, Asmussen E: *Scand J Dent Res* 101:115-119, 1993.)

Conclusion.—The radiometers examined in this study are not totally reliable; however, if calibrated along with the curing units tested, they may be very helpful for monitoring output from a curing unit.

▶ One of the major problems associated with a successful placement of posterior composite resins is adequate polymerization of the composite resin. In the case of the photo-cured systems, the entire polymerization potential is based on the ability of the light to penetrate the surface of the composite resin. The extent or degree of penetration of the light in part is dependent on the intensity of the light. As the intensity decreases, consequently so does the degree of polymerization. The actual light intensity can be reduced by a number of factors, including degradation of the light source, contamination of the exit window, or in the case of fiber optic systems, fracture of the glass rods. It is therefore necessary to monitor the light intensity on a frequent basis.—K.F. Leinfelder, D.D.S., M.S.

Assessing the Long-Term Effect of a Surface-Penetrating Sealant
Dickinson GL, Leinfelder KF (Med College of Georgia, Augusta; Univ of Ala-

bama, Birmingham)
J Am Dent Assoc 124(7):68–72, 1993   105-94-13-13

Introduction.—Because subsurface microdefects develop in composite resin restorations, a surface-penetrating sealant may reduce wear on the occlusal surface of posterior composite restorations.

Study Design.—Fortify, a sealant designed to control viscosity and wetting, was evaluated in experimental class I and class II restorations of BIS-FIL I composite resin. The filler particle was diphasic strontium glass, which has a porous surface. The restorations were placed in 13 patients during a 2-month period. Conservative amalgam-type preparations were made in all cases. Sealant was applied to half the restorations and polymerized with visible light.

Results.—After 1 year, sealed restorations had lost a mean of 14 μ compared with 25 μ for unsealed restorations. At 5 years, the respective figures were 45 and 54 μ. The wear rates remained lower for sealed restorations throughout the study (Fig 13–6). At 5 years, 92% of sealed restorations, but only 67% of the unsealed ones, were rated alfa for marginal integrity (Fig 13–7). Regarding surface texture, the unsealed restorations more often had alfa ratings up to the fifth-year recall (Fig 13–8).

Conclusion.—Application of a low-viscosity, surface-penetrating sealant is a simple means of improving the quality of posterior composite resin restorations.

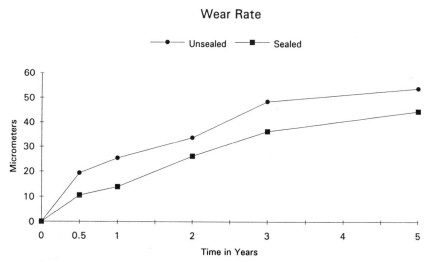

Fig 13–6.—Wear rate of sealed vs. unsealed restorations. (Courtesy of Dickinson GL, Leinfelder KF: *J Am Dent Assoc* 124(7):68–72, 1993.)

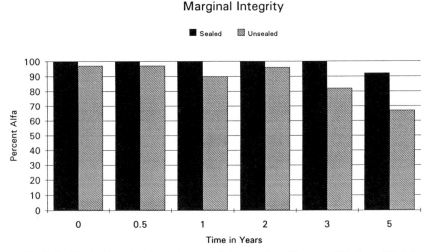

Fig 13–7.—Marginal integrity of sealed vs. unsealed restorations. (Courtesy of Dickinson GL, Leinfelder KF: *J Am Dent Assoc* 124(7):68–72, 1993.)

▶ Microcracks approximating 2 to 5 μ in diameter and perhaps 20 μ in length are commonly created on the surface of a composite resin as a result of the finishing process. Such defects may also be created by normal wear when the restoration is placed in occlusion. These types of defects are commonly associated with posterior composite resins in which the filler particle size is greater than 1 μ. Surface penetrating sealants have the potential for penetrating these defects and sealing them. After polymerization, the microstructure continuity of the surface is regained. Surface penetrating sealants

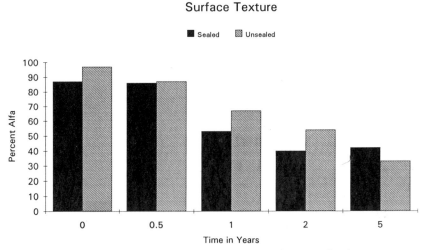

Fig 13–8.—Surface texture of sealed vs. unsealed restorations. (Courtesy of Dickinson GL, Leinfelder KF: *J Am Dent Assoc* 124(7):68–72, 1993.)

are also very effective in penetrating the restoration tooth interface, thereby enhancing marginal integrity.—K.F. Leinfelder, D.D.S., M.S.

Localized Three-Body Wear of Six Types of Composite Resin Veneering Materials

Matsumura H, Leinfelder KF (Nagasaki Univ School of Dentistry, Japan; Univ of Alabama, Birmingham)
J Prosthet Dent 70:207–213, 1993   105-94-13-14

Background.—Extensive research has been done to estimate occlusal wear for posterior restorative materials, but only limited data are available on the occlusal wear response of laboratory-cured composite resin veneering materials.

Objective and Methods.—In vitro wear resistance was estimated for 6 types of light-cured composite resin materials designed for use in fixed prosthodontic veneering procedures. A 3-body wear-testing device was used to quantify the resistance of the various materials in areas of heavy occlusal contact.

Results.—The light-activated composite resin veneering materials had average wear values of 85–160 μm after 100,000 cycles of localized loading (table). All exhibited substantially less wear than did polymethylmethacrylate (PMMA). Viso-Gem was less wear-resistant than the other materials. Scanning electron micrographs indicated surface indentations having well-defined, symmetrical margins associated with Dentacolor,

Wear-Testing Results of Light-Activated Composite Veneering Materials

Material	Wear (μm) x̄	SD
New Metacolor	85.0	2.6
Thermoresin LC	86.5	1.9
Dentacolor	88.7	5.9
Cesead	101.3	10.7
Elcebond	104.5	6.4
Visio-Gem	160.0	10.6
PMMA	352.5	28.0

Note: Vertical lines in same lane indicate that values are not statistically significant at the $P < .01$ level.

Analysis of variance: $df = 6$ and 21, $ss = 227346.6$ and 3295.3, $ms = 37891.1$ and 156.9, F-*value* $= 241.5$, and P-value $= .0001$.

(Courtesy of Matsumura H, Leinfelder KF: *J Prosthet Dent* 70:207-213, 1993.)

New Metacolor, Visio-Gem, and PMMA. Cesead, Elcebond, and Thermoresin LC exhibited irregular intentations with marginal fractures. The surface of PMMA appeared smoother than that of any of the composite resin materials.

Implications.—Composite resin veneering materials should not be used in areas of heavy occlusal contact. They may be used on the occlusal table only if heavy occlusal contacts are on the metal substructure.

▶ Most clinical studies deal with the generalized wear of a composite resin. However, there is not enough discussion about localized wear, which may be even more important from a clinical point of view. Actually, the localized wear is created by the presence of the antagonistic cusp, and it can be significantly greater than that associated with generalized wear.—K.F. Leinfelder, D.D.S., M.S.

Amalgam

An In Vitro and In Vivo Study of the Release of Mercury Vapor From Different Types of Amalgam Alloys
Berglund A (Univ of Umeå, Sweden)
J Dent Res 72:939–946, 1993   105-94-13–15

Objective.—The release of mercury vapor from various types of dental amalgam was quantified in vitro (in air and in air during cyclic dipping into aqueous media) and in vivo from clinical restorations. The in vivo restorations were made from the same batches as were analyzed in the in vitro trial.

In Vitro.—The in vitro trial compared rates of mercury vapor release from dental amalgam specimens in air and in air during cyclical dipping in isotonic saline solution or Fusayama solution. The rate of release of vapor declined rapidly in air (Fig 13-9). In air during cyclical dipping into saline solution, release was most marked for new Dispersalloy and for both new and old Indiloy (Fig 13-10). During dipping into Fusayama solution, values were highest for new Indiloy (Fig 13–11).

In Vivo.—Estimates of mercury vapor release before and after placement of amalgam restorations in 8 patients revealed very small differences. Preprocedure and postprocedure values were very close to background. No changes in salivary or urinary mercury levels were noted after amalgam placement.

Conclusion.—The release of mercury vapor from amalgam restorations in the oral cavity may be far more complex than is apparent from in vitro laboratory studies.

▶ Most current research demonstrates that amalgam restorations do release vapor immediately after brushing or chewing. This mercury vapor can remain elevated for as long as an hour and a half before it returns to baseline values.

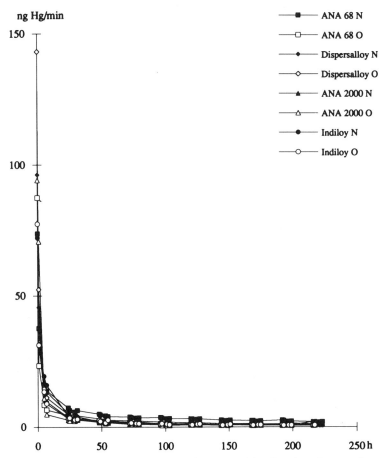

Fig 13–9.—The rate of release of mercury vapor from exposed dental amalgam during 10 days in air. (Courtesy of Berglund A: *J Dent Res* 72:939–946, 1993.)

This type of result has been documented in human and in animal studies. It should be pointed out, however, that although the vapor level does increase and may result in some absorption, the level of mercury is far below that which is considered to be biologically hazardous. The average mercury level in humans runs up to 2 to 3 μg of mercury per liter of urine. Generally, it is considered that 25 μg or more is necessary before any detectable clinical symptom can be observed.—K.F. Leinfelder, D.D.S., M.S.

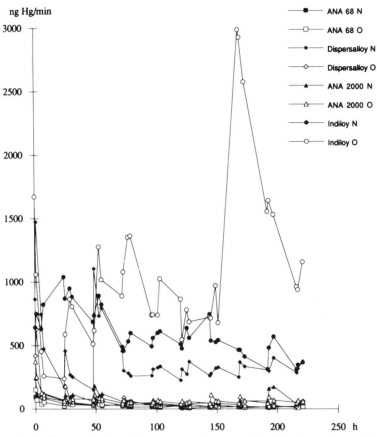

Fig 13–10.—The rate of release of mercury vapor from exposed dental amalgam during cyclic dipping into isotonic saline solution during 10 days. (Courtesy of Berglund A: *J Dent Res* 72:939–946, 1993.)

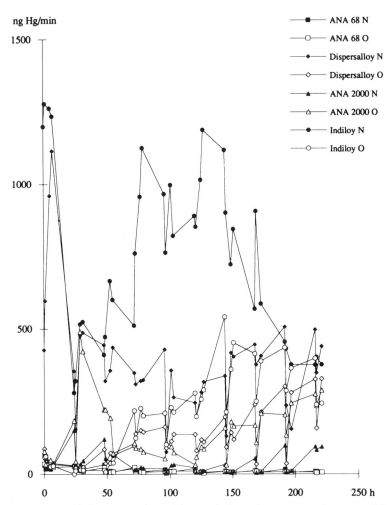

ng Hg/min

──■── ANA 68 N
──□── ANA 68 O
──♦── Dispersalloy N
──◇── Dispersalloy O
──▲── ANA 2000 N
──△── ANA 2000 O
──●── Indiloy N
──○── Indiloy O

Fig 13–11.—Modified Fusayama solution. The rate of release of mercury vapor from exposed dental amalgam during cyclic dipping into modified Fusayama solution during 10 days. (Courtesy of Berglund A: *J Dent Res* 72:939–946, 1993.)

Number of Amalgam Fillings in Relation to Cardiovascular Disease, Diabetes, Cancer and Early Death in Swedish Women

Ahlqwist M, Bengtsson C, Lapidus L (Univ of Gothenburg, Sweden)
Community Dent Oral Epidemiol 21:40–44, 1993   105-94-13–16

Introduction.—Several studies have examined the possible relationship between amalgam restorations and various health problems. The influence of amalgam fillings on cardiovascular disease, diabetes, cancer, and overall death was analyzed in a random sample of women from Gothenburg, Sweden.

Methods.—The 1,462 women were initially examined in 1968–1969 at ages 38, 46, 50, 54, and 60 years. The original sample and the 1,154 women who participated in 12-year follow-up in 1980–1981 underwent a series of medical and dental examinations. End points during the follow-up periods were fatal myocardial infarction, stroke, diabetes, cancer, and death.

Results.—There were 23 cases of myocardial infarction (8 fatal), 13 strokes, and 43 cases of diabetes during the 12-year follow-up period. During 19 years of follow-up, 150 women who were initially free from malignant neoplastic disease had cancer develop. There were 170 deaths during 20 years of follow-up. Women with fewer amalgam fillings had an increased incidence of myocardial infarction, stroke, diabetes, and early death, compared with women with a large number of fillings. When the number of teeth and socioeconomic group were included in multivariate analysis, however, the significant inverse correlations between the number of amalgam fillings and the endpoints studied disappeared.

Conclusion.—Exposure to the mercury in amalgam fillings has been suspected to have negative health effects. The findings of this study provide no evidence for a relationship between the number of fillings and cardiovascular disease, diabetes, cancer, or early death. There is no reason to replace amalgam fillings with those of other materials in symptom-free subjects.

▶ Amalgam as we know it has been used by the dental profession for more than 75 years. In fact, the use of amalgam can be traced back as far as a century and a half. Using special sensing devices, it has been demonstrated that the mercury vapor level over the surface of amalgam restorations increases when the teeth are in function. This early finding tended to initiate the concern by a number of individuals that this vapor deposited in various parts of the body, thereby causing the patient to be susceptible to a number of systemic diseases. Unfortunately, there is no simple way to determine whether restorations of amalgam can contribute to one or more types of diseases. Most immunologic studies, however, suggest strongly that there is little correlation between any specific disease and the presence of amalgam restorations.—K.F. Leinfelder, D.D.S., M.S.

Mercury Sensitization by Amalgam Fillings: Assessment From a Dermatological Viewpoint
Brehler R, Panzer B, Forck G, Bertram HP (Universität Münster, Germany; Universität Witten-Herdecke, Germany)
Dtsch Med Wochenschr 118:451–456, 1993　　　　　105-94-13-17

Introduction.—Because of frequent discussions about the release of mercury from amalgam restorations, patients are increasingly attributing various symptoms to their amalgam restorations and requesting their removal. Patients are also increasingly requesting allergy testing for mercury. Which symptoms can be attributed to mercury allergy was determined.

Patients.—Between 1989 and 1992, 27 men and 61 women, aged 18–68 years, with various symptoms attributed to amalgam restorations underwent patch testing with a series of mercury-containing compounds. The oral mucosa was also examined. Twenty-two patients complained of headaches and facial neuralgia; 26 had oral symptoms, including stomatitis, gingivitis, and burning sensations; 3 had perioral dermatitis; 8 had gastrointestinal symptoms; 9 had joint pain; 5 had atopic dermatitis; 8 had rhinoconjunctivitis; 6 had aphthous ulcers; 3 had oral lichen planus; and 7 had eczematous dermatitis of the hands. Skin tests were read 24, 48, and 72 hours after application of the allergens.

Results.—Seven of the 88 patients were clearly allergic to mercury, including 5 patients with oral mucosal symptoms. Of the 3 patients with perioral dermatitis, 2 had complete resolution of symptoms after the removal of their amalgam restorations. Oral symptoms in 2 patients disappeared after the removal of their amalgam restorations. Two patients got worse after the removal of their amalgam restorations: one had perioral eczema, and the other had diarrhea.

Conclusion.—Because the symptoms of allergy to mercury from dental amalgam vary greatly between individuals, there is no reason to advise against or to prohibit their use. Furthermore, replacement of amalgam with other metal alloys or composite resins may well lead to other types of allergy.

▶ Because of the potential for mercury sensitivity, it has been suggested by some that amalgam restorations should be avoided. It has also been suggested that removal of existing amalgams may reduce or even eliminate the system of certain systemic diseases. Unfortunately, however, no clinical study has ever demonstrated any relationship between amalgam restorations and certain diseases. It should be pointed out that there are some patients who are sensitive to mercury. This number is, however, far less than .1%. —K.F. Leinfelder, D.D.S., M.S.

Factors Influencing Mercury Evaporation Rate From Dental Amalgam Fillings
Björkman L, Lind B (Karolinska Institutet, Stockholm)
Scand J Dent Res 100:354–360, 1992   105-94-13-18

Background.—Recent research has demonstrated that mercury evaporates from amalgam fillings in the mouth. Mechanical factors may in-

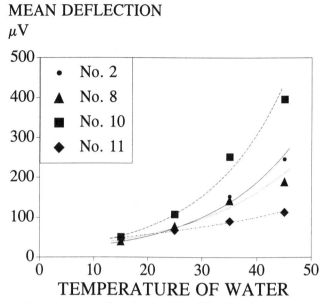

MEAN DEFLECTION
μV

Fig 13–12.—Mercury evaporation from dental amalgam fillings for volunteers no. 2 (age 31), no. 8 (age 34), no. 10 (age 25), and no. 11 (age 38) after rinsing with 30 mL of water of different temperatures (15, 25, 35, and 45°C). The mean for 3 samplings for each test subject and temperature was determined. Mercury evaporation was expressed as the mean recorder deviation (μV) during the 1-minute sampling. (Courtesy of Björkman L, Lind B: *Scand J Dent Res* 100:354–360, 1992.)

crease the evaporation rate. The factors influencing mercury evaporation from dental amalgam fillings were investigated.

Methods.—Eleven volunteers participated in the study. For 1 minute, air was drawn from the oral cavity and analyzed continuously with a mercury detector.

Findings.—The median unstimulated evaporation rate in 6 volunteers was .1 ng Hg/s. After gum chewing for 5 minutes, the highest evaporation rate was 2.7 ng Hg/s. Chewing paraffin wax increased the rate minimally. Changes in airflow rates between 1.5 and 2.5 L/min during the 1-minute test did not affect the amount of mercury drawn from the oral cavity. When sampling with different mouthpieces and closed mouth was compared with open mouth sampling with a thin plastic tube, the latter method was found to result in lower values in some volunteers because of simultaneous mouth breathing. When individual plastic teeth covers were placed in the mouth, the intraoral evaporation of mercury immediately dropped by 89% to 100% of previous levels. Mouth rinsing with heated water for 1 minute increased the mean evaporation rate by a factor of 1.7 when the temperature of the water increased from 35°C to 45°C (Figs 13-12 and 13-13).

Conclusion.—The intraoral evaporation rate of mercury from dental amalgam fillings in this study was generally consistent with those previ-

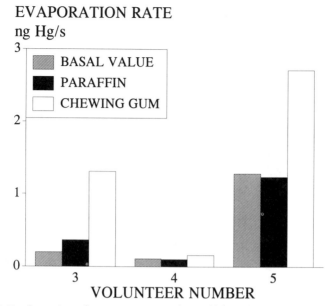

EVAPORATION RATE
ng Hg/s

Fig 13–13.—Comparison of mercury evaporation (ng Hg/s) from dental amalgam fillings for test subjects nos. 3, 4, and 5 after no chewing stimulation, chewing paraffin wax or gum for 5 minutes. *Shaded bar* indicates basal value; *solid bar,* paraffin; *open bar,* chewing gum. (Courtesy of Björkman L, Lind B: *Scand J Dent Res* 100:354–360, 1992.)

ously reported. Daily variations in the levels of mercury evaporation in the oral cavity need to be studied further.

▶ Because of the interest in possible mercury release from existing amalgam restorations, a number of clinical studies have been conducted. Most of them have demonstrated that there is a relationship between the amount of mercury vapor and the number of restorations in the patient's mouth. In general, the greater the number of restorations, the greater the level of mercury vapor. It should be pointed out, however, that regardless of the level and number of amalgam restorations, there is no correlation between these conditions and biological diseases.—K.F. Leinfelder, D.D.S., M.S.

Clinical Evaluation of Four Dental Amalgams Over a Two Year Period
van der Merwe WJ (Med Univ of Southern Africa, Medunsa)
J Dent Assoc S Afr 47:521–525, 1992   105-94-13–19

Background.—The clinical durability of the new amalgams, Amalgaphase and Amalga 43, manufactured by Amalgam Alloys-South Africa, has not been established. These 2 amalgams were compared with Permite C and Dispersalloy in a clinical study.

Marginal Integrity (Alpha Ratings)

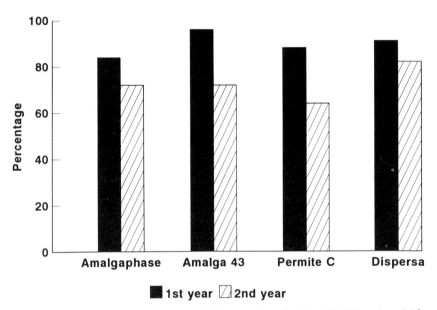

Fig 13–14.—Marginal integrity (alpha ratings). (Courtesy of van der Merwe WJ: *J Dent Assoc S Afr* 47:521–525, 1993.)

Methods.—One class II cavity in each of 82 patients was restored with Dispersalloy, which served as the control. All the other class II cavities were randomly assigned to restoration with Amalgaphase, Amalga 43, or Permite C. Color photographs were taken 24 hours later, and the restorations were assessed.

Findings.—At the 2-year assessment, the 4 brands of amalgam restorations did not differ significantly except for gloss category. The 2 South African products compared well with the imported ones. In the second year, the marginal integrity and surface texture of Amalgaphase compared well with those of Permite C (Fig 13–14). Dispersalloy and Permite C exhibited more deterioration in anatomic form than Amalgaphase and Amalga 43. Amalgaphase was the only product displaying no bulk fracture within 2 years. The performance of Amalgaphase was better in the gloss category than the other 3 amalgams (Fig 13–15). A weighted product calculation showed that Amalgaphase was the best of the 4 amalgams studied, followed by Dispersalloy, Amalga 43, and Permite C.

Conclusion.—The 2 South African amalgams compared well with the 2 imported products. Amalgaphase was judged to be the best amalgam on the basis of the criteria used in this investigation.

Evaluation of High Gloss (Alpha Ratings)

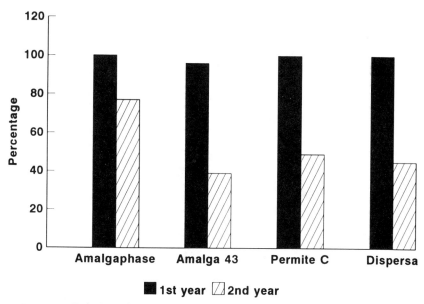

Fig 13–15.—Evaluation of high gloss. (Courtesy of van der Merwe WJ: *J Dent Assoc S Afr* 47:521–525, 1993.)

▶ Because no laboratory data will predict the relative clinical performance of a given amalgam restorative material, it is necessary to conduct well-controlled clinical studies. Today, there are certain methods of evaluation that allow the investigator to determine significant differences among amalgam alloy systems in short periods of time. A review of the literature indicates that there are appreciable differences in the clinical performance of amalgam materials. Undoubtedly, the high-copper amalgams are superior to those of conventional or traditional composition.—K.F. Leinfelder, D.D.S., M.S.

Dentin Adhesive

Hybridizing Dentin: A New Concept in Treating Dentinal Surfaces
Leinfelder K (Univ of Alabama, Birmingham)
Dent Economics 83:96–97, 1993   105-94-13–20

Introduction.—Sensitivity may be a problem with all types of restorative materials, but it is seen more often with zinc phosphate cement and amalgam restorative systems. Posterior composite resins also have produced sensitivity. Branstromm and others have shown that slight fluid pressure changes can cause marked pain responses by the odontoblastic

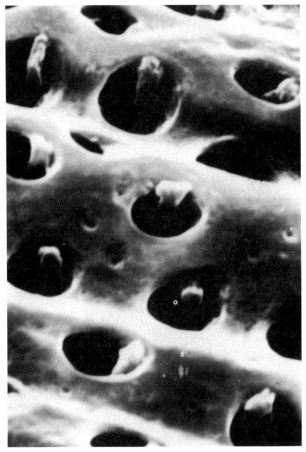

Fig 13–16.—A magnification (×4,200) of etched dentin, showing opened dentinal tubules containing odontoblastic processes. (Courtesy of Leinfelder K: *Dent Economics* 83:96–97, 1993.)

processes (Fig 13-16). The pressure changes may result from fluctuations in temperature, ionic solutions, or drying of the dentinal surface.

Countermeasures.—It now is possible to impede odontoblastic fluid flow and thereby prevent postoperative sensitivity. Nakabayshi developed a method of infiltrating resin into the cut dentin surface to seal the tubules and all the surfaces. A solution of 10% citric acid and 3% ferric chloride was used. Once hydroxyapatite is removed to a depth of about 5 μm, the ferric chloride tends to denature or deproteinize the collagen fibers and the resin flows between the fibers, encapsulating them and forming a "hybrid" layer that prevents fluid and organisms from entering the tubules.

Applications.—This procedure can be recommended for all types of cavity preparation before the restorative stage. It is especially helpful in posterior composite resin procedures. Hybridizing dentin also is useful in amalgam restorations, especially those that are fairly large. Removal of extensive tooth structure raises the likelihood that postoperative sensitivity will occur. Hybridizing should be considered for use in full-crown preparations and when large castings are to be cemented, particularly when zinc phosphate cement is used in conjunction with crown and bridge cementation.

▶ There is no doubt that the area of dentin adhesives represents one of the most exciting advances in restorative dentistry. In addition to exhibiting very high bonding strengths to dentin, the new adhesive systems are capable of hybridizing the dentin. In other words, the bonding agent becomes an integral part of the dentin itself by replacing the hydroxyapatite on the surface and in the tubules. Consequently, not only is there an increase in bond strength, but there is also an excellent mechanism for the protection of the pulp from microbial invasion. Coincidentally, this process also has been very effective in eliminating postoperative sensitivity.—K.F. Leinfelder, D.D.S., M.S.

Evaluation of the Syntac Bonding System
Retief DH, Mandras RS, Russell CM, Denys FR (Univ of Alabama, Birmingham)
Am J Dent 6:17–21, 1993   105-94-13–21

Introduction.—Lack of adherence of polymeric restorative resins to mineralized dental tissues is a major problem in restorative dentistry and is associated with microleakage of salivary components and bacteria at the tooth-restoration interface as well as marginal breakdown and secondary caries. The Syntac Enamel-Dentin Bonding System is a third-generation dentin bonding system.

Objective and Methods.—The shear bond strength of Syntac to dentin was measured after exposing the superficial dentin of the occlusal surfaces of human mandibular permanent molar teeth and applying Syntac Primer and Syntac Adhesive. Microleakage was quantified in class V preparations having dentin restored with the Syntac system. Penetration of resin into the dentin tubules was assessed by scanning electron microscopy.

Observations.—Shear bond strengths of test specimens stored in saline for 24 hours were significantly greater than for specimens removed 1 minute (rather than 15 minutes) after final cure. The mean microleakage after restoring class V preparations with the Syntac System was 2.57 μg dye/restoration. The resin penetrated deeply into the dentin tubules.

Implication.—The high shear bond strength observed after 24 hours indicates that preparations restored with the Syntac Enamel-Dentin

Bonding Agent/Heliomolar system may be effectively retained in the clinical setting.

▶ It is generally recognized that for a dentin adhesive to successfully bond to dentin clinically, the shear bond strength must be at least 10 MPa. Many of the fourth-generation adhesives now exhibit shear bond strengths of between 15 and 20 MPa. A recently completed 3-year clinical study of Syntac in which no mechanical preparation was generated revealed a retention value of 100%.—K.F. Leinfelder, D.D.S., M.S.

Effect of Eugenol-Containing Endodontic Sealer on Retention of Prefabricated Posts Luted With an Adhesive Composite Resin Cement
Tjan AHL, Nemetz H (Loma Linda Univ, Calif)
Quintessence Int 23:839–844, 1992   105-94-13–22

Background.—A reliable luting agent must be used to cement posts to prevent premature failure of a restoration from dislodgment of the posts. A new composite resin cement, Panavia EX, is a quartz-filled bis-GMA composite containing a phosphate monomer as an adhesive promoter. It is reported to bond chemically as well as mechanically to tooth structure and dental alloys.

Objectives.—An attempt was made to determine the effect of residual eugenol in the postspace on the retention of Para-Post dowels luted with Panavia EX composite resin cement. A cleansing procedure also was sought to counter the adverse effects of eugenol.

Methods.—Seventy extracted human mandibular premolars were used in the study. Post spaces 8-mm deep were prepared to accommodate a no. 4 vented, serrated Para-Post dowel. The post spaces were contaminated with eugenol and stored for a week before cementing the posts with Panavia EX resin cement or zinc phosphate cement. In addition to water, the contaminated post spaces were irrigated with ethyl alcohol, 25% citric acid solution, and acetone.

Results.—The presence of eugenol compromised the retention of posts luted with Panavia EX cement. Retention was enhanced by irrigating the post space with ethyl alcohol. Failures occurred mainly at the tooth-cement interface. Etching with phosphoric acid gel also promoted retention of the posts, but irrigating with alcohol produced more consistent results. Cementing posts with Panavia was more effective than using zinc phosphate cement when the post space was effectively cleansed.

▶ It is generally agreed that eugenol-containing materials will inhibit the polymerization of composite resins or various types of resin cements. It is further speculated that such a condition will result in a substantial reduction in bond strength values between the dentin and cement. This study indicates that removal of the residual eugenol layer on the surface of the dentin will effectively eliminate the effects of this agent if used during the restorative process.—K.F. Leinfelder, D.D.S., M.S.

Repair of High-Copper Amalgam With and Without an Adhesive System: In Vitro Assessment of Microleakage and Shear Bond Strength
Hadavi F, Hey JH, Ambrose ER, ElBadrawy HE (Univ of Saskatchewan, Saskatoon, Canada; Univ of Alberta, Edmonton, Canada)
Gen Dent 41:49–53, 1993   105-94-13-23

Background.—Microleakage and bond strength at the repaired junction are 2 important parameters for assessing a repaired restoration. Microleakage and shear bond strength of intact amalgam and amalgam repaired with and without an adhesive material were assessed.

Methods.—Two types of molds were created for the microleakage study. The first was used to make an amalgam cylinder with both sides open, and the second consisted of a mounted positioning rod. Amalgam was condensed in the first mold and filled with amalgam. Twenty amalgam cylinders were made with both sides open; 10 more were made after the mold was altered to serve as controls. After 10 days of storage, the lower part of the inner surface of the 20 amalgam cylinders was roughened. An adhesive system (Amalgambond) was applied to the roughened surfaces of 10 specimens; the remaining 10 were not treated. A 2-mm amalgam base was condensed to the treated inner surface using the same method. The junction was then refined with a sharp instrument. The 10 samples in each of the 3 groups were divided in half, and 5

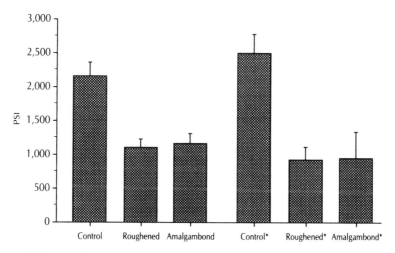

*With thermocycling

Fig 13–17.—Shear bond strength in the different test groups with and without thermocycling. (Courtesy of Hadavi F, Hey JH, Ambrose ER, et al: *Gen Dent* 41:49–53, 1993.)

samples were thermocycled for 6 hours at 4°C and 60°C. For the shear bond strength assessment, a 2-piece Delrin mold connected by mortices assembled in a supporting Delrin frame was used to make a rectangular amalgam rod. Twenty amalgam rods were made; 10 served as controls, and 10 were hemisectioned, roughened, and repaired.

Findings.—None of the thermocycled or nonthermocycled samples in the control of Amalgambond groups demonstrated leakage after centrifuging. Microleakage occurred only in the group repaired without the adhesive system. Nonsignificant differences were found in microleakage among the control, roughened, and Amalgambond groups. In the shear bond strength study, differences between the corresponding groups repaired with or without thermocycling were nonsignificant. Intact specimens had a higher shear bond strength after thermocycling than nonthermocycled intact specimens. They also had a significantly higher strength than repaired specimens in the thermocycled and nonthermocycled groups (Fig 13–17).

Conclusion.—Microleakage occurred in the specimens repaired without the adhesive system, whereas the Amalgambond group did not show leakage. However, between-group differences were nonsignificant. The shear bond strengths of the Amalgambond test groups were 37.8% and 53.3% of intact controls with and without thermocycling, respectively. Differences between the test groups repaired with and without the adhesive system were nonsignificant.

▶ One of the advantages of the new types of dentin bonding systems is that they are considerably more versatile in their application than are their predecessors. Specifically, the fourth-generation bonding agents can be used to bond composite to composite, composite to metal, and composite to amalgam surfaces. Some of the systems, in fact, can actually be used to bond amalgam to the surface of the dentinal walls of the cavity preparation.—K.F. Leinfelder, D.D.S., M.S.

Effect of a Resin Lining and Rebonding on the Marginal Leakage of Amalgam Restorations
Dutton FB, Summitt JB, Chan DCN, Garcia-Godoy F (Univ of Texas Health Science Ctr, San Antonio)
J Dent 21:52–56, 1993   105-94-13–24

Background.—The idea of rebonding restorations to seal marginal gaps was suggested in a 1987 microleakage evaluation with resin composite. The rebonding procedure involved applying an unfilled resin bonding agent over the margins of the finished restoration. The use of amalgam in conjunction with resin composite has been proposed to create restorations that conserve tooth structure and enhance restoration performance. Microleakage in class V amalgam restorations was compared with 3 different lining agents and with no lining agent, with and without resin rebonding of the margins in an in vitro study.

Methods and Findings.—Eight groups of 10 molars each were divided into 4-group pairs. Class V preparations were produced in the facial surfaces of each molar, with the occlusal margin in enamel and the gingival margin in dentine. Preparations in 1 group pair received no lining agent, and preparations in the rest of the group pairs were lined with Copalite, Universal Bond 3 (UB3) Primer and Adhesive, or UB3 Primer. In 1 of each pair of groups, restoration margins were treated with 37% phosphoric acid gel, and UB3 Adhesive was applied over the amalgam and tooth margins and rebonded. At the enamel margins, microleakage in the nonrebonded Copalite and all the rebonded specimens was less than the other nonrebonded groups. Significantly less microleakage occurred at enamel margins in the group lined with the UB3 Primer only and rebonded compared with all other groups except those lined with Copalite and rebonded. Restorations lined with UB3 Primer and rebonded had significantly less microleakage at the cementum/dentine margins than the other groups.

Conclusion.—This study suggests that rebonded enamel and dentinal margins of class V amalgam restorations that have been treated with UB3 Primer as a cavity liner have significantly less microleakage than nonrebonded margins; the results support previous conclusions that rebonding reduces the degree of microleakage in vitro.

▶ One of the problems associated with amalgam as a restorative material is that it undergoes microleakage for days to several weeks. Such a condition normally results in postoperative sensitivity. Copalite has been recommended for the purpose of eliminating or reducing postoperative sensitivity. However, a review of the literature indicates there is little agreement as to the effect of copalite in carrying out this objective. In this regard, it has been suggested that the use of the newer dentin bonding agents may reduce or eliminate postoperative sensitivity by developing a seal of the dentin. Under such conditions, the cavity varnish would not be needed.—K.F. Leinfelder, D.D.S., M.S.

Effect of Powder/Liquid Ratio on Physical and Chemical Properties of C&B Metabond
Myers ML, Caughman WF, Rueggeberg FA, O'Connor RP (Med College of Georgia, Augusta)
Am J Dent 6:77–80, 1993   105-94-13-25

Introduction.—The resin cement C&B Metabond has the ability to bond to nonnoble alloys, enamel, and dentin. Because the manufacturer supplies this cement as a powder and as a liquid system, there may be some variability in the degree and rate of curing. The effect of 3 powder-

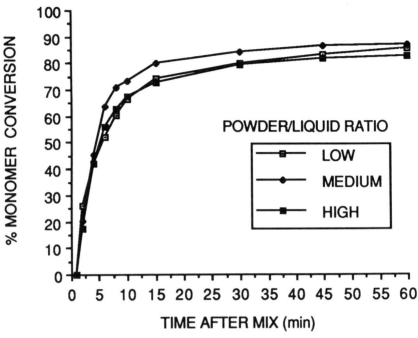

Fig 13–18.—Monomer conversion as function of various postmix times for 3 powder-liquid ratios tested. (Courtesy of Myers ML, Caughman WF, Rueggeberg FA, et al: *Am J Dent* 6:77–80, 1993.)

liquid (P/L) ratios on the physical and chemical properties of C&B Metabond was investigated.

Methods.—The specific properties of the system that were evaluated included film thickness, retentive force of cemented crowns, tensile strength of Ni-Cr-Be rods bonded to etched enamel, and the monomer conversion of the resin. Crown retentive force and film thickness were tested on freshly extracted and nonrestored human molars. Bovine teeth were used to test enamel bond strength. The cure of various P/L mixtures was monitored by observing changes in the infrared spectrum of test specimens as they cured.

Results.—There was no significant difference in retentive force of the cemented crowns when the 3 different P/L ratios were used. The high P/L ratio (2/1) gave significantly greater film thickness than either the medium (1.5/1) or low (1/1) P/L ratios. No significant differences in film thickness were observed between the low and medium P/L ratios. The 3 mixtures did not vary significantly in strength of the Rexillium enamel bond. Within the range of P/L ratios studied, there were no significant differences in rate of monomer conversion and total conversion (Fig 13–18). The majority of the polymerization occurred within 5 minutes after mixing and was almost complete after 10 minutes.

Conclusion.—The hypothesis tested here, that varying the ratio of powder to monomer would result in varied polymer networks with different physical properties, did not prove to be the case. Extremes, however, with very high P/L ratios, would probably result in a considerably weaker polymer network. The medium ratio is recommended for adequate physical and chemical properties and acceptable handling characteristics.

▶ The development of 4-META has been significant improvement in adhesive systems. Developed nearly 20 years ago, this material has proved to be highly adhesive and quite stable under clinical conditions. This particular chemical agent is an integral part of the Metabond and Amalgambond systems.—K.F. Leinfelder, D.D.S., M.S.

Use of Phosphoric Acid Etchants With Scotchbond Multi-Purpose
Swift EJ Jr, Denehy GE, Beck MD (Univ of Iowa, Iowa City)
Am J Dent 6:88–90, 1993   105-94-13-26

Introduction.—The manufacturer of Scotchbond Multi-Purpose and various researchers have claimed that the new dentin-enamel adhesive has a bond strength of 27 MPa to enamel. However, tests at 1 laboratory have suggested that the enamel bond strength of Scotchbond is in the range of 13–17 MPa. Whether using phosphoric acid in place of maleic acid as a dentin conditioner would improve the product's enamel bond strength was investigated.

Shear Bond Strengths of Scotchbond Multi-Purpose (Primer and Adhesive) and Restorative Z100 to Dentin Etched with Different Acids

Etchant	Mean bond strength (MPa)*	Duncan grouping†
10% maleic acid	17.3 (6.2)	A
10% phosphoric acid	17.2 (5.6)	A
35% phosphoric acid	15.2 (4.6)	A
32% phosphoric acid	13.6 (5.1)	A
Etch 'N' Seal	5.2 (3.8)	B

* Standard deviations are listed in parentheses.
† Means with same letter are not significantly different.
(Courtesy of Swift EJ Jr, Denehy GE, Beck MD: *Am J Dent* 6:88–90, 1993.)

Methods.—Various agents were tested on 50 intact extracted human molars. The specimens were randomly assigned to 5 treatment groups of 10 molars each. Proximal dentin surfaces of the molars were etched for 15 seconds with Scotchbond Multi-Purpose Etchant (10% maleic acid; the control), Scotchbond Etching Gel (35% phosphoric acid with silica thickener), Uni-Etch (32% phosphoric acid; polymer thickener), All-Etch (polymer-thickened 10% phosphoric acid), or Etch 'N' Seal (25% phosphoric acid with aluminum oxalate crystals). Scotchbond Multi-Purpose Primer and Adhesive were applied as directed and composite posts were bonded to the dentin.

Results.—The highest mean shear bond strength, 17.3 MPa, was in the control group; samples etched with Etch 'N' Seal had the lowest mean bond strength, 5.2 MPa (table). The first 4 etchants did not differ significantly from each other in mean shear bond strength, but their strength was significantly greater than that of Etch 'N' Seal. The latter etchant was the only 1 to coat the surface with a precipitate, which occluded the dentin tubules.

Conclusion.—Some types of phosphoric acid etchants may be used in place of 10% maleic acid with the Scotchbond Multi-Purpose adhesive system. Such a modification may achieve a more predictable enamel bonding and comparable dentin bonding. The higher concentrations of phosphoric acid (30% to 40%) may be the better choice.

▶ There are a number of acids that may be used to condition the dentin for use in conjunction with the fourth-generation dentin bonding systems, including citric, maleic, phosphoric, and nitric acids. In some commercial formulations, EDTA is also used. It should be pointed out that the concentration of these acids is approximately 10%, compared with the 35% to 37% used to etch enamel. It has been demonstrated that the 10% concentration is sufficient not only to etch the dentin for enhancing the bond of the resin to its surface, but also for effectively acid etching the enamel.—K.F. Leinfelder, D.D.S., M.S.

Microleakage of Amalgam Restorations Using Amalgambond and Copalite

Edgren BN, Dehehy GE (Univ of Iowa, Iowa City)
Am J Dent 5:296–298, 1992   105-94-13–27

Background.—New resin materials have been produced that can bond metal to tooth structure. Amalgambond, a commercial product, contains 4-META as the active ingredient. The efficacy of Amalgambond as a liner under amalgam restorations to reduce microleakage was evaluated.

Methods and Findings.—Amalgambond was compared with Copalite in the reduction of microleakage in amalgam class V restorations. Retentive traditional and nonretentive cavity preparations with gingival cavo-

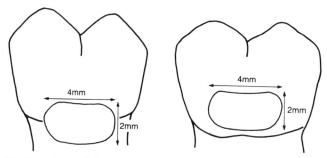

Fig 13–19.—Dimensions and shape of cavity preparations showing cementoenamel junction and enamel locations. (Courtesy of Edgren BN, Dehehy GE: *Am J Dent* 5:296–298, 1992.)

surface margin locations in enamel and dentin were used. Cavity preparations were restored, thermocycled, and stored in erythrosin red stain for 10 days. The samples were then sectioned, and microleakage was assessed. Significantly more microleakage occurred with the nontraditional cavity design and cavity margins in dentin. As a cavity liner, Amalgambond significantly reduced microleakage compared with Copalite (Figs 13–19, 13–20, and 13–21).

Conclusion.—Amalgambond can be used to reduce microleakage with class V amalgam restorations. Microleakage at the cavosurface margins of an amalgam restoration was significantly greater with a nontraditional cavity preparation design than with a traditional design.

▶ This particular study demonstrates that Amalgambond, which is a fourth-generation adhesive material, is considerably more effective in reducing microleakage than is Copalite, which was used as a control. The results are not surprising, because Amalgambond totally seals the dentin, preventing an out-

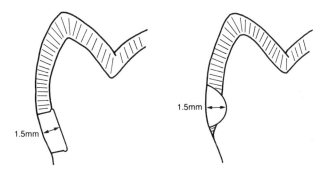

Traditional Preparation
CEJ Location

Non-Traditional Preparation
Enamel Location

Fig 13–20.—*Abbreviation: CEJ*, cementoenamal junction. Cross-sectional view of traditional and nontraditional cavity preparations showing different examples of cavity location. (Courtesy of Edgren BN, Dehehy GE: *Am J Dent* 5:296–298, 1992.)

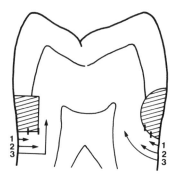

Fig 13–21.—Scoring criteria for the determination of the degree of microleakage with bold traditional and nontraditional cavity restorations. (Courtesy of Edgren BN, Dehehy GE: *Am J Dent* 5:296–298, 1992.)

ward flow of the odontoblastic fluids. Copalite, on the other hand, does not totally seal or fill in the tubules, and in addition, it is quite porous. An increasing number of clinicians are now using dentin adhesives for the purpose of sealing the tubules and the cut dentin rather than using a cavity varnish. This particular procedure has considerably reduced or eliminated the postoperative sensitivity normally associated with amalgam placement.—K.F. Leinfelder, D.D.S., M.S.

Shear Bond Strengths of 10 Dentinal Bonding Restorative Systems
Mandras RS, Retief DH, Russell CM (Univ of Alabama, Birmingham; Ctrs for Disease Control and Prevention, Atlanta, Ga)
Gen Dent 41:133–137, 1993   105-94-13–28

Background.—Most dentists currently use third-generation dentinal bonding systems that interact with chemically altered dentin surfaces. The shear bond strengths of 10 third-generation dentinal bonding restorative systems were compared in an in vitro study.

Methods and Findings.—The systems studied were Tenure Solution Dentin Bonding System, Mirage Bond, Gluma Bonding System, Scotchbond 2 Light Cure Dental Adhesive, XR-Bonding System, Tripton Universal Visible Light-Cured Bonding System, Clearfil Photo-Bond, Super-Bond, Prisma Universal Bond 2, and Optec Pentra Bond II Universal Dentin Adhesive. Super-Bond had the highest mean shear bond strength after 24 hours of storage in physiological saline at 37°C; Mirage Bond had the lowest mean shear bond strength (table). Differences among groups were highly significant. The shear bond strengths of Super-Bond, XR-Bonding System, and Tripton were significantly greater than those of the other 7 systems.

Conclusion.—Most information on dentinal bonding agents comes from laboratory testing. However, the clinical performance of these re-

Shear Bond Strengths of Third-Generation Dentinal Bonding Restorative Systems

Bonding system	No. of Specimens	Shear bond strength (MPa)			
		Mean	SD	Range	C of V %
A. Super-Bond Silux	20	18.3	3.8	9.2-24.0	21
B. XR-Bond Herculite XR	20	15.4	3.7	9.2-21.5	24
C. Tripton Opalux	20	12.8	3.4	7.5-19.6	26
D. Gluma Lumifor	20	10.5	4.6	4.4-22.4	43
E. Prisma UB 2 Prisma AP.H.	20	10.4	2.5	6.6-14.6	24
F. Scotchbond 2 Silux	20	8.5	3.3	4.5-14.9	38
G. Clearfil PB Photo CF Bright	20	8.5	2.2	5.6-12.8	26
H. Tenure Solution Perfection	15	8.0	4.0	4.2-18.0	50
I. Optec Pentra Bond II Pentrafil II	20	7.2	2.0	4.5-11.1	27
J. Mirage Bond Mirage Resin	20	6.6	1.7	3.7-9.7	26

Note: Means linked by vertical lines were not significantly different.

(Courtesy of Mandras RS, Retief DH, Russell CM: *Gen Dent* 41:133–137, 1993.)

storative agents ultimately determines their success or failure. Nonetheless, laboratory studies can help screen experimental dentinal bonding systems before in vivo assessments are done.

▶ Because of the apparent success of the fourth-generation bonding systems, an increasing number of materials has been introduced to the dental profession. As would be expected, the mean shear bond strength values for these systems vary considerably. Nearly all of those that are truly fourth-generation bonding systems, however, exhibit values between 15 and 20 MPa. Current ongoing clinical studies demonstrate that these newer systems are significantly more adhesive to tooth structure in the absence of mechanical undercuts on the surface of the cavity preparation.—K.F. Leinfelder, D.D.S., M.S.

Bond Strengths of Scotchbond Multi-Purpose to Moist Dentin and Enamel

Swift EJ Jr, Triolo PT Jr (Univ of Iowa, Iowa City)
Am J Dent 5:318–320, 1992   105-94-13-29

Background.—The total-etch method for dentin bonding has gained popularity in the United States. Scotchbond Multi-Purpose Universal Dental Adhesive is a new total-etch system that uses 10% maleic acid instead of phosphoric acid for etching dentin and enamel. The shear bond strengths of the Scotchbond Multi-Purpose system were compared with dry and visibly moist dentin and enamel.

Methods and Findings.—Extracted human molars were used in this in vitro study. The teeth were etched and the surfaces were either dried with compressed air or blotted with tissue paper, leaving them visibly moist. Primer, adhesive, and resin composite posts were applied, and the specimens were thermocycled. An Instron universal testing machine was used to determine shear bond strengths. Mean shear bond strengths for both enamel and dentin were higher when the surface was left visibly moist after etching. Bond strength to moist dentin was 21.8 MPa and to dry dentin, 17.8 MPa; enamel strengths were slightly lower, with respective values of 17.0 and 14.2 MPa (table).

Conclusion.—The Scotchbond Multi-Purpose adhesive system provides stronger bonds to both enamel and dentin when tooth surfaces remain visibly moist after etching. Dentinal bond strengths with Scotchbond were very high and consistent in this study, exceeding those of enamel bond.

▶ With the introduction of the fourth-generation bonding agents, there has been a change in attitude as related to how dry the surface of the prepared dentin should be. It was previously recommended that the surface of the dentin be as dry as possible. With the development of these newer dentin adhesive systems, however, it is now suggested that the surface should re-

Shear Bond Strengths of Scotchbond Multi-Purpose/Z100 to Dry and Moist Enamel and Dentin

Substrate	Condition	Bond strengths (MPa)			
		Mean	S.D.	High	Low
Enamel	Dry	14.2	2.3	17.5	10.6
Enamel	Moist	17.0	5.3	25.6	10.3
Dentin	Dry	17.8	5.4	28.0	7.8
Dentin	Moist	21.8	2.7	25.6	16.3

(Courtesy of Swift EJ Jr, Triolo PT Jr: *Am J Dent* 5:318–320, 1992.)

main slightly moist. The main reason for this is that after acid etching of the dentin, the exposed collagenous fibers will collapse on themselves if no moisture is present. Consequently, overdrying of the surface of the dentin before the application of the adhesive will result in a significantly reduced bond strength. It should be pointed out that there are limited exceptions to this rule. Consequently, the manufacturers' recommendations should be followed carefully.—K.F. Leinfelder, D.D.S., M.S.

Bonding of Enamel-Dentin Crown Fragments After Crown Fracture: An Experimental Study Using Bonding Agents
Andreasen FM, Steinhardt U, Bille M, Munksgaard EC (Univ of Copenhagen)
Endodont Dent Traumatol 9:111–114, 1993   105-94-13–30

Introduction.—Enamel-dentin crown fragments reattached with dentin bonding agents may achieve a fracture strength only 50% to 60% of the strength of intact teeth. Thus refracture, and the need for repeated bonding, occurs frequently. In this experimental study, researchers tested the strength of 2 newer bonding agents, All-Bond 2 and Scotchbond MP.

Methods.—The study used central and lateral incisors from sheep, with the testing machine used to evaluate the strength of the bond. The newer bonding agents and an older agent (Gluma) were used to reattach crown fragments to the remaining portion of the sheep incisors. The force in newtons at which the tooth was fractured was noted, and the fracture strength calculated in MPa using the actual area of the fracture surface of the experimental tooth.

Results.—The mean fracture strength of rebonded fractured incisors on loading at a speed of 1 mm/min ranged from 1.5 with Gluma and resin I (1 of 4 resins used with Gluma) to 6.8 with Scotchbond MP. Analysis of the results with Duncan's Multiple-Range tests revealed no significant differences between Gluma/resin III, Gluma/Danbond, All Bond 2, and Scotchbond MP. In a second study, fragments were bonded with Scotchbond MP and loaded at various speeds. Fracture strength was found to decrease exponentially with increased loading speed. The bonding resin was concluded to be the weak link in the bond between the tooth fragment and the remaining tooth structure.

Conclusion.—All Bond 2 and Scotchbond MP did not appear to improve fracture strength relative to the older bonding agents when used to attach crown fragments. Given the stress demands, resin bonding of fragments is a realistic treatment alternative to composite resin buildup.

▶ With the development of these newer and stronger adhesives, it has been possible to carry out a wider range of clinical operations. One interesting application of these systems has been the recementing and rebonding of fragmented portions of fractured teeth.—K.F. Leinfelder, D.D.S., M.S.

Endodontic Dowel Retention With Resinous Cements

Standlee JP, Caputo AA (Univ of California, Los Angeles)
J Prosthet Dent 68:913–917, 1992   105-94-13-31

Background.—Endodontic dowel designs are passive or active. Passive designs do not contact the channel wall; active designs mechanically engage the channel wall. Although active dowels are retentive, they can cause stresses during installation and functional loading (Fig 13-22). Recent research on cementation of endodontic dowels suggests that improvement may be possible by removing the smear layer in the prepared channel to permit the luting agent access to the dentinal tubules (Fig 13-23). The dislodgment resistance of 3 commercial dowel cementation systems that use micromechanical and adhesive methods was investigated.

Methods and Findings.—All systems studied incorporated some form of smear-layer removal on the dentin of the endodontic channel. The systems studied were the Unity Post regimen, the Boston Post regimen, and the C&B Metabond systems. The Unity regimen, which had a methyl ethyl ketone drying agent, provided inadequate clinical resistance to dislodgment (5.4 DaN). The Boston Post, a cementing system using only smear layer removal, was able to resist loads at 54.7 DaN. The C&B

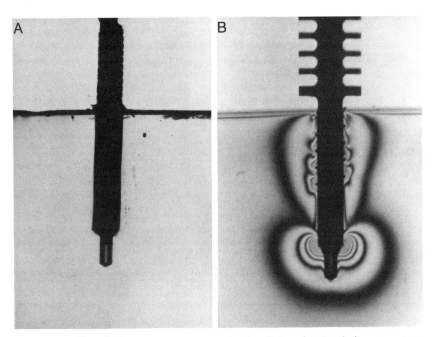

Fig 13–22.—Photoelastic stress patterns generated at installation of .060-inch diameter posts at 8-mm embedment depth. **A,** parallel-sided cemented dowel. **B,** parallel-sided threaded dowel in tapped channel. (Courtesy of Standlee JP, Caputo AA: *J Prosthet Dent* 68:913–917, 1992.)

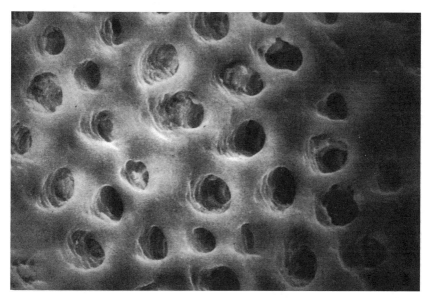

Fig 13–23.—Scanning electron micrograph of cut nonvital dentin without smear layer and tubules opened before placement of composite resin. (Courtesy of Standlee JP, Caputo AA: *J Prosthet Dent* 68:913-917, 1992.)

Metabond regimen included a surface-initiated dentinal adhesive and smear layer and had a retention of 77.4 DaN.

Conclusion.—Cementation of endodontic dowels with resins after removal of the smear layer can be one of the most retentive dowel systems. The Boston Post and C&B Metabond systems appear to be clinically promising.

▶ The composite resin type of cements or luting agents has become increasingly more popular. The reason for this is that they offer the potential for doing as much as other cements and even more. It is the only type of material, for example, that can be used in conjunction with a hybridizing technique. Most other cements depend primarily on mechanical retention rather than on bonding to the dental surface.—K.F. Leinfelder, D.D.S., M.S.

Compressive and Diametral Tensile Strengths of Current Adhesive Luting Agents
White SN, Yu Z (Univ of Southern California, Los Angeles)
J Prosthet Dent 69:568–572, 1993   105-94-13-32

Objective.—Because strength is a very important parameter in selecting a luting agent, compressive and diametral tensile strengths were com-

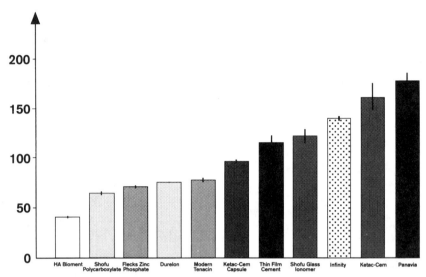

Fig 13–24.—Compressive strength means and standard errors in MPa ($n = 10$). (Courtesy of White SN, Yu Z: *J Prosthet Dent* 69:568–572, 1993.)

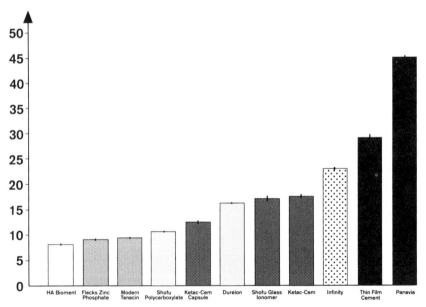

Fig 13–25.—Diametral tensile strength, menas, and standard errors in MPa ($n = 10$). (Courtesy of White SN, Yu Z: *J Prosthet Dent* 69:568–572, 1993.)

pared for 6 classes of new adhesive luting agents (ALAs), using zinc phosphate as a control. Eleven different materials were tested.

Results.—The highest compessive strength values were obtained for Panavia, Ketac-Cem, and Infinity (Fig 13–24). Two of these materials, Panavia and Infinity, were among the 3 with the highest diametral tensile strengths (Fig 13–25). On compessive strength testing, hydroxyapatite, zinc phosphate, and polycarboxylate fractured into a number of small fragments. Glass ionomer ALAs often fractured along their long axes into several large fragments. The composite resin materials usually did not form separate fragments, but circumferential rupture lines were noted.

Conclusion.—A number of ALAs based on composite resin and glass ionomer materials exhibit greater compressive and diametral tensile strength than do zinc phosphate cements.

▶ Compared with the conventional cements such as zinc phosphate and polycarboxylate, the resin cements are considerably stronger. When used in conjunction with the hybridizing process, these materials offer significantly higher retention values than do their predecessors. The use of the newer cements is very useful in solving the problems of loose crowns associated with short or extremely tapered preparations.—K.F. Leinfelder, D.D.S., M.S.

Call Mosby Document Express at **1 (800) 55-MOSBY** to obtain copies of the original source documents of articles featured or referenced in the YEAR BOOK series.

14 Restorative Dental Materials: Indirect Systems

Introduction

Glass ionomer continues to be an extremely popular material in the dental armamentarium. These agents have been improved to the point that they are now being used for a wide variety of purposes. At the present time, they are successfully being used as a luting agent for prosthetic appliances and orthodontic bands. The advantage to this particular system is that it provides fluoride ion release. These ions are then absorbed by the adjacent tooth structure. Consequently, it is anticipated that the caries rate will be considerably lower than that associated with other cements such as polycarboxylate and zinc phosphate. Glass ionomers are also being used as liners and bases in conjunction with composite resin and amalgam restorations, as core buildup materials, and for cementing endodontic post systems.

Perhaps the greatest advancement in glass ionomers came about with the introduction of the photo-cured technique. Such a condition allows the clinician ample working time for placing the glass ionomer. It also accelerates the setting time considerably. Maximum compressive strengths are attained within minutes, whereas in the conventional chemically cured systems, this property is not achieved for at least 24 hours.

Glass ionomers have become increasingly popular for a number of reasons. In addition to their ability to release fluoride into the adjacent dental surfaces, they tend to reduce or inhibit microleakage. Finally, release of the fluoride from the glass ionomer has been shown to be effective in reducing microbial activity.

As a result of the problems associated with the placement of posterior composite resins, esthetic inlays have been recommended. Because they can be created outside the oral cavity, there is better potential for generating the appropriate proximal contact and contour as well as for marginal adaptation. Recent clinical studies have demonstrated that inlays offer the potential for reducing secondary caries and, quite importantly, reduce the potential for postoperative sensitivity. Although it has been recommended that postcuring heat treatment will optimize the mechanical characteristics of the material, recent clinical studies have demonstrated that under most conditions the resistance to generalized wear is not enhanced appreciably. On the other hand, resistance to localized wear after the additional heat treatment can be increased considerably.

Perhaps one of the major problems associated with the esthetic inlay/onlay systems is that there has been very little information in the literature concerning critical interfacial gap dimensions. Recent clinical studies, however, demonstrate that once the interfacial gap on the occlusal surface exceeds 150 μ there is a significantly increased potential for secondary caries. These studies also demonstrate that the wear rate of the cement is linear during the first year and then tapers off so that no additional wear will occur. It is also interesting to note that the wear rate of the cement is dependent on particle size. The smaller the particle size, the greater the wear resistance. Therefore, cements exhibiting the greatest wear resistance are those that are either microfilled or those that contain particles that are submicron in size.

Karl F. Leinfelder, D.D.S., M.S.

Glass Ionomers

Release of Fluoride and Other Elements From Light-Cured Glass Ionomers in Neutral and Acidic Conditions

Forss H (Univ of Kuopio, Finland)
J Dent Res 72:1257–1262, 1993   105-94-14–1

Background.—A number of new light-cured glass-ionomer cements have been described for use as cavity liner and base materials. These cements are known to gradually erode in the oral environment, but it is not

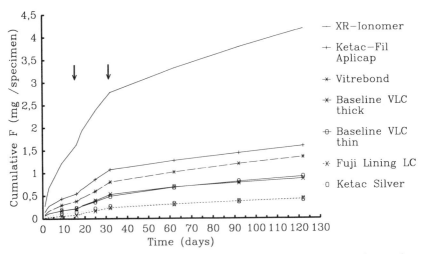

Fig 14–1.—The mean amounts of cumulative fluoride release in long-term immersion (*arrows* show the period of acidic immersion). (Courtesy of Forss H: *J Dent Res* 72:1257–1262, 1993.)

Mean Weight Change of the Specimens During Immersion

	32*		92		122	
Baseline VLC thick mix	+3.1†		+4.0		+6.1	
Baseline VLC thin mix	+6.8		+9.0		+12.2	
Fuji Lining LC	+1.4	A‡	+1.2	A	+3.6	
Vitrebond	-0.5	B	-1.6	B	+0.4	
XR-Ionomer	-0.4	BC	-2.3	B	-1.2	
Ketac-Fil Aplicap	+0.3	CD	+0.2	C	+1.4	A
Ketac-Silver	+0.8	AD	+0.9	AC	+1.4	A

* Immersion time (days).
† % Change of the original weight.
‡ Weight changes in groups marked with the same letter were not significantly different (*P* < .01).
(Courtesy of Forss H: *J Dent Res* 72:1257–1262, 1993.)

clear whether they are more susceptible to erosion than are conventional materials.

Study Design.—Five light-cured glass ionomers were compared with one another and with control materials with respect to the release of fluoride, sodium, silicon, calcium, strontium, and aluminum under neutral and acidic conditions. The materials included Baseline VLC thick mix, Baseline VLC thin mix, Fuji Lining LC, Vitrebond, and XR-Ionomer. The control materials were Ketac-Fil Aplicap, a conventional glass ionomer, and Ketac-Silver, a silver-reinforced glass ionomer. The specimens were stored for 16 days in deionized water; for 16 days longer in .01 mol/L lactic acid at pH 4; and finally in deionized water for up to 122 days.

Results.—The light-cured glass ionomers exhibited considerable variation in the release of fluoride (Fig 14–1) and other elements. All the cements eluted matrix-forming cations, aluminum, and calcium or strontium under acidic conditions. Weight gain was most marked for Baseline VLC (table).

Conclusion.—The new light-cured glass ionomer cements vary considerably in chemical composition and behavior, making it necessary to evaluate them from as many aspects as possible.

▶ At the present time, there are no fewer than 20 different brands of glass ionomers on the market. Furthermore, each company usually fabricates several types. Because fluoride release is one of the important characteristics of the glass ionomer, it is important to know which materials are most effective in this regard. A review of the literature reveals that there is a significant difference in the amount of fluoride release from one material to the next.—K.F. Leinfelder, D.D.S., M.S.

A Comparative Study of Three Glass Ionomer Base Materials

Burgess JO, Barghi N, Chan DCN, Hummert T (Univ of Texas Health Science Ctr, San Antonio)
Am J Dent 6:137–141, 1993   105-94-14-2

Introduction.—Visible light-cured (VLC) glass ionomer base materials have eliminated some of the handling problems encountered with chemically cured materials. Fluoride release by these materials is significantly greater than by conventional glass ionomer preparations.

Objective and Methods.—Three glass ionomer base materials, Fuji Lining LC, Vitrebond, and Ketac-Bond, were compared in vitro with respect to shear bond strengths to dentin and resin composite; compressive strength and modulus, diametral tensile strength; marginal gap; and fluoride release. The materials were applied to the facial surfaces of human molar teeth.

Results.—In general, the VLC base materials Vitrebond and Fuji LC outperformed the autopolymerizing glass ionomer base Ketac-Bond (Figs 14-2 to 14-5). Compressive modulus values were significantly less for the VLC materials. Fuji LC exhibited the highest diametral tensile strength and compressive strength, and it had the firmest bonds to dentin and composite resin. Fluoride release by Vitrebond was greater than the release by other materials. The marginal gap at the tooth/base interface was the least for Fuji LC.

Conclusion.—The VLC glass ionomer base materials are a significant advance compared with conventional chemically cured glass ionomer

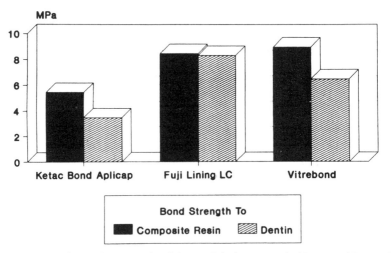

Fig 14–2.—Bond strength to enamel and dentin of the base materials. (Courtesy of Burgess JO, Barghi N, Chan DCN, et al: *Am J Dent* 6:137–141, 1993.)

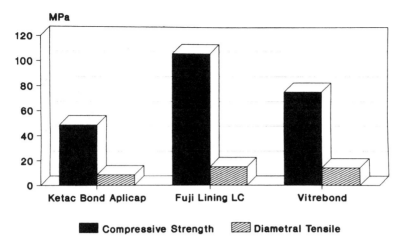

Fig 14–3.—Mechanical properties. Compressive and diametral tensile strength of the base materials. (Courtesy of Burgess JO, Barghi N, Chan DCN, et al: *Am J Dent* 6:137–141, 1993.)

materials. Their superior handling and mechanical properties make them preferable for clinical use.

▶ Because there are so many proprietary glass ionomers available to the clinician, it is obvious that there is also the potential for a wide variation in properties. For example, it has been demonstrated that the coefficient of thermal expansion associated with the light-cured glass ionomers is somewhat higher than that associated with the conventionally cured systems. However, this differential does not seem to have any clinically significant effect.—K.F. Leinfelder, D.D.S., M.S.

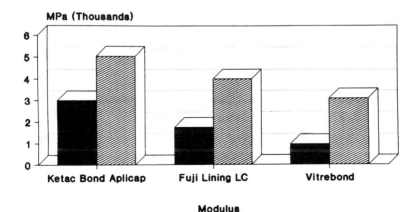

Fig 14–4.—Modulus. Compressive and diametral tensile strengths of the base materials. (Courtesy of Burgess JO, Barghi N, Chan DCN, et al: *Am J Dent* 6:137–141, 1993.)

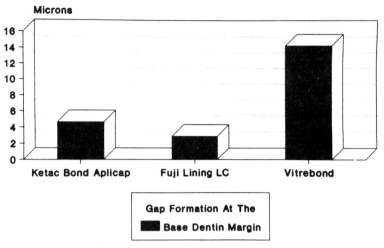

Fig 14–5.—Marginal gap formation of the base materials. (Courtesy of Burgess JO, Barghi N, Chan DCN, et al: *Am J Dent* 6:137–141, 1993.)

Marginal Leakage of Visible Light-Cured Glass Ionomer Restorative Materials

Crim GA (Univ of Louisville, Ky)
J Prosthet Dent 69:561–563, 1993   105-94-14-3

Introduction.—Glass-ionomer cements, introduced during the 1970s, have many advantages as a restorative material. Negative characteristics of these cements, however, have included prolonged setting time, sensitivity to moisture during initial hardening, dehydration, rough surface texture, and opaqueness. Two recently developed visible light–cured (VLC) glass ionomer materials have overcome some of these problems. The sealing of 2 VLC glass ionomer restorative materials and a conventional glass ionomer was examined.

Methods.—Extracted human molar teeth were divided into groups and class V cavity preparations were completed at the cementoenamel junction on the facial and lingual surfaces. Cavity preparations were restored with VariGlass VLC, GC Fuji II LC, or GC Fuji II glass ionomer cements. When enamel crazing was found to occur with VariGlass glass ionomer cement, 2 additional groups of 3 teeth each were added to determine whether a different technique would result in less crazing. In the first group, the enamel margin was not etched before the primer was applied; in the second group, a short enamel bevel (.5 mm to .75 mm) was placed with a no. 170 bur before the cavity preparation was restored.

Results.—None of the specimens showed measurable leakage at the restoration/preparation interface, enamel, or dentin. Six of the VariGlass ionomer cement specimens had staining of the enamel adjacent to the restoration. In each case, microleakage penetrated the crazed enamel and progressed to the dentoenamel junction. The crazing was eliminated by addition of an enamel bevel.

Conclusion.—VariGlass VLC and Fuji II LC glass ionomer cements both controlled microleakage in these extracted teeth. With VariGlass, however, cavity preparation with an enamel bevel may be needed to minimize enamel crazing.

▶ A basic advantage of the glass ionomers is that they tend to inhibit, or at least substantially reduce, microleakage between the material and the adjacent tooth structure. This reduction in microleakage, of course, can be related to similarities in coefficient of thermal expansion. It should be pointed out that the thermal expansion of the photo-cured systems is somewhat higher and therefore may undergo a higher degree of leakage. This difference, however, may not be clinically significant because both systems effectively release fluoride ions that in turn tend to discourage microbial growth.—K.F. Leinfelder, D.D.S., M.S.

The Effect of Dentine Conditioning With Polyacrylic Acid on the Clinical Performance of Glass Ionomer Cement
Tyas MJ (Univ of Melbourne, Australia)
Aust Dent J 38:46–48, 1993   105-94-14–4

Introduction.—Although many manufacturers of glass-ionomer cements recommend that dentine surfaces be pretreated with polyacrylic acid (PAA) to enhance bond strength, there is no evidence that such conditioning improves the long-term clinical performance of glass ionomer cements. Restorations using PAA conditioning were compared with those in which the pretreatment was not used.

Methods.—Forty caries-free class V abrasion lesions in 15 patients were selected for restoration. All lesions were cleaned for a few seconds with pumice and water on a rubber cup; 20 were then lightly scrubbed with Ketac Conditioner (25% PAA) for about 10 seconds. Ketac-Fil GIC was used for the restoration. All patients received at least 1 PAA restoration and 1 non-PAA restoration. The restorations were photographed at baseline and after 1 year.

Results.—At 1-year follow-up, all restorations placed with PAA conditioning were present. One non-PAA restoration was partially lost. The mean marginal staining score at 1 year was .26 for PAA-conditioned restorations and .55 for non-PAA restorations, a difference that was not statistically significant. Marginal staining was not clinically significant in any of the restorations.

Conclusion.—After 1 year, no difference was found in terms of retention rates or marginal staining in GIC restorations of class V abrasion lesions pretreated with PAA and those cleaned with pumice and water alone.

▶ A number of efforts have been made to make the glass ionomer more adhesive to the surface of the dentin. It has been shown that because glass ionomers are basically hydrophilic in nature, they tend to bond better to a surface that is slightly moist rather than one that is perfectly dry. It should also be pointed out, however, that glass ionomers bond better to the surface of the dentin if the smear layer has been removed. This is of particular significance when dealing with abfracted or cervically eroded lesions.—K.F. Leinfelder, D.D.S., M.S.

Glass-Ionomer–Silver-Cermet Interim Class I Restorations for Permanent Teeth
Croll TP, Killian CM (Doylestown, Pa)
Quintessence Int 23:731–733, 1992   105-94-14–5

Introduction.—Since 1985, Ketac-Silver, a glass-ionomer–silver-cermet cement, has been used as an interim restorative material for partly erupted permanent first and second molars with caries. These lesions are frequent in the permanent first molars of children aged 5 to 8 years and in the second molars at ages 10 to 14 years. In addition to providing longer-lasting results compared with zinc oxide-eugenol, cermet material can be cut down and left in place as a dentinal replacement.

Technique.—After removing caries with appropriate burs, a cavity is prepared as it would be for a silver amalgam restoration, except that the internal line angles do not have to be sharp. The preparation is not extended into noncarious grooves. The smear layer is removed with polyacrylic acid before injecting Ketac-Silver into the cavity preparation using a Centrix syringe. The preparation is overfilled and, after hardening, the excess is removed. Varnish or resin glaze do not have to be applied to the cement surface.

Results.—These restorations have held up well for as long as 6 years in primary teeth in non–stress-bearing areas. Cermet cement performs similarly well in class I preparations of permanent teeth and in primary teeth.

▶ Metals such as pure silver or silver alloys have been added to glass ionomer for the purpose of enhancing its radiopacity as well as its strength. The gray appearance of these agents makes it possible to differentiate between the core material and the tooth. It should be pointed out that although the compressive strength of the metal-filled glass ionomer may be somewhat higher than conventional glass ionomers, there may be a tendency toward a reduction in fluoride release.—K.F. Leinfelder, D.D.S., M.S.

A Comparison of the Shear Bond Strengths to a Resin Composite of Two Conventional and Two Resin-Modified Glass Polyalkenoate (Ionomer) Cements

Chadwick RG, Woolford MJ (The Dental School, Dundee, Scotland)
J Dent 21:111–116, 1993   105-94-14–6

Objective.—Resin composite does not bond directly to dentine, which has limited its clinical usefulness. The so-called laminate technique, in which glass polyalkenoate cement is placed on the dentine and covered with a resin composite, may be useful in dealing with this problem. In addition to dentinal adherence, the cement also provides micromechanical attachment to the composite. Resin-modified glass polyalkenoate cements (RMCs) may now make it possible to chemically unite the cement and the composite.

Methods.—The shear bonding strength of P-50 resin composite to 4 different glass polyalkenoate bonding materials was evaluated. Half of the specimens were prepared with and half without the use of Scotchbond 2 intermediate bonding agent. The cements tested included 2 RMCs (Vitrebond and XR-Ionomer) and 2 conventional base materials (Baseline and Ketac-Bond).

Results.—The strongest and most consistent bond existed between P-50 and Vitrebond. This was true regardless of the presence of Scotchbond 2. The bonding strength of all 3 of the other materials was increased significantly with Scotchbond 2. For some unknown reason, adhesive failure was much more common than cohesive failure with Vitrebond, with and without Scotchbond 2 (table).

Breakdown of Specimen Failure Mechanisms		
Mode of failure material	*Adhesive failures (no.)*	*Cohesive failures (no.)*
BL/P50	30	0
BL/SB2/P50	13	16
KB/P50	17	0
KB/SB2/P50	26	2
VB/P50	0	30
VB/SB2/P50	29	1
XR/P50	18	11
XR/SB2/P50	4	25

(Courtesy of Chadwick RG, Woolford MJ: *J Dent* 21:111–116, 1992.)

Conclusion.—These results show a stronger and more dependable bond between Vitrebond and P-50 composite resin than with the other materials studied, regardless of whether an intermediate bonding agent is used. When conventional glass polyalkenoate cements are used, an effective intermediate bonding agent should always be used as well.

▶ As a rule, the bond strength between the composite resin and the glass ionomer is less than that between the glass ionomer and tooth structure, particularly in the case of the photo-cured systems. The bond strength of the composite resin to the glass ionomer is strictly a mechanical one and normally does not exceed 500 psi (3 MPa). It is probable that the bond strength between the composite resin and the glass ionomer depends on the type of ionomer investigated. As a rule, those that are photo-cured should exhibit a higher bond strength than those that are conventionally chemically cured or set. This study demonstrates that the bond strength of the composite resin to the glass ionomer can be improved if a bonding agent is used.—K.F. Leinfelder, D.D.S., M.S.

The Short-Term Fluoride Release of a Hand-Mixed vs. Capsulated System of a Restorative Glass-Ionomer Cement

Verbeeck RMH, De Moor RJG, Van Even DFJ, Martens LC (Univ of Gent, Krijgslaan, Belgium; Univ of Gent, De Pintelaan, Belgium)
J Dent Res 72:577–581, 1993   105-94-14–7

Introduction.—The use of glass-ionomer cements has increased in dental operations and in some types of restorations because of the materials' ability to adhere to both dentin and enamel and to produce long-term fluoride release. The variability in fluoride release by a glass-ionomer cement capsular system was compared with that from a hand-mixed system.

Methods.—Fuji II glass-ionomer cement restorative filling material was used in powder/liquid and capsule forms. Five operators prepared 5 disks of each type of glass-ionomer cement filling. After 1, 2, 3, 7, and 14 days from equilibrium, the disk was moved from 1 liquid to another for continued equilibration, with the equilibration fluid analyzed for fluoride by ion chromatography.

Results.—The variances found in fluoride release with time appeared homogeneous. Only the mean fluoride release after 3 days for the Fuji II glass-ionomer cement samples differed significantly from the other measured mean values for samples of the other operators. Because of this lack of variability, the fluoride release values were pooled for both Fuji II and Fuji Cap II materials. A regression analysis of the data indicated no variability in fluoride release values. The Fuji Cap II demonstrated significantly higher cumulative fluoride release than Fuji II material.

Conclusion.—The mixing process for glass-ionomer cement for dental restorations dramatically alters the short- and long-term release of fluoride. The reason for this mixing effect on fluoride release requires further study.

▶ Although never documented through clinical studies, it is generally accepted that the fluoride release from glass ionomers is effective in resisting secondary caries. Studies have shown, however, that the fluoride release is very effective in inhibiting microbial activity. Assuming that the fluoride release from the glass ionomer is an important function, one must select the cement and method of handling that will provide the optimum condition.—K.F. Leinfelder, D.D.S., M.S.

The Tunnel Restoration: Nine Years of Clinical Experience Using Capsulated Glass Ionomer Cements. Case Report
Knight GM (Brighton, Victoria, Australia)
Aust Dent J 37:245–251, 1992   105-94-14–8

Background.—The tunnel restoration was introduced several years ago as a conservative alternative to the conventional class II preparation for initial carious lesions. Since then, the method has been modified to incorporate a composite overlay on the occlusal surface. Evidence suggests that the technique is a viable restorative procedure. A 9-year experience with the tunnel restoration using capsulated glass ionomer cements was reviewed, and a case was reported.

Technique.—A young adult was treated using the modified "T" tunnel restoration for mesial caries on tooth 16. Rubber dam was applied to control moisture, and the broken-down amalgam on the occlusal surface was removed. Using a cylindrical diamond bur, the cavity was prepared to the width of the marginal ridge parallel to and about 2 mm from the margin. The central fissure was removed to form the neck of the T. Carious dentine was removed with a bur and small excabators accessing the lesion at each "T" extension. The smear layer was removed with a weak acid solution, and the preparation was washed and dried. A matrix band was then placed and firmly wedged. Capsulated Ketac-Bond, a type III glass ionomer cement, was used to restore the tooth to the level of the dentino-enamel junction on the occlusal surface. When the glass ionomer cement became gelatinous, it was further compacted with a ball burnisher to eliminate voids and maximize the integrity of the proximal margin. Excess glass ionomer cement was trimmed, and the cement was removed to the depth of the dentino-enamel junction. The glass ionomer and enamel were then etched with 37% phosphoric acid for 15 seconds. Enamel bond was brushed over the occlusal and interproximal surface. A small increment of posterior composite resin was put into the preparation, spread thinly, and light-cured for 20 seconds. Later, another increment of posterior composite was placed to fill the preparation and cured for 40 seconds. The restoration was then contoured.

Conclusion.—The tunnel restoration technique appears to provide a viable long-term restoration that has many benefits over a conventional class II preparation for the initial lesion. Continuing improvements in dental materials will enable further advancements in the strength and predictability of this method.

▶ Although the concept of the tunnel preparation has been available to the dental profession for at least 10 years, very little information related to clinical performance has been presented in the literature. As a result, there has been relatively little interest in this particular concept. It now appears, however, on the basis of recent clinical studies that there is enough information available to defend this treatment modality.—K.F. Leinfelder, D.D.S., M.S.

Effect of Mixing Speed on Mechanical Properties of Encapsulated Glass-Ionomer Cements
Gee D, Pearson GJ (Inst of Dental Surgery, London)
Br Dent J 174:65–68, 1993   105-94-14–9

Introduction.—Glass-ionomer cements have become the material of choice for dentists performing esthetic restorations. Studies indicate that the strength of encapsulated glass-ionomer cements depends on the speed of mixing in a mechanical vibrator. The variations in the mixing speeds must consider the setting time and short- and long-term mechanical properties of these materials.

Methods.—Three encapsulated glass-ionomer cements were evaluated to determine the effects of 4 different mixing speeds on the working and setting times and the compressive strength measures at 24 hours and 7 days. The weights of the powder and the liquid in the capsules were measured by disassembling the capsules.

Results.—The working and setting times did not change with the different mixing speeds. The Opusfil brand demonstrated the longest setting time, and the Ketac-fil type had the shortest setting time. The Opusfil and Chemfil brands showed a slight rise in compressive strength at 24 hours, but the Ketac-fil brand had a significant increase in strength after 1 day. No consistent strength differences occurred after 7 days. The greatest differences in the powder/liquid ratio occurred with the Opusfil capsules, which demonstrated an 11.6% underfill. The Chemfil II brand showed a 6% overfill.

Conclusion.—Varying the mixing speed does not appear to alter the outcome of encapsulated glass-ionomer cements for either early or extended compressive strength. However, some differences in compressive strength occurred in 2 of the encapsulated materials, suggesting that changes in the materials occur when trying to obtain a satisfactory encapsulation mix. These alterations in the composition of the materials may decrease the strength of the hand-mixed substances.

▶ A review of the literature indicates that variations in trituration time can have a significant effect on the setting time of dental amalgam. Spherical particle amalgams, however, are less affected. Until recently, there was no information available about mixing time on the compressive strength and setting time of glass ionomers. On the basis of this study, it appears that the compressive strength and setting time of the glass ionomers are relatively unaffected by changes in mixing time. All of this work was done using pre-measured capsulated mixes of glass ionomer.—K.F. Leinfelder, D.D.S., M.S.

Sealing Effectiveness of Light-Cured Glass Ionomer Cement Liners
Sidhu SK (Natl Univ of Singapore)
J Prosthet Dent 68:891–894, 1992   105-94-14–10

Introduction.—A goal of restorative dentistry is to control intraoral marginal leakage around the cavity walls and interfacial gaps. The microleakage largely depends on the type of restorative material used. Glass-ionomer cements harden quickly, adhering to the enamel and dentin. The dentin bonding and microleakage of 2 light-cured glass-ionomer lining materials were measured.

Methods.—Extracted teeth with a gingival cavosurface margin of dentin served as the base for wedge-shaped cervical cavities. They were randomly assigned to 3 groups: 2 experimental groups filled with 2 light-cured glass-ionomer cements and a control group cured chemically. Thermocycling and dye immersion methods produced a level of dye penetration, which became the final measure of microleakage from the gingival cavosurface margin to the base of the cavity preparation.

Results.—The specimen teeth in the experimental groups demonstrated some leakage from the gingival areas, but the control specimens did not. A comparison of the 3 groups found a significant difference for the microleakage. The microleakage levels appeared similar before and after the thermocycling, but further analysis of the data indicated a significant difference between the 2 experimental groups and the control teeth; however, the 2 experimental groups did not differ significantly from each other.

Conclusion.—Although glass-ionomer cements produce good restorations, the creation of a hermetic seal with this material can be a problem because incomplete seals occur in cervical wedge-type cavities. Light-cured glass-ionomer liners bonded to the dentin, but this bond was slightly disrupted at times.

▶ Light-cured glass ionomers have a greater potential for bonding to the dentin than conventional chemically cured glass ionomers. However, any potential advantage of one over the other may be offset by the difference in coefficient of thermal expansion. From a clinical point of view, it is probable that neither of these have any clinically significant effect when used as an intermediate material underneath the restoration. However, in the case of abfracted or cervically eroded lesions, it is suggested that the photo-cured glass ionomer be considered because of its greater potential for bonding to the dentinal subsurface.—K.F. Leinfelder, D.D.S., M.S.

Prosthetic Materials

A New All-Ceramic Crown: A Dense-Sintered, High-Purity Alumina Coping With Porcelain

Andersson M, Adén A (Univ of Umeå, Sweden; Karolinska Inst, Huddinge, Sweden)
Acta Odontol Scand 51:59–64, 1993   105-94-14-11

Introduction.—Dental ceramic materials are increasingly used for both anterior and posterior restorations as esthetics become a more important consideration. In alumina-reinforced dental porcelain, feldspathic porcelain is strengthened by dispersed crystals of high-strength alumina in the feldspathic matrix. Highly pure alumina is biocompatible and has served as an implant material for nearly 3 decades.

Objective.—A new technique for making an individual all-ceramic crown combined a coping of dense-sintered, high-purity alumina with dental porcelain. The microstructural studies were used to evaluate this product.

Findings.—During sintering, the alumina particles form a grain-like structure in which crystalline planes are clearly evident. The mean grain size of dense-sintered alumina, estimated from polished and thermal-etched cross-sections of sintered copings, was 4 μm. The phase boundary between the dense-sintered alumina and porcelain lacked pores and other defects. The density of the sintered copings was 3.9 μm, and the measured flexural strength was 601 MPa.

Conclusion.—This method makes it possible to produce individual dental copings from biocompatible implant material. The density, grain size, and flexural strength of the alumina are within the limits of requirements in ISO 6474-1981 "Implants for surgery, ceramic materials based on alumina."

▶ Never before has the dental profession witnessed so many different types of porcelain for use in practice. The materials available today are considerably better than they were just 10 years ago. For example, some of the porcelains no longer contain quartz, containing instead a softer material that reduces the potential for scratching of the antagonistic enamel cusp. Other materials may be castable, such as Dicor, and others are injectable. The Empress system is a good example of this type. Recently, there has been a trend toward restoring anterior teeth with all ceramic crown restorations. The advantage to these new systems is that they are more natural looking than are the conventional porcelain-fused-to-metal type, which have a tendency to be somewhat opaque.—K.F. Leinfelder, D.D.S., M.S.

Recent Developments in Restorative Dental Ceramics

Anusavice KJ (Univ of Florida, Gainesville)
J Am Dent Assoc 124(2):72–84, 1993   105-94-14–12

Introduction.—Dental ceramics come in varied types for use in (porcelain-fused-to-metal (PFM) restorations. All-ceramic crowns continue to have less strength than PFM crowns. The important advances in dental ceramic materials during the past 2 decades were reviewed.

Discussion.—Porcelain-fused-to-metal restorations first appeared in 1962 when patents were awarded for a gold alloy formulation and feldspathic porcelain to ensure adequate bonding. The Rochette bridge, a large-holed metal or PFM prosthesis, appeared in 1973 but had a bonding failure rate of 52%. The initial failure rate decreased when a Ni-Cr alloy was used. The newer resin-bonded prostheses usually fail because of design, judgment, and manipulation errors. In 1974, dentists began to use more economical Au-Pd-Ag and Pd-Ag alloys. The PFM restorations became more esthetic in the 1980s because of thinner Ni-Cr and Ni-Cr-Be copings and the introduction of the PFM crown with a porcelain margin. Biocompatible pure titanium then followed as a coping and framework metal for these restorations. The longevity of the various restorations and crown types depends on the materials used, with glass-ceramics representing a late development. High-strength feldspathic ceramic and alumina core ceramic continue to promote the esthetic appearance and increase the strength of restorations.

Conclusion.—The material and techniques used influence the success of ceramic and PFM restorations. New materials continue to promote esthetic outcome and strength.

▶ Since the introduction of the porcelain jacket crown in the early 1900s, the materials and the systems by which they are fabricated have been modified so substantially that they have the same inherent esthetic properties of natural enamel. Although in the past it has been difficult to establish exacting margins, some of the newer ceramic systems replicate detail so well that interfacial gaps of 15 to 20 μ are becoming the norm. It is anticipated that in the not-too-distant future all-ceramic crowns will be a substitute for the conventional PFM restoration.—K.F. Leinfelder, D.D.S., M.S.

The Practical Dental CAD/CAM in 1993

Duret F (Univ of Southern California, Los Angeles)
J Can Dent Assoc 59:445–453, 1993   105-94-14–13

The Concept.—The so-called CAD/CAM systems, available for the past 3 years, are able to produce dental prostheses with robots or computers. The systems use palpation devices or cameras to make impressions. Then they either transmit the data to directly produce the die, the counter die, or some intermediate elements, or they use the computer to reconstruct the prosthesis on a monitor. The CAD/CAM systems are based on the premise that the data, or impression, from the patient's mouth are digitized as rapidly as possible. In this way, most, if not all, of the hazards associated with using material impressions to collect data are avoided. Reproducing the patient's mouth using CAD/CAM rests on a known volume depicted on a computer monitor rather than on a plaster or wax model.

Existing Systems.—The Celay system, not intended as a CAD/CAM system, is geared toward robotization. It consists of 1 unit that palpates a piece to read all its surfaces and another that manufactures it in a ceramic block by following the manual motion of the sensor. The Procera system is a more complex version of the Celay system that combines pantographic reproduction with electro-erosion manufacturing to produce titanium crowns for ceramic coating. The DCS Titan system digitizes data which are fed into a computer to guide the manufacturing unit. The Cerec system is an optical impression technique which models line by line using isoplans, rather than on surface, to manufacture the internal elements of ceramic inlays, onlays, or facets. The Sopha Dental CAD/CAM system involves optical impression-taking, surface construction and modeling of the future prosthesis, and manufacturing using a numerically controlled machine tool.

Systems in Development.—The Cicero system, based on the Sopha CAD/CAM system, produces a special die from data recorded by a laser-driven optical sensor moving along the margins. The Dens system consists of a very fast optical sensor and a device that can work titanium.

▶ Undoubtedly, the introduction of the CAD/CAM system for electronically designing and mechanically milling porcelain restorations represented one of the major breakthroughs for clinical dentistry. Although several systems have been introduced, it is anticipated that many more will follow. Each system brings about improvement for the clinician and a promise for even better results. Presently, however, CAD/CAM systems are now are being used for the purpose of successfully restoring teeth with inlays/onlays and veneers. Long-term clinical studies have demonstrated that restorations placed by this technique are highly acceptable. During a 4-year period, for example, none of the restored teeth exhibited any secondary caries.—K.F. Leinfelder, D.D.S., M.S.

An Analysis of Multiple Failures of Resin-Bonded Bridges
Creugers NHJ, Käyser AF (Univ of Nijmegen, The Netherlands; TRIKON Inst for Dental Research, Nijmegen, The Netherlands)
J Dent 20:348–351, 1992   105-94-14–14

Introduction.—Several recent reports suggest that resin-bonded bridges are clinically effective, but a substantial number of failures continue to occur. A 7.5-year follow-up of 203 resin-bonded bridges (RBBs) identified the variables that influence their survival.

Methods.—Sixty-two dislodged and rebonded RBBs were included in the study. Thirty-two bridges that dislodged a second time were replaced by another type of RBB. The cementation materials used were Clearfil F, Panavia Ex, Silar, and Conclude. The bridges were a combination of nonprecious metal and acrylic resin. Five dentists provided the bridges, which replaced 1 or 2 missing teeth. In all cases, 2 abutment teeth were used for retention. Anterior teeth were replaced by 166 RBBs and posterior teeth by 37.

Results.—Rebonded bridges survived less well than those that were originally bonded. Original RBBs that failed within 1 year of placement were more than twice as likely to fail again, compared with those failing more than 1 year after placement. Rebonded RBBs had a median survival of 2.1 years. More than 40% of dislodgements of original RBBs were total failures, and RBBs that had failed a number of times had a median survival of only 1 year.

Implications.—It seems wise to rebond failed RBBs, because the procedure is relatively easy and inexpensive. After multiple failures, a new RBB is warranted only if clear design improvements are possible. These findings may not apply to designs that entail relatively extensive tooth preparation.

▶ Ten years ago, the Maryland Bridge was considered to be a major breakthrough in the area of fixed prosthetics. However, as time went on it became evident that these bridges were subject to failure. It has now been determined that the techniques associated with their use need to be somewhat more detailed than had previously been thought. However, now that many of the problems associated with the clinical techniques have been resolved, the retention rate and clinical success have been much higher.—K.F. Leinfelder, D.D.S., M.S.

The Effect of Finish Line Form and Luting Agent on the Breaking Strength of Dicor Crowns

Bernal G, Jones RM, Brown DT, Munoz CA, Goodacre CJ (Indiana Univ, Indianapolis)
Int J Prosthodont 6:286–290, 1993   105-94-14–15

Objectives.—Selection of a luting agent influences the strength of all-ceramic restorations, as do restoration and tooth precementation procedures. Whether different luting agents produce varying all-ceramic restoration strengths, and whether the use of resin cement and related bonding procedures counteracts the negative effect of some finishing line designs was determined.

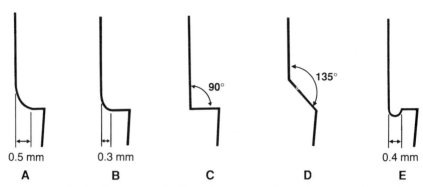

Fig 14–6.—Finishing line forms: **A,** shoulder with a .5-mm rounding of the axiogingival line angle; **B,** shoulder with a .3-mm rounding of the axiogingival line angle; **C,** shoulder with a 90-degree axiogingival line angle; **D,** shoulder with a 135-degree cervical slope and sharp axiogingival line angle; **E,** shoulder with a .4 mm wide axiogingival groove. (Courtesy of Bernal G, Jones RM, Brown DT, et al: *Int J Prosthodont* 6:286–290, 1993.)

Methods.—Five different finish line forms were used in preparing human maxillay first molars (Fig 14–6). All preparations had a total occlusal convergence angle of 10 degrees and a finish line depth of 1.2 mm. Dicor crowns were luted using zinc phosphate, glass-ionomer, and resin cements. The crowns were thermocycled and subjected to fracture loading.

Results.—Restorations luted with visible light-activated resin cement were significantly stronger than those luted with glass-ionomer or zinc phosphate cement. No differences in strength were evident between the various finish line designs when light-activated resin cement and associated bonding procedures were used (table).

Effect of Finish Line on Restoration Strength ($n = 15$)

Group*	Finish line, axiogingival line angle form	Cement *	Breaking strength (kg)	SD
D	135-degree cervical slope, sharp axiogingival line angle	VLAR	148.47	21.11
C	90-degree shoulder, sharp axiogingival line angle	VLAR	145.20	21.50
B	Shoulder with 0.3 mm of axiogingival rounding	VLAR	142.73	21.68
E	Shoulder with axiogingival groove	VLAR	141.00	26.56
A	Shoulder with 0.5 mm of axiogingival rounding	VLAR	129.13	29.57

Note: Groups designated in accordance with **Figure 14–6,** listed in decreasing order of restoration strength.
* Visible light-activated resin, VLAR.
Values connected by vertical line are not significantly different at the 95% confidence level (Newman-Keul's test).
(Courtesy of Bernal G, Jones RM, Brown DT, et al: *Int J Prosthodont* 6:286–290, 1993.)

Conclusion.—The use of resin cement or associated procedures appears able to counteract the negative effect of a sloping finish line.

▶ The traditional method for cementing porcelain crowns has been by means of zinc phosphate or polycarboxylate cement. Because of the ability for bonding to dentin, the composite resin luting agents have recently grown in popularity. Using this system, it is possible to hybridize the dentin, thereby decreasing the potential for microbial invasion and postoperative sensitivity. Also, the retentive value of the crown can be enhanced significantly. At least one recent study (1) has demonstrated that the resin cement in conjunction with the hybridizing process increases the retention rate 3.5 times that associated with zinc phosphate cement.—K.F. Leinfelder, D.D.S., M.S.

Reference

1. Sadig WM: *Evaluation of enhancing crown retention using resin cement and silicoating (MSC Thesis).* University of Alabama, 1992.

Effect of Fluoride Prophylactic Agents on Titanium Surfaces
Pröbster L, Lin W, Hüttemann H (Eberhard-Karls-Univ, Tübingen, Germany)
Int J Oral Maxillofac Implants 7:390–394, 1992   105-94-14–16

Background.—Titanium, the material of choice for dental implants, is quickly becoming the material of choice for conventional restorative procedures as well. Endosseous titanium implants are usually treated with a fluoride solution before they are placed in the bone cavity. It has been reported that this treatment results in a blue discoloration of the titanium surface. Titanium surface changes resulting from commonly used prophylactic fluids and gels containing fluorides were described.

Methods and Findings.—Titanium specimens were cast and subjected to several fluoride agents. Fluocal, Oral B mouthrinse, Elmex fluid, Blendamed Fluor-Gel, and Duraphat lacquer caused no visible changes in titanium surfaces. Although no change was visible at 1 minute after treatment with Elmex gelee, increasing gloss reduction was observed later. Septogel and Oral B Fluor-Gel resulted in severe surface changes appearing after 1 minute as dull gray spots where drops were placed. One percent hydrofluoric acid produced a severe etching effect after 1 minute. One percent phosphoric acid had no destructive effect on the titanium surface. None of the substances tested left a blue coloration of the titanium surfaces. Profilometry showed that surface roughness was significantly increased with exposure time to Septogel, Oral B Fluor-Gel, and hydrofluoric acid. Scanning electron microscopy further demonstrated the corrosive effects of the acidic agents. Elmex gelee was increasingly destructive, with pitting corrosion visible after 5 minutes of exposure. Septogel and Oral B Fluor-Gel had severe destructive effects on polished titanium surfaces. An implant stored for 24 hours in Oral B gel had massive corrosion.

Conclusion.—Titanium, which is well known for its corrosion resistance, cannot withstand the effects of certain acidic fluoride prophylactic agents. When using fluoride preparations in patients with titanium implants or restorations, clinicians must examine the effects of the agent on titanium to prevent restoration damage.

▶ Although titanium has become a very important element for the fabrication of implant material, it has become obvious through clinical studies and clinical experience that scratching of its surface will cause an accelerated corrosion process. Consequently, many clinicians are now using specially designed instruments for scaling and cleaning the surfaces of the titanium implant. It has also been demonstrated that acidic fluoride prophylactic agents have undesirable effects on the surface of the titanium.—K.F. Leinfelder, D.D.S., M.S.

Evaluation of Tin Plating Systems for a High-Noble Alloy
Imbery TA, Davis RD (Plattsburgh AFB, NY; Osan AFB, Korea)
Int J Prosthodont 6:55–59, 1993   105-94-14–17

Introduction.—In contrast to the bond between Panavia EX and base-metal alloys, the bonding of the material to noble alloys is significantly enhanced by tin plating.

Objective and Methods.—The tensile bond strength of Panavia EX to a high-noble alloy prepared by abrasive spraying and 1 of 2 tin-plating systems was measured. Disk-shaped specimens were cast in type III gold, abrasive-sprayed with aluminum oxide, and then tin plated using either a Kura Acte Mini unit or a Micro Tin unit. Control specimens were not plated. Disks within each group were luted to one another with Panavia EX. The specimens then were thermocycled and tested in tension.

Results.—There were no significant differences in strength between the tin-plated groups, but each luting bond was significantly stronger than in control specimens. The Micro Tin plating unit produced solitary spheres of tin on the alloy surface while preserving the basic surface contour. The Kura Ace Mini unit produced dendritic crystal growth that covered the abraded surface.

Conclusion.—Tin plating of a noble alloy significantly enhances the tensile bond to Panavia EX resin, compared with abrasive spraying with aluminum oxide alone.

▶ It is commonly known that the adhesion of resin to the surface of metal can be enhanced significantly by sandblasting the metal surface. However, after a period of time, the bond strength drops dramatically. This reduction in bond strength can be attributed to the ability of water to penetrate the interfacial regions. Consequently, sandblasting by itself does not have a long-term clinical effect on the bonding of resins to metals when used as the only technique. It has been known for a considerable period, however, that tin plating of gold alloys increases the bond strength considerably. By fusing into the surface of the gold, the outgrowing crystals of tin act as a lock to bond the resin to its surface mechanically.—K.F. Leinfelder, D.D.S., M.S.

Comparison of the Adhesive Strength of a BIS-GMA Cement to Tin-Plated and Non–Tin-Plated Alloys
Gates WD, Diaz-Arnold AM, Aquilino SA, Ryther JS (Univ of North Carolina, Chapel Hill; Univ of Iowa, Iowa City)
J Prosthet Dent 69:12–16, 1993   105-94-14–18

Objective.—Investigators compared the bond strength of a single Bis-GMA adhesive cement with 4 different alloys for restorations of porcelain fused to metal. Two alloys were predominantly base metal, the third was a noble alloy, and the fourth was a high noble alloy. The noble and high noble alloys were tested with and without tin plating with the use of 2 different tin platers.

Methods.—Cylinders of the 4 alloys were bonded end to end with the adhesive cement and thermocycled for 24 hours. Panavia Op, the Bis-GMA resinous cement, was mixed according to the manufacturer's instructions and placed on the prepared surface of each cylinder. After storage in distilled water for 27 days, a testing machine was used to evaluate the tensile bond strength of the alloys.

Results.—The lowest mean tensile bond strengths were recorded with the noble alloy specimens; the remaining groups showed no statistically significant differences. The greatest mean tensile bond strength (45.95 MPa) occurred with the cobalt-chromium alloy. The lowest mean tensile bond strength of the tin-plated samples (37.33 MPa) was seen in the palladium noble alloy with the Micro Tin tin plater. Macroscopic examination showed failure of the bond in an adhesive-cohesive mode in the nickel-chromium-beryllium and cobalt-chromium specimens. Adhesive failures were noted in the non–tin-plated Olympia and PTM-88 specimens. Failures in the tin-plated specimens appeared similar to those of the nickle-chromium-beryllium and cobalt-chromium alloys.

Conclusion.—The most difficult variable to control was the consistency of the mixture of cement. This factor could be the primary cause of the range of tensile strengths. Nevertheless, the mean tensile bond strength of non–tin-plated noble and high noble alloys was significantly lower than both the tin-plated noble and high noble alloys and the non–tin-plated base metal alloys. There were no significant differences in mean tensile bond strength for tin-plated alloys and base metal alloys or for different tin platers.

▶ Bonding resins to the surface of metals without mechanical undercuts, loops, or beads has always been a difficult challenge for the laboratory technician. The use of tin plating or placing a thin layer of flexible glass on the surface have been 2 excellent methods for bonding resins to metal. This study again demonstrates that the use of tin plating on the surface of the casting significantly increases the retention of the composite resin.—K.F. Leinfelder, D.D.S., M.S.

Optimization of Surface Micromorphology for Enhanced Osteoblast Responses In Vitro
Bowers KT, Keller JC, Randolph BA, Wick DG, Michaels CM (Univ of Iowa, Iowa City)
Int J Oral Maxillofac Implants 7:302–310, 1992   105-94-14–19

Introduction.—Titanium is the material of choice for uncoated implants because it is biologically compatible with bone. The micromorphologic structure of the implant surface also affects the success of a dental implant. Surface profilometry measurements were taken to assess the response of osteoblast-like cells to titanium surfaces with varied surfaces.

Methods.—After cutting commercially pure titanium into disks and etching them with solvent, a surface profilometer quantified the surface roughness of the implants. An in vitro cell attachment measured the effects of titanium surfaces on the cells, and electron microscopy determined the morphologic characteristics of the cells as a function of the surfaces and time intervals for attachments.

Results.—Scanning electron microscopy showed that the grinding and polishing with SiC grit metallographic papers followed by nitric acid application produced regular morphologies. Polishing with finer grade papers resulted in smaller defects and a smoother surface. Profilometry measurements demonstrated that grinding with 60-grit SiC metallographic papers or sandblasting with a 600-grit surface created the highest average roughness values. In vitro cell measures indicated that no significant differences occurred in osteoblast-like cell attachment at 15 minutes, but sandblasting of the surface significantly increased the percentage of cell attachment for all 30-minute intervals thereafter. Scanning electron microscopy showed the attached cells maintained similar morphology on all surfaces except the sandblasted surface.

Conclusion.—The type of titanium surface roughness appears to affect the first biological responses of cells, including attachment and spreading. The sandblasted irregular rough surface favored the attachment process. Implants with roughened surfaces at the bone attachment sites may have increased success.

▶ The information in the literature related to tissue implant surfaces has been rather meager. During the past 2 years, a number of investigations have contributed to our knowledge considerably. Interestingly, this study demonstrated that sandblasted surfaces of titanium implants favored the attachment process.—K.F. Leinfelder, D.D.S., M.S.

Tissue Response to the Implantation of Two New Machinable Calcium Phosphate Ceramics
Smith KG, Franklin CD, van Noort R, Lamb DJ (Univ of Sheffield, England)
Int J Oral Maxillofac Implants 7:395–400, 1992   105-94-14–20

Background.—Most clinicians working with hydroxyapatite (HA) would like to have an implant material in block form that could be readily and accurately trimmed to the required shape at the time of operation. Two new materials that satisfy these requirements better than currently available materials have been developed. The early response of

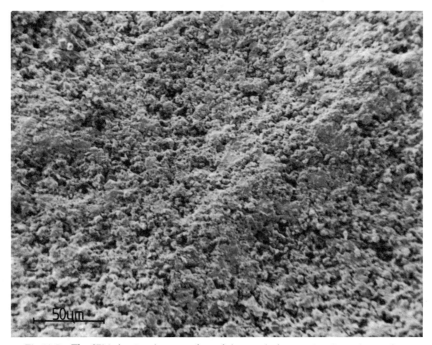

Fig 14–7.—The SEM showing the cut surface of the new hydroxyapatite. Original magnification, ×320. (Courtesy of Smith KG, Franklin CD, van Noort R, et al: *Int J Oral Maxillofac Implants* 7:395–400, 1992.)

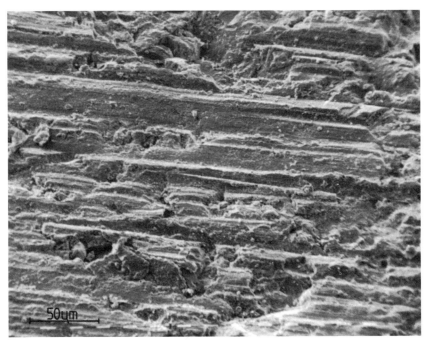

Fig 14–8.—The SEM showing the cut surface of the machinable glass ceramic. Original magnification, ×320. (Courtesy of Smith KG, Franklin CD, van Noort R, et al: *Int J Oral Maxillofac Implants* 7:395–400, 1992.)

these new materials, which have not been used previously as implants, to implantation in bone was investigated.

Methods and Findings.—The machinable calcium phosphate ceramics were investigated in a rat model (Figs 14–7 and 14–8). One of the materials was a machinable form of HA, and the other was a new machinable glass ceramic. One month after the materials had been implanted, new bone was found growing onto the surface of both implants. More bone deposition and remodeling occurred in the next 2 months.

Conclusion.—The new form of HA seems to be as biocompatible as other forms of HA; it should prove to be a valuable asset to oral and maxillofacial surgery. Unlike dense HA, the new HA is microporous, enabling it to be carved. The pore size is very small. Further study is needed to confirm that long-term use of this new HA is not problematic before it can be used clinically. The glass ceramic material is machinable and appears to be biocompatible in bone. New bone clearly formed around the implant. However, the strength of the bone-ceramic bond resulting after implantation has to be determined.

▶ The field of dental implantology has grown considerably during the last several years. The introduction of new materials and techniques have provided the clinician with an increased promise of success. This study offers some new light into the relationship between HA and the adjacent bone surface. The use of a microporous hydroxyapatite with a very small particle size renders the material carvable. Clinical studies will have to be conducted, however, before such a system can be recommended for clinical practice.—K.F. Leinfelder, D.D.S., M.S.

Esthetic Inlay/Onlay Systems

Marginal Adaptation and Fit of Adhesive Ceramic Inlays
Krejci I, Lutz F, Reimer M (Zurich Univ, Switzerland)
J Dent 21:39–46, 1993   105-94-14-21

Background.—There is minimal long-term quantitative data on the behavior of adhesive ceramic inlays. The marginal adaptation of CAD/CAM and laboratory-made ceramic inlays before, during, and after loading was compared in an in vitro study.

Methods and Findings.—Six MOD inlay preparations of standardized design with 1 cervical margin in dentine and the other in enamel were prepared for each inlay type. They were CAD/CAM fabricated MGC-glass ceramic inlays, CAD/CAM fabricated feldspathic porcelain inlays, laboratory-made glass ceramic inlays, and laboratory-made feldspathic porcelain inlays. Appropriate luting composite materials were applied. Restored teeth were then subjected to occlusal loading, thermal cycling, toothbrush and toothpaste abrasion, and chemical degradation in vitro. Marginal adaptation was determined quantitatively along the length of the cavosurface margin and selected sections of the margin using SEM after in vitro testing corresponding to 0, .5, 1, 2.7, and 5 years of clinical service. The marginal fit of the cemented inlays was also assessed in the SEM (Fig 14–9). All groups had excellent initial marginal adaptation in enamel. Significant marginal discrepancies occurred after in vitro testing in all groups. There was a high percentage of marginal openings, notably

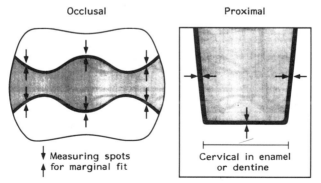

Fig 14–9.—Schematic representation of the marginal sections of an MOD inlay, which were rated separately in the scanning electron microscope. In addition, the measuring spots for marginal fit are depicted. (Courtesy of Krejci I, Lutz F, Reimer M: *J Dent* 21:39-46, 1993.)

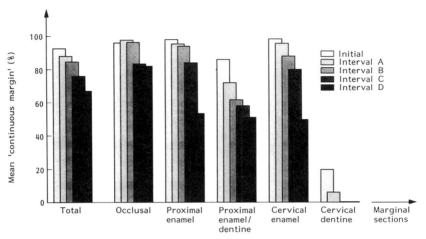

Fig 14–10.—The mean percentages of "continuous margin" at the interface between tooth and cement in group 1 (Dicor, laboratory made). (Courtesy of Krejci I, Lutz F, Reimer M: *J Dent* 21:39–46, 1993.)

in the cervical parts of the margins, in both enamel and dentine (Figs 14-10 to 14-14).

Conclusion.—The ceramic inlays tested had excellent initial marginal adaptation in enamel, irrespective of the fabrication method used. No dentinal sealing was possible, however, without dentinal adhesives. Thermal, mechanical, and chemical testing resulted in disintegration of the marginal adaptation of ceramic inlays, regardless of marginal fit.

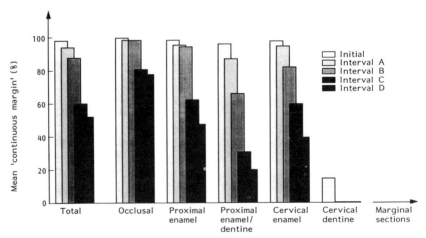

Fig 14–11.—The mean percentages of "continuous margin" at the interface between tooth and cement in group 2 (Dicor MGC, CAD/CAM). (Courtesy of Krejci I, Lutz F, Reimer M: *J Dent* 21:399–46, 1993.)

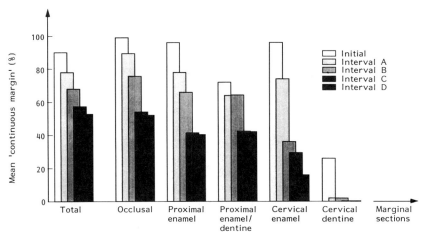

Fig 14–12.—The mean percentages of "continuous margin" at the interface between tooth and cement in group 3 (Biodent, laboratory made). (Courtesy of Krejci I, Lutz F, Reimer M: *J Dent* 21:39–46, 1993.)

▶ Ceramic and composite resin inlays have been used by the dental profession at a growing rate. Such a technique permits the esthetic restoration of a tooth with minimal problems of proximal contour/contact marginal adaptation microleakage and secondary caries. One of the areas now receiving a considerable amount of attention is the horizontal gap dimension between the restoration and the cavosurface margin of the cavity preparation. This in vitro study compared the marginal adaptation of laboratory-made ceramic inlays and those generated by the CAD/CAM after various times of loading.

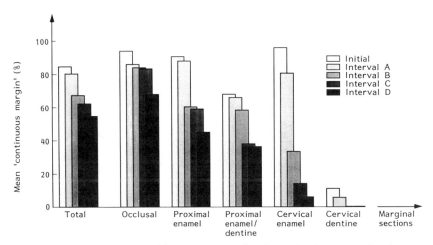

Fig 14–13.—Mean percentages of "continuous margin" at the interface between tooth and cement in group 4 (CEREC Vita Mk I, CAD/CAM). (Courtesy of Krejci I, Lutz F, Reimer M: *J Dent* 21:39–46, 1993.)

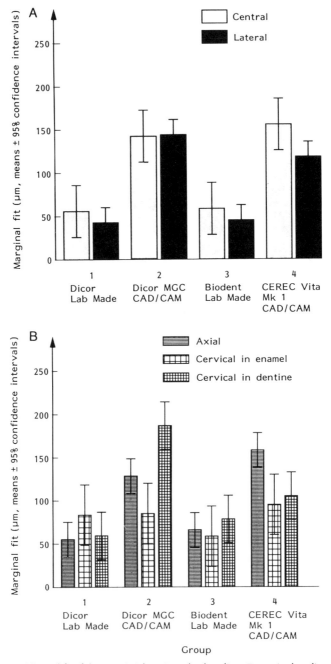

Fig 14–14.—Marginal fit of the ceramic inlays. **A,** occlusal readings. **B,** proximal readings. (Courtesy of Krejci I, Lutz F, Reimer M: *J Dent* 21:39–46, 1993.)

The authors found that the marginal adaptation depended to a great extent on the location of the interface.—K.F. Leinfelder, D.D.S., M.S.

Wear of Ceramic Inlays, Their Enamel Antagonists, and Luting Cements

Krejci I, Lutz F, Reimer M, Heinzmann JL (Zurich Univ Dental Inst, Switzerland)
J Prosthet Dent 69:425–430, 1993   105-94-14-22

Background.—A number of ceramic inlays are being used today because of their versatile color shading and good occlusal morphology, but few quantitative data are available on their wear resistance and, in particular, their abrasiveness against antagonistic enamel cusps.

Study Design.—The wear of laboratory-made ceramic inlay materials and antagonistic enamel cups was examined in vitro. Inlays were adhesively cemented in extracted human mandibular first molars, using castable glass ceramic, pressed glass ceramic, and feldspathic porcelain as inlay materials. A microfilled composite and a fine hybrid composite served as luting agents. The restorations were exposed to wear corresponding to about 5 years in clinical service, and wear in the occlusal contact area was quantified using a 3-dimensional scanner.

Results.—Occlusal contact wear was significantly less for glazed and polished pressed glass ceramic than for porcelain and castable glass ceramic. Enamel wear was comparable in the polished and glazed groups.

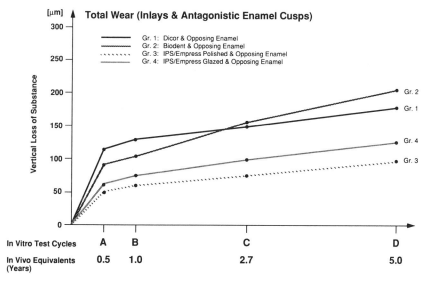

Fig 14–15.—Total vertical loss of substance in occlusal contact point region of ceramic inlays tested (in microns; means). (Courtesy of Krejci I, Lutz F, Reimer M, et al: *J Prosthet Dent* 69:425–430, 1993.)

Total wear was least for the pressed glass ceramic (Fig 14–15). The microfilled composite wore less than the fine hybrid material, but the difference was not significant.

Conclusion.—All the ceramic materials examined were highly wear-resistant. Wear resistance is not critical for these materials, because it is in the range of enamel. More resistant luting composite materials are needed.

▶ Although interfacial gap dimension seems to be the most frequently investigated characteristic of inlays/onlays, little information is available concerning the wear of the inlay itself or the antagonistic cusp. This particular study was of a great deal of interest because it demonstrated that there was a difference in results relating to type of material when measured as a combination of tooth wear and restoration wear. The IPS/Empress system seemed to be the most ideal.—K.F. Leinfelder, D.D.S., M.S.

Clinical Evaluation of a Heat-Treated Resin Composite Inlay: 3-Year Results

Wendt SL Jr, Leinfelder KF (Univ of Connecticut, Farmington; Univ of Alabama, Birmingham)
Am J Dent 5:258–262, 1992   105-94-14–23

Objective.—Heat-treated composite resin inlays of Occlusin were placed in class I and class II inlay cavity preparations, and their clinical performance was followed for 3 years.

Methods.—Sixty Occlusin restorations were placed in premolar and molar teeth. Half were fabricated by direct, bulk placement of composite with intramural light curing. The others involved the direct, bulk placement of an inlay that was light-cured and then subjected to dry heat as a secondary curing method; they were heat-treated at 125°C for 7.5 minutes. The cavity design consisted of a conventional gold inlay preparation. A glass ionomer liner was applied to the dentin, and the enamel margins were etched with 37% phosphoric acid gel. All the inlays were cemented using a light-cured enamel bonding resin.

Results.—More of the light-cured inlays compared with the heat-treated restorations deteriorated in color. There was no interfacial staining during 3 years of study, and no secondary caries were reported. Three light-cured inlays were sensitive for the first 3 months. The resin matrix of the light-cured inlays appeared coarser and less contiguous than that of the heat-treated inlays. Indirect wear measurements indicated no significant differences between the 2 types of inlay (table).

Conclusion.—Heat-treated composite inlays of composite resin have exhibited better marginal integrity than exclusively light-cured composite

Means for Indirect Evaluation of Wear on Resin Composite Inlays

Type	Baseline	3 months	6 months	12 months	24 months	36 months
Light-cured	7.3 ± 13.3	27.5 ± 23.4	43.0 ± 27.4	48.0 ± 27.4	54.0 ± 30	66.4 ± 39
Heat-treated	8.3 ± 12.7	27.5 ± 24.2	39.4 ± 26.3	48.8 ± 27.9	57.6 ± 42	69.0 ± 47

Note: All groups were not significant at the P < .05 level.
(Courtesy of Wendt SL Jr, Leinfelder KF: *Am J Dent* 5:258–262, 1992.)

inlays. Wear resistance depends on the type of composite used rather than on heat treatment.

▶ Most clinicians assume that a postcure heat treatment after first curing with light will substantially increase the wear resistance of resin inlay/onlays. This particular clinical study, however, demonstrated that during a 3-year period no differences in wear could be detected between the light-cured only and the light-cured plus heat-treated inlay systems. These results were quite surprising, because a laboratory test conducted in the same manner provided different results. Specifically, the heat treatment after light-curing enhanced the wear resistance of the systems. The differences in the results between the clinical and the laboratory tests have not been delineated. However, it is possible that the heat-treating process may have partially degraded the silane coupling agent, which then offset the positive effects incurred by the enhancement of polymerization generated by the additional heat-curing process. Additional clinical studies will have to be conducted to fully understand the importance of the postcure heat treatment.—K.F. Leinfelder, D.D.S., M.S.

15 Dentoalveolar Surgery and Ambulatory Anesthesia

Introduction

The nature of the office practice of oral and maxillofacial surgery continues to change. The reasons for this change include an advancing state of knowledge in areas such as facial pain, the increased sophistication in monitoring techniques, and the ever-increasing cost efficiencies that accompany office procedures when compared with the same procedure performed in the hospital. Patient expectations, competition, and managed-care programs are demanding that care be provided in the safest, most expeditious, and cost-efficient manner. This is all good for the long term, but modifying behavior in the short term can be difficult. This chapter discusses some of these issues. The use of steroids to hasten recovery after extractions, surgical treatment of HIV-infected patients, current management technique for office sedation and anesthesia, and a presentation of the agents used to treat trigeminal neuralgia are included. As a practicing surgeon, I applaud these changes. I now have populations of patients (such as those with facial pain) that I follow on a long-term basis, which gives me a gratification not experienced with the usual short-term episodic patient relationship.

Steven M. Roser, D.M.D., M.D.

Dentoalveolar Surgery

Evaluation of Dexamethasone for Reduction of Postsurgical Sequelae of Third Molar Removal
Neupert EA III, Lee JW, Philput CB, Gordon JR (Naval Hosp, Portsmouth, Va; USS Enterprise CUN-65; Naval Dental Ctr, Bethesda, Md)
J Oral Maxillofac Surg 50:1177–1182, 1992   105-94-15–1

Background.—Reducing postoperative discomfort from exodontia is of concern to clinicians and patients. The effect of dexamethasone on decreasing postsurgical sequelae after third molar extraction was investigated in a controlled clinical study.

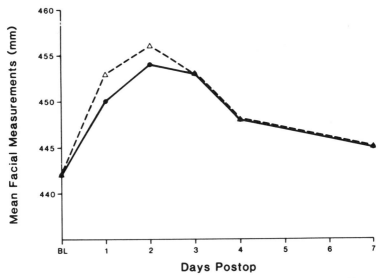

Fig 15–1.—Comparison of facial swelling in experimental and control groups. *Dotted line,* water; *solid line,* steroids. (Courtesy of Neupert EA III, Lee JW, Philput CB, et al: *J Oral Maxillofac Surg* 50:1177–1182, 1992.)

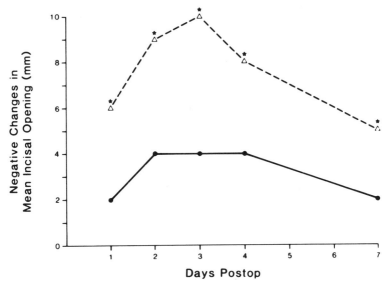

Fig 15–2.—Comparison of trismus in experimental and control groups. *Dotted line,* water; *solid line,* steriods. *Statistically significant. (Courtesy of Neupert EA III, Lee JW, Philput CB, et al: *J Oral Maxillofac Surg* 50:1177–1182, 1992.)

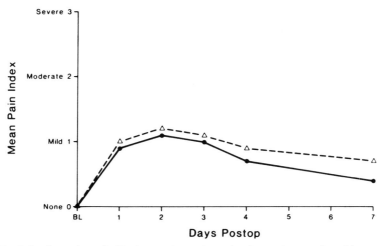

Fig 15–3.—Comparison of subjective pain in experimental and control groups. *Dotted line,* water; *solid line,* steroids. (Courtesy of Neupert EA III, Lee JW, Philput CB, et al: *J Oral Maxillofac Surg* 50:1177–1182, 1992.)

Methods.—Sixty patients with bilaterally symmetrical impacted third molars participated in the study. Each patient's surgery was staged by side of mouth in 2 appointments 5–6 weeks apart. A preoperative dose of 4 mg of dexamethasone was given intravenously by random assignment to side of the mouth and surgical appointment. Thus, the subjects served as their own controls. The other side of the mouth was given sterile water at the other appointment. Facial swelling, pain, and trismus were recorded.

Findings.—There were no significant differences in swelling or daily pain (Fig 15–1). However, the steroid significantly affected trismus and global pain (Fig 15–2). Patients had a daily postoperative increase in incisal opening of 4 to 6 mm on the steroid treated side when compared with the control side. When asked to indicate which side was least painful, patients chose the steroid side by a 4:1 margin (Fig 15–3). Steroid administration did not increase the rate or type of complications.

Conclusion.—Global pain and trismus were positively affected by the administration of dexamethasone. The greatest concern about steroid use in third molar surgery is suppression of the hypothalamus-pituitary-adrenal axis (HPA). However, research indicates that short-term, high-dose steroids do not significantly impair the HPA. The use of dexamethasone during third molar surgery has objective and subjective benefits.

▶ This article reports the benefits of using a single dose of steroids before third molar extraction to decrease pain and swelling after extraction. Although there are reports of no benefit, the majority of investigators agree that steroids do reduce pain and swelling of extraction. The article describes statistically significant benefit only in reduction of global pain and more rapid return to normal interincisal opening. By using a more sensitive pain scale and including less area of the face that is not affected by third molar swelling, greater differences might have been appreciated in the groups. Additionally, 4 mg of dexamethasone equal to 80 mg of hydrocortisone, is a low dose of steroid compared with what has been used for other studies and what is used clinically (I use 125 mg of methylprednisolone, which is equal to 600 mg of hydrocortisone). The low dose may be subtherapeutic and may account for the lack of difference in swelling and pain between the steroid and the control groups. As the authors state in the discussion, studies should be undertaken using combinations of glucocorticoids, nonsteroidal anti-inflammatory drugs, and long-acting local anesthetics that will lead to establishing a protocol for maximum effectiveness in reducing postextraction discomfort.—S.M. Roser, D.M.D., M.D.

Long-Term Clinical and Radiologic Evaluation of Autotransplanted Teeth

Schatz JP, Joho JP (Univ of Geneva, Switzerland)
Int J Oral Maxillofac Surg 21:271–275, 1992   105-94-15–2

Background.—Reports of long-term assessment of autotransplantation were uncommon until recent methodologic advances allowed precise radiologic screening of pulp and periodontium healing of a transplant. A study was done to identify root growth potential and related factors, such as pulp and periodontal survival, in autotransplanted molars and premolars.

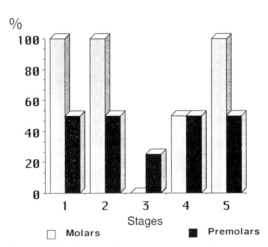

Fig 15–4.—Replacement resorption rates (in percentages), according to stages of root formation. (Courtesy of Schatz JP, Joho JP: *Int J Oral Maxillofac Surg* 21:271-275, 1992.)

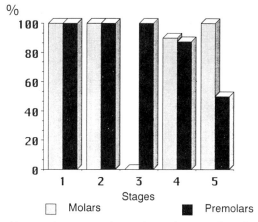

Fig 15–5.—Pulp obliteration (in percentage), according to the stages of root formation. (Courtesy of Schatz JP, Joho JP: *Int J Oral Maxillofac Surg* 21:271-275, 1992.)

Methods.—Forty teeth transplanted in 34 patients between 1979 and 1990 were included in the study. The patients were followed up for up to 11.3 years. The mean length of radiographic follow-up was 6.2 years.

Findings.—Pocket depth was normal in all but 6 cases (Fig 15-4). Pulp obliteration occurred in all transplanted molars at all stages, except for 1 tooth at stage 4, in which pulp necrosis necessitated endodontic treatment (Fig 15-5). In patients with molar transplant, 123% of root growth at stage 1, 80% at stage 2, 16% at stage 4, and 6% at stage 5 was observed (Fig 15-6). For premolar transplantation, growth was 285% at stage 1, 172% at stage 2, 93% at stage 3, 14% at stage 4, and 5% at stage 5.

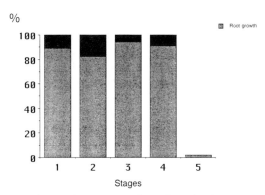

Fig 15–6.—Root growth, according to stages of root formation, in percentage of expected root length (premolar sample). (Courtesy of Schatz JP, Joho JP: *Int J Oral Maxillofac Surg* 21:271-275, 1992.)

Discussion.—Persistence of pulp vitality and continuous root development were observed in this study. However, in most cases replacement root resorption followed. These findings, consistent with previous studies, indicate an ideal developmental stage for molar and premolar transplantation to ensure pulpal and periodontal survival.

▶ The investigators of this study evaluated periodontal healing, pulp healing, and root growth of 40 transplanted teeth in 34 individuals to determine an ideal developmental stage for molar and premolar transplantation to ensure pulpal and periodontal survival. Their findings that transplantation at stage 3 or 4 (half to three fourths root development) is most successful is consistent with other studies. The authors raise questions that merit further investigation concerning factors that affect the success of autotransplantation and the etiology of replacement resorption.—A. Schreiber, D.M.D., and S.M. Roser, D.M.D., M.D.

Changing Methods of Preventing Infective Endocarditis Following Dental Procedures: 1943 to 1993
Hupp JR (Univ of Medicine and Dentistry of New Jersey, Newark)
J Oral Maxillofac Surg 51:616–623, 1993   105-94-15–3

Purpose.—Despite the great advances in understanding the relationship between dental procedures and bacterial endocarditis, controversy remains as to whether this is a true cause-and-effect relationship and whether patients at risk of endocarditis should receive antibiotics. The changing approaches to preventing infective endocarditis after dental procedures since the pioneering report by Northrop and Crowley in 1943 were reviewed.

Dental Procedures and Bacteremias.—Previous reports paved the way for Northrop and Crowley; for example, those of O'Kell and Elliot, which found a 64% incidence of bacteremia after tooth extraction. In 1944, Northrop and Crowley established that preoperative sulfathiozole could reduce the incidence of immediate postextraction bacteremia from 16% to 4%. Others found that bacteremias did indeed occur after extractions in children and after multiple suture removal.

Antibiotic Reduction of Bacteremias.—Thoma was the first to call for antimicrobial prophylaxis in patients with valvular heart disease in 1948, and in 1955 the American Heart Association issued its first statement on the issue. The standards have been revised several times, each time becoming more complex, until the 1984 standard, which limited prophylaxis to a single dose of penicillin 1 hour before operation and another 6 hours later. By 1990, amoxicillin had been substituted for penicillin in some patients. All of these complex regimens still fail to match the simplicity of the single preoperative dose used by Northrop and Crowley.

Dental Procedures and Endocarditis.—Ethical considerations and the limited knowledge of the incubation period of endocarditis inhibit definitive studies of the link between dental procedures and endocarditis. Even studies of cases in which prophylaxis fails to prevent endocarditis fail to prove that the bacteremia does not result from some other factor. The debate continues as to whether the benefits of preventing endocarditis outweigh the costs of universal use of prophylaxis in patients at risk, including the possibility of a serious hypersensitivity reaction. The risk-benefit ratio appears to be poor. leading to the conclusion that although many cases of infective endocarditis are preventable, many more and possibly most are not.

Questions also persist regarding which antibiotic to administer and how it should be given. The important factor of the patient's level of oral hygiene may be addressed by preprocedure brushing and irrigation with chlorhexidine. It is of interest to note that the incidence of bacterial endocarditis has not declined recently and may even be increasing.

Discussion.—Since the original report of Northrop and Crowley, the knowledge about antibiotic prophylaxis to prevent bacterial endocarditis and the interaction between dental procedures and bacteremias has increased greatly. However, it remains to be established once and for all whether such prophylaxis yields significant reductions in the incidence of endocarditis.

▶ The author effectively documents the evolution of antibiotic prophylaxis for dental procedures in patients at risk of developing endocarditis. Additionally, the author discusses a few issues that usually do not receive attention. These include the poor risk-benefit ratio of antibiotic prophylaxis, the occurrence of endocarditis despite antibiotic prophylaxis, and the increasing incidence of endocarditis. Should the question of antibiotic prophylaxis be revisited?—S.M. Roser, D.M.D., M.D.

Complications of Dental Surgery in Persons With HIV Disease
Porter SR, Scully C, Luker J (Univ of Bristol, England)
Oral Surg Oral Med Oral Pathol 75:165–167, 1993   105-94-15–4

Background.—Infective complications after tooth extraction in HIV-infected persons have occasionally been reported. However, little information is available on the frequency of such complications and the need for antibiotic prophylaxis. In addition, the frequency of postextraction bleeding in HIV-infected persons who may have thrombocytopenia is not known.

Methods.—Thirty-eight patients in stages 2-4 of HIV infection were studied to determine the frequency of postextraction complications. Twenty-six matched, seronegative subjects from patient groups commonly at risk of HIV infection were also studied. A total of 100 teeth was extracted in 40 clinical procedures in the HIV-positive persons, and 68 teeth were extracted in 30 procedures in the noninfected group.

Findings.—There were 3 episodes of delayed postextraction healing in the infected group and 2 in the noninfected group, a nonsignificant difference. Only 1 episode of severe postextraction bleeding occurred in an HIV-positive patient. This patient was a hemophiliac who bled despite factor VIII prophylaxis. The bleeding, which occurred 7 days after extraction, was stopped with tranexamic acid and additional factor VIII. There were no episodes of severe postextraction bleeding in the control group.

Conclusion.—Postextraction complications apparently are uncommon in patients with HIV infection. Routine antibiotic prophylaxis seems unnecessary.

▶ There is a tendency to prescribe prophylactic antibiotics for medically compromised patients for extractions because of a fear of postextraction infection and a subsequent worsening of the underlying medical conditions. In most of these situations, there is no support for the use of antibiotics; however, there is little help for the dentist who chooses not to use prophylactic antibiotics. This small study provides just such support, and a larger study would be welcomed.—S.M. Roser, D.M.D., M.D.

Drugs Used in the Management of Trigeminal Neuralgia
Zakrzewska JM, Patsalos PN (Eastman Dental Hosp, London; Natl Hosp for Neurology and Neurosurgery, London)
Oral Surg Oral Med Oral Pathol 74:439–450, 1992   105-94-15–5

Introduction.—Trigeminal neuralgia is a sudden, severe, brief, stabbing recurrent pain limited to the distribution of the fifth cranial nerve. It was first described in the first century A.D. Only 3% of the cases are bilateral, and involvement of the right side is more common. Episodes occur periodically for a few weeks or months and are followed by a period of complete pain remission. Since the 17th century, more than 40 different preparations have been used to treat trigeminal neuralgia (Table 1).

Drug Management.—The introduction of phenytoin in 1942 heralded a new era in the drug management of trigeminal neuralgia. In 1962, carbamazepine was shown to be more effective than phenytoin with fewer side effects. The successful use of clonazepam in 1975 and baclofen in 1980 expanded the treatment options. Carbamazepine is currently the drug of choice.

Pharmacokinetics.—The most common reason for therapeutic failure is inadequate dosage. The pharmacokinetic characteristics of each drug were used to formulate dosage recommendations (Table 2). The high specificity of carbamazepine in relieving the pain of trigeminal neuralgia

TABLE 1.—Treatments Used for Trigeminal Neuralgia

Drug	Trade name	First report
Early treatments, 1677-1940[2]		
Purgatives	—	1677
Hemlock and quinine	—	1773
Ferrous carbonate	—	1824
Gelseminum powder	—	1874
Galvanic therapy	—	1875
Radiation and x-ray therapy	—	1897
Trichloroethylene	—	1918
Thiamine hydrochloride	—	1940
Treatments recently abandoned*		
Cyanocobalamin	Cytacon	1952[91]
Stilbamidine	—	1953[92]
Mephenesin	Tolseral	1958[93]
Tizanindine	—	1986[95]
Tocainide	Tonocard	1987[95]
Pimozide	Orap	1988[96]
Mexiletine	Mexitil	1989[97]
Current treatments		
Phenytoin	Dilantin or Epanutin	1942[4]
Antihistamines	—	1948[98]
Carbamazepine	Tegretol	1962[5]
Clonazepam	Clonopin or Rivotril	1975[6]
Baclofen	Lioresal	1980[7]
Valproic acid	Depakene or Epilim	1980[71]
L-Baclofen	—	1987[60]
Oxcarbazepine†	Trileptal	1987[99]

* Withdrawn because of low efficacy or unacceptable side effects.
† Drug currently undergoing development but unavailable as a licensed drug in a number of countries.
(Courtesy of Zakrzewska JM, Patsalos PN: Oral Surg Oral Med Oral Pathol 74:439-450, 1992.)

and no other type of facial pain makes it a useful diagnostic indicator. Dosages should initially be kept small, e.g., 100 mg given twice daily to minimize side effects. A dose increase of 100 mg every 48 hours should be effected until pain control is achieved. The target therapeutic range for serum concentration of carbamazepine is 24 to 43 μmol/L. An average effective dose is 200 mg 4 times a day. Proportionately more of the drug should be taken at night to achieve adequate serum concentrations for early morning pain control. Complete pain control should be maintained for a month followed by withdrawal of the drug at a rate of 100 mg every 48 hours. Drug withdrawal is the only way to determine whether a remission has been achieved. Investigations of a new drug, ox-

TABLE 2.—Pharmacokinetic Characteristics of Currently Used Antineuralgic Drugs

Drug	Nature (acid/base)	Bioavailability (%)	Time to maximum concentration (hr)	Bound to albumin (%)	Half-life (hr)	Time to steady-state concentration (days)*	Therapeutic target range (µmol/L)
Baclofen	Acid	—	3-8	—	3-4	2	—
Carbamazepine†	Neutral	>70	2-8	70-80	11-27	5‡	24-43
Clonazepam	Base	100	1-2	80-85	24-36	12	0.08-0.24
Oxcarbazepine	Neutral	100	1-2	40-45§	8-11	3	35-110
Phenytoin	Acid	98	4-8	90-92	15-20‖	14	20-80
Valproic acid†	Acid	99	1-4	90-92	8-10	3	200-700

* Earliest time to achieve and therefore measure steady state serum concentrations after start of a dosage regimen.
† Carbamazepine and valproic acid exhibit significant diurnal variations; sampling time in relation to dose is critical.
‡ Twenty days if the drug has been introduced for the first time.
§ Binding of 10,11-dihydroxycarbazepine metabolite.
‖ Variable because of saturation kinetics.
(Courtesy of Zakrzewska JM, Patsalos PN: Oral Surg Oral Med Oral Pathol 74:439–450, 1992.)

carbazepine, suggests efficacy similar to carbamazepine with a better tolerability profile. An average effective dose is 1,200 mg/day. Phenytoin can be used as an adjunct to carbamazepine or oxcarbazepine therapy or in patients allergic to carbamazepine. Baclofen can be used first in new cases of trigeminal neuralgia or in patients with hypersensitivity to carbamazepine. Clonazepam is used only occasionally, usually when carbamazepine is contraindicated.

Conclusion.—There are several options for therapeutic drug management of trigeminal neuralgia with antineuralgic drugs. Inadequate dosage is the most common reason for therapeutic failure.

▶ This article provides a historical overview of the medications used to treat trigeminal neuralgia, as well as a detailed description of the pharmacokinetics of the medications currently in use. The common side effects, drug interactions, and rationale for dosages and timing are all presented. Carbamazepine remains the drug of choice. A need for more double-blind studies comparing the efficacy of various alternative drugs is cited by the authors. Agents that may be promising in the future include oxcarbazepine and the ʟ form of baclofen.

Other approaches and new innovations to therapy of trigeminal neuralgia such as peripheral neurectomy, peripheral radiofrequency thermoneurolysis, and microvascular nerve root decompression were not addressed in this article.—A. Schreiber, D.M.D., and S.M. Roser, D.M.D., M.D.

Restoring Sensation After Trigeminal Nerve Injury: A Review of Current Management

Colin W, Donoff RB (Massachusetts Gen Hosp, Boston; Harvard School of Dental Medicine, Boston)
J Am Dent Assoc 123(12):80–85, 1992   105-94-15–6

Background.—Paresthesia or altered sensation of the lower lip and anterior part of the tongue may result from inferior alveolar or lingual nerve injury after injection injuries, endodontic therapy, malposed dental implants, displaced mandible fracture, maxillofacial surgery, tumor resection, or third molar removal. Paresthesia was the most common cause of litigious action for oral and maxillofacial procedures from 1983 to 1987. The best management of trigeminal nerve injuries is early referral and intervention.

Nerve Microstructure.—The neuron is the fundamental unit of the trigeminal nerve and all of the peripheral nervous system. The 3 parts of the neuron are the nerve cell body, various dendrites, and an axon which may be several feet in length. The axon may or may not be invested in a myelin sheath. Several layers of connective tissue, the endoneurium, perineurium, epineurium, and mesoneurium provide vascular supply, support, and protection for the peripheral nerves. A fascicle is a group of nerve fibers surrounded by a perineurium. Within a nerve trunk, 1 or more fascicles are arranged in 1 of 3 patterns: unifascicular, oligofascicular, and polyfascicular (Fig 15–7). After resection or transection, these layers must be aligned accurately to prevent sensory disturbances. The major pathophysiologic categories of peripheral nerve injuries are neuro-

- *UNIFASCICULAR*

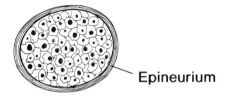

Epineurium

- *OLIGOFASCICULAR*

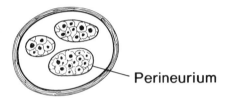

Perineurium

- *POLYFASCICULAR*

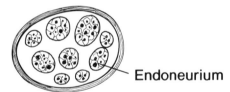

Endoneurium

Fig 15–7.—Connective tissue layers and fascicular patterns of peripheral nerves. (Courtesy of Colin W, Donoff RB: *J Am Dent Assoc* 123(12):80–85, 1992.)

praxia, axonotmesis, and neurotmesis. The resulting abnormal sensations include anesthesia, paresthesia, and dysesthesia.

Microsurgical Intervention.—Neural lesions with anesthesia or severe nerve parasthesias persisting for at least 2 months and dysesthetic injuries that have been relieved by a nerve block may be indications for microsurgical intervention (Figs 15-8 and 15-9). An extraoral approach may be used for exploration of the inferior alveolar nerve. The lingual nerves may be explored through a transoral approach. Typical findings include extraneural compressive scar bands or foreign objects, nerve collaterals, traumatic neuromas, or complete transection.

Conclusion.—A knowledge of anatomy and careful technique will minimize the risk of trigeminal nerve injuries. The results of microsurgical intervention for trigeminal nerve injuries are variable with the best results achieved when surgery is performed within 6 months of injury. Beyond 1 year, the prognosis for peripheral nerve repair is poor.

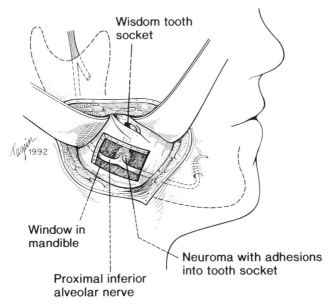

Fig 15–8.—Surgical approach and exposure of the lateral aspect of the mandible for inferior alveolar nerve explorations. (Courtesy of Colin W, Donoff RB: *J Am Dent Assoc* 123(12):80–85, 1992.)

▶ Trigeminal nerve injury with associated sensory disturbance may occur unavoidably as a result of mandible fracture and tumor resection or, unfortunately, secondary to a myriad of dentoalveolar procedures, including third molar extractions, implant placement, and local anesthetic injections.

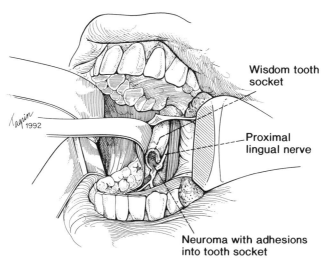

Fig 15–9.—Surgical approach and exposure of the floor of the mouth for lingual nerve explorations. (Courtesy of Colin W, Donoff RB: *J Am Dent Assoc* 123(12):80–85, 1992.)

This article provides an excellent overview of the biology of peripheral nerve microanatomy, injury, and regeneration. The indications and timing for microsurgical intervention and surgical approaches for nerve repair are discussed. Of significance to every practitioner is the comprehensive description of the protocol for evaluation of dysfunction of the trigeminal nerve. Although the results of microsurgical nerve repair are variable, the best outcomes rely on early recognition, referral, and intervention.—A. Schreiber, D.M.D., and S.M. Roser, D.M.D., M.D.

Ambulatory Anesthesia

The Use of Intravenous Anesthesia and Sedation Techniques in Oral and Maxillofacial Surgery
Dembo JB (Univ of Kentucky, Lexington)
J Oral Maxillofac Surg 51:346–351, 1993   105-94-15–7

Background.—The concept of performing surgery in anesthetized patients with a nonintubated airway has endured for decades. Four milestones have had a significant impact on the practice of intravenous anesthesia in the past 50 years.

Discussion.—Office anesthesia changed substantially when lidocaine was introduced. The action of barbiturates was predictable but relatively nonspecific. Anxiolysis, amnesia, and sedation were identified as desirable in oral surgery patients, but no single drug could provide all these effects until diazepam was introduced in the mid-1960s. In the 1980s, midazolam, which did not have many of the undesirable characteristics of diazepam, was introduced. Most recently the introduction of a benzodiazepine antagonist, flumazenil, has undoubtedly further increased the safety of office anesthesia. There are now antagonists for almost all commonly used medications that may need reversal, except methohexitol.

In the 1980s, the first reports of the benefits of pulse oximetry appeared. The pulse oximeter represents a major breakthrough in patient safety, because hypoxia is still the main cause of unanticipated morbidity and mortality.

Increased public and professional awareness of dental safety issues have resulted in state-level anesthesia legislation. By 1991, a total of 45 states regulated the use of general anesthesia and 43 regulated the use of parenteral sedation.

Many of the office anesthetic practices used by oral and maxillofacial surgeons are also now being used by other health-care providers. There has been a general increase in the use of conscious sedation and co-medication.

Conclusion.—Future progress in the field of office anesthesia will rely greatly on neuropharmacologic research and the development of new drugs, such as new ultra-short-acting, sedative-hypnotic drugs. Incremental bolus techniques may be replaced by continuous infusion methods so that a specific serum level can be achieved easily and maintained predictably. In addition, automatic drug-delivery systems are currently being assessed.

▶ This article summarizes the changes and progress that have occurred in the area of office anesthesia during the past 50 years. The safety record for anesthesia administered in oral and maxillofacial surgery offices has been remarkable, with mortality rates reported between 1 in 1–3 million. The increasing demand for general anesthesia by the surgical patient has been met by the development of safer sedation agents and better monitoring techniques. The establishment of state regulations regarding qualifications of the provider and office equipment used for monitoring and anesthesia has helped to set standards in the area. Office anesthesia should become even more popular as health-care reform measures are implemented and more surgery moves away from expensive hospital settings.—S.M. Roser, D.M.D., M.D.

16 Orthognathic Surgery

Introduction

The techniques of orthognathic surgery continue to be refined. The benefits of orthognathic surgery in the growing child, which permit better function and, ultimately, better form, and the consistent reduction of symptoms in patients with temporomandibular disorders have been reported. Skeletal and soft tissue cephalometric norms and surgical management protocols have been established for black and Asian patients. Simplified bone grafting techniques have prompted the use of this material more often than alloplastic materials, which have recently received adverse publicity as the result of the silicone and the TMJ implant problems. Stability remains as one of the most frequently debated issues. This chapter presents discussions on maxillary stability after superior repositing done for vertical maxillary excess (gummy smile); inferior respositing done for vertical maxillary deficiency (shows no upper teeth); and surgically assisted rapid palatal expansion. Even though orthognathic surgery has a modern history of more than 20 years, the difficulty in obtaining standardized images on a long-term basis for controlled prospective populations of patients who are to undergo controlled surgery has left us still debating the issue of stability. The articles presented represent some of the best attempts to look at stability. The use of rigid fixation has added hundreds of dollars in plate and screw costs to each case. If rigid fixation does not increase stability in a particular situation, it should not be used.

An article on obstructive sleep apnea syndrome (OSAS) is included in this chapter. This syndrome has received increased attention. A variety of management protocols are available, including orthognathic surgery. In its severe form, OSAS is well defined and requires treatment. Management of less severe forms of OSAS remains to be determined.

Steven M. Roser, D.M.D., M.D.

Superior Repositioning of the Maxilla Combined With Mandibular Advancement: Mandibular RIF Improves Stability
Forssell K, Turvey TA, Phillips C, Proffit WR (Turku, Finland; Univ of North Carolina, Chapel Hill)
Am J Orthod Dentofacial Orthop 102:342–350, 1992   105-94-16-1

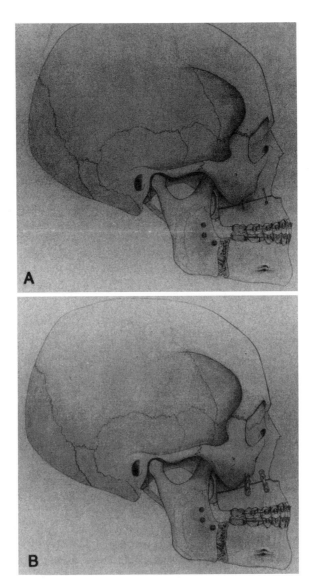

Fig 16–1.—A, diagrammatic representation of fixation with mandibular rigid internal fixation and wire fixation in maxilla. **B,** fixation with bone plates in the maxilla and screws in the mandible. (Courtesy of Forssell K, Turvey TA, Phillips C, et al: *Am J Orthod Dentofacial Orthop* 102:342–350, 1992.)

Background.—In patients with skeletal open bite and mandibular deficiency, mandibular surgery alone has a high potential for relapse, and maxillary surgery alone fails to correct the mandibular deficiency. Combined osteotomies produce satisfactory clinical results. Improved stabil-

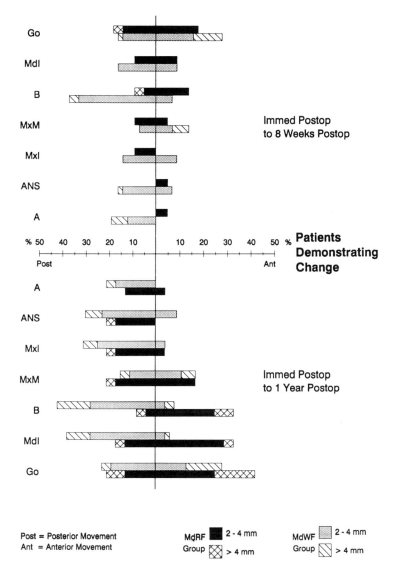

Fig 16–2.—Bar graph showing percentage of patients in MMF and RIF groups who had horizontal changes greater than 2 mm. (Courtesy of Forssell K, Turvey TA, Phillips C, et al: *Am J Orthod Dentofacial Orthop* 102:342-350, 1992.)

ity has been reported when rigid internal fixation is used rather than conventional wire fixation and maxillomandibular fixation (MMF). This study reports the long-term stability of combined osteotomies using either rigid internal fixation or conventional wire fixation and MMF.

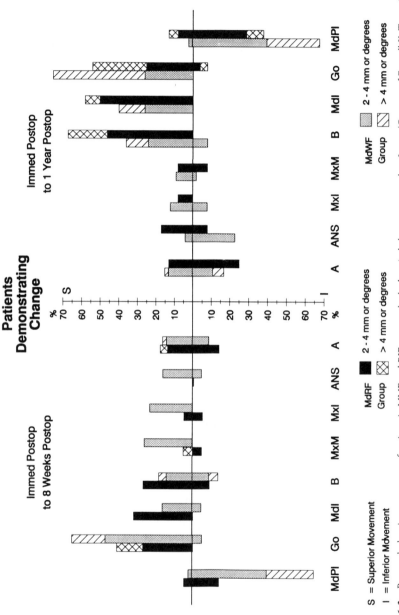

Fig 16-3.—Bar graph showing percentage of patients in MMF and RIF groups who had vertical changes greater than 2 mm. (Courtesy of Forssell K, Turvey TA, Phillips C, et al: *Am J Orthod Dentofacial Orthop* 102:342–350, 1992.)

Methods.—Stability and clinical outcome were compared in 77 patients treated with superior repositioning of the maxilla and mandibular advancement. Twenty-four patients had rigid internal fixation (RIF) to stabilize the sagittal osteotomy, with wires or plates to stabilize the maxilla (Fig 16–1). The remaining 53 patients had the same surgery but with osseous suspension wires and 8 weeks of MMF. Results were evaluated at the patients' 1-year follow-up visits. Descriptive, computer-generated cephalometric data were subjected to repeated measures analysis of variance to assess the effect of type of fixation, time, and the interaction between them.

Results.—At 8 weeks, the MMF group had a greater mean posterior mandibular relapse than the RIF group. The MMF group also had a higher percentage of patients with significant vertical and horizontal change. At follow-up, the MMF group had some additional mean relapse, 2 mm or more in 42% of the patients (Fig 16–2). Forward repositioning of the mandible was more likely than posterior repositioning in the RIF group, with one third of the patients having at least 2 mm of forward movement. Short-term vertical stability was also better in the RIF group (Fig 16–3). Ninety-six percent of the patients in the RIF group were deemed to have an excellent clinical outcome, compared with only 60% of the MMF group.

Conclusion.—Two-jaw surgery and mandibular RIF produces better short-term and long-term stability than wire fixation. This presumably results from the greater ability of bone screws to resist muscle pull and/or the forces of stretched soft tissues, although absence of condylar displacement and early jaw mobilization may also play a role. Early function may play a role in the improved clinical results.

▶ The etiology and factors associated with stability and relapse of maxillary and mandibular movements are only partially known. The authors, using a large number of available long-term patients managed at 1 institution, undertook a retrospective study of 2 groups of patients treated with combined osteotomies for correction of skeletal open bite deformity. They concluded that rigid fixation of the mandible significantly decreased the relapse when compared with a similar group in which wire fixation and MMF was used. They postulated that early mandibular function and better seating of the condyle in the fossa were the most important factors involved in preventing relapse. The reader is reminded that this is a retrospective, multisurgeon study in which the patients received surgery over a period of time (not indicated). The results should be interpreted accordingly.—S.M. Roser, D.M.D., M.D.

Long-Term Stability After Inferior Maxillary Repositioning by Miniplate Fixation

Baker DL, Stoelinga PJW, Blijdorp PA, Brouns JJA (Univ of Washington, Seattle; Rijnstate Hosp, Arnhem, The Netherlands)

Int J Oral Maxillofac Surg 21:320–326, 1992   105-94-16-2

Objective.—Vertical maxillary hypoplasia is a relatively rare deformity as compared with other dentofacial deformities and presents a significant treatment challenge. A high incidence of skeletal relapse has been reported after maxillary repositioning, and a variety of techniques have been proposed to minimize relapse. The short-term and long-term stability of maxillary repositioning were examined by means of Le Fort I osteotomy with miniplate fixation.

Patients and Outcomes.—The subjects were 19 non–cleft palate patients undergoing Le Fort I osteotomy with inferior maxillary repositioning and miniplate fixation. All but 5 patients had bone grafts. In 3, the movement was less than 2 mm; 1 had miniplates alone; and 1 had HA blocks used. They were followed for 12–58 months. Long-term stability was achieved in 14 patients, including 9 patients with no relapse and 5 patients with 12% to 25% vertical or horizontal relapse. Five patients had 30% to 50% vertical relapse (Fig 16–4). Relapse tended to be greater in patients with more than 5 mm of inferior repositioning and in those in whom the Le Fort I osteotomy included concurrent segmentalization (Figs 16–5 and 16–6). In most cases, relapse occurred in the first 3–6 postoperative months. All patients had acceptable long-term dental occlusion.

Conclusion.—On its own, miniplate fixation appears unable to overcome the forces that cause relapse when used for inferior maxillary repositioning. Gaps larger than about 3 mm should be filled with bone grafts. The main force leading to relapse appears to be lengthening of the mandibular elevator muscles.

▶ Vertical maxillary skeletal hypoplasia or deficiency, which produces the appearance of a short face and often mandibular prognathism, occurs far less frequently than other dentofacial deformities. This is fortunate because the surgical correction of this problem has been associated with a relatively high incidence of relapse. In this study, the authors found that half of the surgically treated patients exhibited relapse. Common to the relapse group was more vertical movement at surgery than in the group that did not relapse. Most of the relapse occurred by the first 6 months after operation. The authors attributed the relapse to failure of the miniplates to hold the maxilla in the new position against the mandible and the increased forces of the lengthened levator muscles that occurred as a result of the (inferior) downward positioning of the maxilla and the mandible. The authors reported that despite the relapse, the esthetic and occlusal results were acceptable. The organization of the study, however, suffers from problems common to studies like

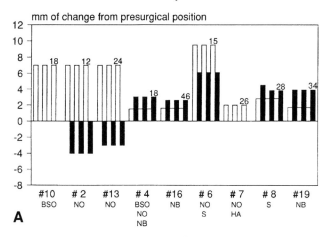

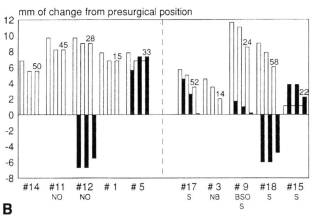

Fig 16–4.—**A,** group 1. **B,** groups 2 and 3. Horizontal axis shows assigned patient numbers (#) for study. Vertical axis shows mm of change from presurgical position measured at Is. *Open bars* represent vertical dimension of movement. *Filled bars* represent horizontal dimension of movement. First bar on left for each patient shows immediate postoperative position. Second bar is 3- to 6-month follow-up position. Last bar is latest follow-up postion, and number of months after surgery is shown above bar. Range of relapse in vertical dimension is shown for each group in parentheses. *Abbreviations: BSO,* patients with bilateral sagittal split setback osteotomies; *S,* patients with 2 or more segments in the maxilla; *No,* no orthodontic treatment; *NB,* no bone graft; *HA,* HA block. (Courtesy of Baker DL, Stoelinga PJW, Blijdorp PA, et al: *Int J Oral Maxillofac Surg* 21:320–326, 1992.)

Category A

less than or equal to 5 mm of vertical lengthening $n = 7$

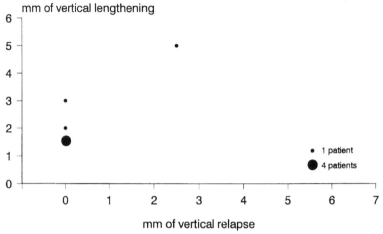

Fig 16–5.—One of 7 patients with 5 mm or less vertical lengthening had vertical relapse. (Courtesy of Baker DL, Stoelinga PJW, Blijdorp PA, et al: *Int J Oral Maxillofac Surg* 21:320-326, 1992.)

Category B

greater than 5 mm of vertical lengthening $n = 12$

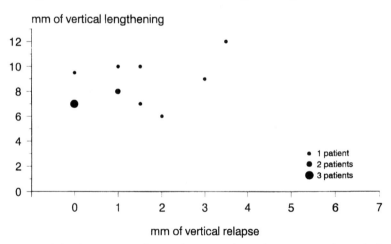

Fig 16–6.—Eight of 12 patients with more than 5 mm of vertical lengthening had vertical relapse. (Courtesy of Baker DL, Stoelinga PJW, Blijdorp PA, et al: *Int J Oral Maxillofac Surg* 21:320-326, 1992.)

this, including it being a retrospective study, surgery was performed by more than one surgeon, and the patients underwent a variety of additional procedures such as mandibular ramus osteotomies. Despite this, the conclusions of the authors are consistent with other reports in the literature.—S.M. Roser, D.M.D., M.D.

Stability of Surgical Maxillary Expansion
Phillips C, Medland WH, Fields HW Jr, Proffit WR, White RP Jr (Univ of North Carolina, Chapel Hill; Queensland, Australia; Ohio State Univ, Columbus)
Int J Adult Orthod Orthognath Surg 7:139–146, 1992   105-94-16-3

Purpose.—A variety of malocclusions include a component of transverse maxillary deficiency, or skeletal crossbite. Although rapid maxillary expansion using an orthodontic appliance alone is usually effective in young patients, adults with skeletal crossbite usually must be managed by

	Transverse Changes at Surgery and Postsurgery						
	Two-piece			Three-piece			
	No.	Mean	SD	No.	Mean	SD	*P*
			Surgery				
Canine	26	1.8	1.4	13	0.2	0.9	.001
First premolar	22	2.6	1.5	6	2.3	1.3	.60
Second premolar	21	3.7	1.7	13	1.9	2.2	.01
First molar	23	4.7	2.4	13	3.5	2.6	.17
Second molar	18	5.7	3.0	13	5.2	3.1	.68
			Postsurgery				
Canine	26	−0.2	1.5	13	0.1	1.2	.53
First premolar	22	−0.7	1.5	6	−0.7	1.8	.97
Second premolar	20	−1.4	1.4	13	−1.1	1.6	.58
First molar	23	−2.0	1.6	13	−1.8	1.4	.70
Second molar	18	−2.7	1.4	13	−2.3	1.5	.40

(Courtesy of Phillips C, Medland WH, Fields HW Jr, et al: *Int J Adult Orthod Orthognath Surg* 7:139-146, 1992.)

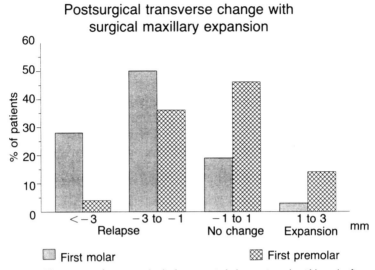

Postsurgical transverse change with surgical maxillary expansion

Fig 16–7.—The percent of patients who had postsurgical changes in arch width at the first molars and first premolars. Relapse at the first molars occurred in two thirds of the patients and was severe (greater than 3 mm) in 20%. At the first premolars, 40% of the patients had some relapse, but only 1 patient had greater than 3 mm of postsurgical change. (Courtesy of Phillips C, Medland WH, Fields HW Jr, et al: *Int J Adult Orthod Orthognath Surg* 7:139–146, 1992.)

surgically assisted rapid maxillary expansion or Le Fort I osteotomy with segments because of the resistance of the maxillary articulations. The transverse stability of the latter operation was evaluated in 39 patients.

Observations.—The average amount of expansion performed was 5.4 mm at the second molars, decreasing to 2.8 mm at the first premolars. The greatest amount of postsurgical relapse was seen at the second molars, where it averaged 2.6 mm. The posterior areas showed the greatest percentage of relapse, averaging 49% at the second molars and 30% at the first premolars (table). Some relapse was seen at the first molars in three fourths of the patients, with more than one fourth having more than 3 mm of relapse. The remaining one fourth of the patients remained stable (Fig 16–7). Arch width at the first molars increased in 62% of the patients (Fig 16–8). Transverse relapse was unrelated to the type of presurgical orthodontic tooth movement, the use of rigid wire fixation, or the use of an auxiliary stabilizing arch wire. Patients undergoing concurrent mandibular surgery had more postsurgical relapse.

Discussion.—The stability after transverse expansion of the maxilla by Le Fort I osteotomy was explored. These results may be improved by using moderate overexpansion at surgery for major transverse changes, using the occlusal splint for a minimum of 6 weeks, and using a lingual or auxiliary labial arch wire to maintain molar width during postsurgical orthodontic treatment. These steps acknowledge the tendency toward maxillary expansion as well as providing a means of compensating for

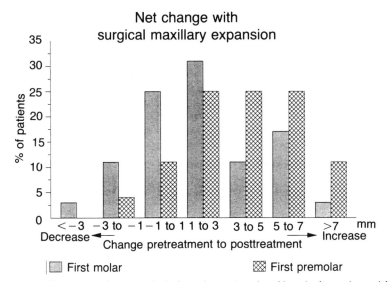

Fig 16–8.—The percent of patients who had net changes in arch width at the first molars and first premolars. Although the initial expansion was greater at the molars, greater relapse there meant that a net increase of greater than 3 mm was more likely across the first premolars than across the molars. (Courtesy of Phillips C, Medland WH, Fields HW Jr, et al: *Int J Adult Orthod Orthognath Surg* 7:139-146, 1992.)

and controlling the change. For adult patients whose skeletal problems are in the transverse plane only, surgically assisted rapid maxillary expansion is indicated.

▶ It is currently accepted treatment to initially overexpand the maxillary arch when correcting a posterior crossbite or transverse arch discrepancy. The relapse that inevitably occurs will then produce the desired occlusion. However, when correcting a transverse arch discrepancy using a Le Fort I osteotomy with segments, it is common to put the maxilla into the desired position or occlusion. Very little information is available in the literature regarding the stability of this surgical procedure. It is not surprising that the authors report it is not stable and that patients relapse after a Le Fort I with segments regardless of the fixation technique used. Their recommendations appear sound and should be considered by all those involved in this type of treatment.—S.M. Roser, D.M.D., M.D.

Obstructive Sleep Apnea Syndrome: A Surgical Protocol for Dynamic Upper Airway Reconstruction
Riley RW, Powell NB, Guilleminault C (Stanford Univ, Calif)
J Oral Maxillofac Surg 51:742–747, 1993   105-94-16-4

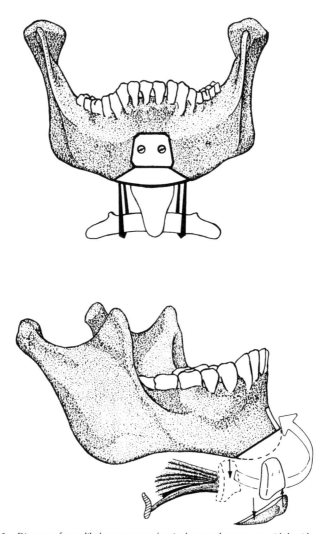

Fig 16–9.—Diagram of mandibular osteotomy/genioglossus advancement with hyoid myotomy/suspension. (Courtesy of Riley RW, Powell NB, Guilleminault C: *J Oral Maxillofac Surg* 51:742-747, 1993.)

Purpose.—Although uvulopalatopharyngoplasty (UPPP), the primary method of treatment of obstructive sleep apnea syndrome (OSAS), remains an excellent method of controlling snoring, recent reviews suggest that it improves OSAS in only half of patients. Multiple upper airway sites appear to play a role in the obstructive process, including the soft palate, pharyngeal walls, and base of the tongue. The use of maxillofacial surgery in conjunction with UPPP was explored to correct these multiple sites of obstruction. The procedure included a mandibular osteotomy/

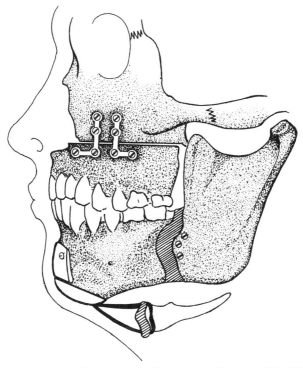

Fig 16–10.—Diagram of maxillary and mandibular osteotomy. (Courtesy of Riley RW, Powell NB, Guilleminault C: *J Oral Maxillofac Surg* 51:742-747, 1993.)

genioglossus advancement with hyoid myotomy/suspension (GAHM) (Fig 16-9) and, when this failed, maxillary and mandibular advancement osteotomy (MMO) (Fig 16-10).

Methods.—Outcomes in 239 consecutively treated patients were evaluated. A presurgical evaluation was done to document the diagnosis and isolate the obstructed areas, including fiberoptic pharyngoscopy, cephalometric analysis, and polygraphic monitoring. Treatment was directed to the obstructive site in a two-phase surgical protocol, beginning with GAHM. If surgical failure was documented at 6 months by polysomnography, MMO was offered (Fig 16-11). The results of this protocol were compared with those of a series of patients using nasal continuous positive airway pressure (CPAP).

Results.—The success rate with phase 1 therapy was 61%; most of those patients required both GAHM and UPPP. Twenty-four patients went on to phase 2 therapy, for which the success rate was 100% (Table 1). Surgery was as effective as nasal CPAP, as reflected by analysis of changes in sleep architecture and sleep-disordered breathing (Table 2). Success rates in phase 1 were almost as high as 80% for patients with mild to moderate OSAS, compared to about 40% for those with severe

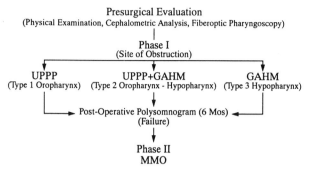

Fig 16–11.—Surgical protocol. (Courtesy of Riley RW, Powell NB, Guilleminault C: *J Oral Maxillofac Surg* 51:742–747, 1993.)

OSAS (Table 3). Postoperative morbidity was low for all surgical procedures.

Conclusion.—The surgical protocol described for treatment of OSAS yields a more than 95% long-term success rate, the highest of any reported protocol. The comprehensive presurgical evaluation, permitting a logical approach to reconstruction of the upper airway, is a vital part of treatment.

▶ The significance of OSAS has only recently received attention. In its mildest form, OSAS is snoring during which an individual will occasionally obstruct the airway and awaken enough to shift position. In its severest form, multiple periods of apnea occur that prevent the individual from any effective sleep. In addition to excessive daytime sleepiness, secondary changes in the cardiovascular system and hypertension can occur that are associated with increased mortality. The diagnostic evaluation and treatment protocol for OSAS described in this article appears to be valid but should not be con-

TABLE 1.—Results of Surgical Protocol

Surgery Groups	Total Patients	Success Rate (%)/No. Patients
Phase 1		
GAHM + UPPP	223	60/133
GAHM	6	67/4
UPPP	10	80/8
Total	239	61/145
Phase 2		
MMO	24	100/24

(Courtesy of Riley RW, Powell NB, Guilleminault C: *J Oral Maxillofac Surg* 51:742–747, 1993.)

TABLE 2.—Phase 1 and Phase 2 Surgical and Nasal Continuous Positive Airway Pressure Results

	Phase 1 (N = 145)			Phase 2 (N = 24)		
	Presurgery	CPAP	Postsurgery	Presurgery	CPAP	Postsurgery
RDI	47.3 (SD 25.8)	7.2 (SD 4.9)	9.5 (SD 9.5)	75.1 (SD 26.7)	8.2 (SD 2.9)	9.6 (SD 2.9)
LSAT (%)	72.3 (SD 12.9)	86.4 (SD 11.0)	86.6 (SD 4.5)	64.0 (SD 15.9)	87.5 (SD 6.9)	86.7 (SD 7.0)
TST	360 (SD 72)	363 (SD 67)	379 (SD 63)	379 (SD 58)	376 (SD 69)	388 (SD 56)
% St 3-4	4.4 (SD 5.6)	11.1 (SD 10.8)	8.5 (SD 7.7)	2.7 (SD 4.3)	11.0 (SD 13.3)	8.2 (SD 6.7)
%REM	11.9 (SD 5.8)	18.3 (SD 7.0)	17.7 (SD 5.6)	8.1 (SD 3.1)	21.2 (SD 8.4)	21.5 (SD 6.1)
SNB (GAHM) (°)	77.5 (SD 5.2)			75.5 (SD 3.1)		79.5 (SD 4.7)
PAS (GAHM) (mm)	5.5 (SD 1.6)		8.5 (SD 2.1)	4.6 (SD 1.7)		9.2 (SD 2.1)
BMI (kg/m^2)	29.2 (SD 5.2)		28.8 (SD 4.9)	31.4 (SD 6.5)		30.9 (SD 6.0)

(Courtesy of Riley RW, Powell NB, Guilleminault C: *J Oral Maxillofac Surg* 51:742–747, 1993.)

TABLE 3.—Phase 1 Results by Severity of Obstructive Sleep
Apnea Syndrome

OSAS Severity	No. Patients	Success Rate (%)/ No. Patients
Mild (RDI < 20, LSAT > 85)	26	77/20
Moderate (RDI 20-40, LSAT > 80)	58	78/45
Moderate-severe (RDI 40-60, LSAT > 70)	51	71/36
Severe (RDI > 60, LSAT < 70)	104	42/44

(Courtesy of Riley RW, Powell NB, Guilleminault C: *J Oral Maxillofac Surg* 51:742–747, 1993.)

sidered for all patients. For instance, the mandibular osteotomies that are part of phase II therapy are not appropriate for the pediatric (growing) patient for whom removal of enlarged tonsils and adenoids should be considered. To put their protocol in better perspective, the authors should have included descriptions with critiques of other treatment protocols (such as the linguoplasty reported by Fujitas, which has been reported to be somewhat successful). The reader should keep in mind that this is a controversial area, and the proposed treatment protocol needs further validation by other groups.—S.M. Roser, D.M.D., M.D.

17 Implantology

Introduction

Until recently, we relied on the long-term data on the use of implants to restore edentulous mouths to base all of what we are accomplishing with implants. This year, 4 studies were published that should add significantly to our knowledge base about other than fully edentulous situations. Two multicenter studies review implants in the partially edentulous situation and the implant-supported overdenture. A retrospective study using rigid evaluation parameters reviews the use of extraoral implants to support auricular and orbital prostheses. The outcome of implants in the previously irradiated mandible and the effect of aging on the healing of hydroxyapatite (HA) implants are also discussed.

An area that is becoming of increasing concern is late implant failure. Soft tissue inflammation around the implant with or without excessive mechanical forces can produce bone loss that weakens the support of the fixture and exposes the HA coating or titanium threads. Accelerated bone loss then occurs, resulting in implant mobility and loss. This chapter includes 2 articles that discuss the salvage of the implant that is beginning to fail. This area will continue to receive more attention as a portion of the large number of implants that have been placed begin to develop problems that were unknown at the time of placement. I expect that as we sort out late implant failure and what can be done about it, we will incorporate modifications into the placement technique.

Steven M. Roser, D.M.D., M.D.

Outcome Studies

The Applicability of Osseointegrated Implants in the Treatment of Partially Edentulous Patients: Three-Year Results of a Prospective Multicenter Study
Henry PJ, Tolman DE, Bolender C (Univ of Western Australia, Perth; Mayo Med Ctr, Rochester, Minn; Univ of Washington, Seattle)
Quintessence Int 24:123–129, 1993   105-94-17–1

Background.—Results of the Brånemark System of osseointegrated implants in edentulous patients are well established. Clinical and conceptual differences make it difficult to extrapolate these results to partially edentulous patients.

Life-Table Analysis of Cumulative Success Rates

Time	Fixtures in situ (No.)	Failed fixtures (No.)	Success for time (%)	Cumulative success (%)
Fixture installation–Prosthesis insertion	558	20	96.4	96.4
Prosthesis insertion–Loaded 1 year	528	3	99.4	95.9
Loaded 1–2 years	494	8	98.4	94.3
Loaded 2–3 years	474	2	99.6	93.9

(Courtesy of Henry PJ, Tolman DE, Bolender C: *Quintessence Int* 24:123–129, 1993.)

Methods.—The 3-year results of a multicenter study of osseointegrated implants in 159 partially edentulous patients were evaluated. The prostheses were all freestanding, with no connections to natural teeth. At least 2 fixtures were placed per prosthesis. Evaluations included Plaque Index, gingivitis, pocket depth, Bleeding Index, tooth mobility, prosthesis stability, and stomatognathic function, with bone height changes measured radiographically.

Results.—At 3 years, the study included 460 fixtures supporting 174 fixed prostheses in 139 patients. Cumulative fixture survival rate was 94% (table). The failure rates were higher for fixtures in the 7-, 10-, and 13-mm lengths. Cumulative failure rate was 8% for maxillary vs. 5% for mandibular fixtures. There was no significant gender difference in failure rates. Most failures occurred in patients with a relatively high preplacement Plaque Index. A significant number of fixtures showed increased marginal bone height. Fracture of the occlusal surface material was the most common technical complication, followed by loosening of prosthesis-fixation screws.

Conclusion.—The use of Brånemark osseointegrated implants in the partially edentulous arch was supported. Follow up for 5 years is planned. Acceptable plaque control can be maintained on the titanium abutments; implant failure is most common in patients with more plaque accumulation. A good passive fit is easier to achieve on a short-span, partial denture than on the cross-arch framework of an edentulous patient, accounting for the low number of fixture losses after prosthesis insertion in partially edentulous patients.

▶ In traditional Brånemark terms, this is a preliminary report, because the study lasted for less than 5 years. Findings such as a higher maxillary implant failure and a 4% incidence of paresthesia from posterior mandibular implants are similar to the results of previous studies. An advantage to this multicenter study at the 5-year mark will be that it will be an analysis of management at different centers. It seems strange that we await the results of this study, which is about something being done daily, until it is remembered that all of the original investigative work was done in the edentulous patient before the implants were available for clinical use. We are now doing the reverse by undertaking the science to justify our clinical success.—S.M. Roser, D.M.D., M.D.

A Multicenter Study of Overdentures Supported by Brånemark Implants

Johns RB, Jemt T, Heath MR, Hutton JE, McKenna S, McNamara DC, van Steenberghe D, Taylor R, Watson RM, Herrmann I (Univ of Sheffield, England; Univ of Göteborg, Sweden; Royal London Hosp; et al)
Int J Oral Maxillofac Implants 7:513–522, 1992   105-94-17–2

Introduction.—The Brånemark System is based on nonremoveable fixed prostheses, but the need for facial support in patients with advanced ridge resorption is better met by a removable, flanged prosthesis. Such prostheses can be supported by fewer implants, and when the opposing prosthesis is supported by a resorbed jaw, greater stability may be obtained by denture occlusion. Overdentures supported by implants impart stability to the denture, good support for the facial soft tissues, and easy removal for denture cleaning. However, experience with such overdentures is limited.

Methods.—In a prospective, multicenter study, the efficacy of overdentures supported by Brånemark osseointegrated fixtures was evaluated. The initial study sample included 133 patients at 9 centers with a total of 117 maxillary and 393 mandibular implants. Fifty-nine percent of the patients were women, and the mean age of the entire group was 57 years. This analysis extends to the 1-year follow-up visit.

Results.—Overdentures were provided for 127 patients, including 29 maxillary and 98 mandibular. Two hundred seventy-nine activated implants were stable and supporting overdentures at follow-up (Table 1). Thirty-two mobile implants were removed and another 29 were lost to follow-up. The failure rate was higher for maxillary than for mandibular implants, 8% vs. 2%, before prosthesis placement. Maxillary implants were also more likely to show unfavorable mucosal reactions. Most of the differences between the fixed and the present overdentures in the maxilla were based on differences in patient selection and bone quality (Table 2).

Conclusion.—This 1-year follow-up study reports promising short-term results with implant-supported removable overdentures in the

TABLE 1.—Implant Status From Surgical Placement Through 1-Year Follow-up

Implant placement

	Placed	Withdrawn
Maxilla	117	—
Mandible	393	4
Total	510	4

Abutment connection/overdenture placement

	Loaded	Failure	Sleeper	Withdrawn
Maxilla	100	9	7	1
Mandible	198	7	170	14
Total	298	16	177	15

1-year follow-up

	Loaded	Failure	Activated sleeper	Sleeper	Withdrawn Connected	Withdrawn Sleeper
Maxilla	89	12	1	6	—	—
Mandible	190	4	1	164	5	5
Total	279	16	2	170	5	5

(Courtesy of Johns RB, Jemt T, Heath MR, et al: *Int J Oral Maxillofac Implants* 7:513–522, 1992.)

edentulous mandible. The results are comparable to those for fixed prostheses supported by more implants. Mucosal problems and implant failures are more common in the maxilla. There is need for further reports to clarify the role of implant-supported overdentures in the maxilla and the mandible.

▶ This is the largest overdenture study available. It is a prospective study. Standardized outcome criteria were used. The success rate for the mandibular overdenture was excellent and similar to that demonstrated for implants supporting fixed bridges. However, maxillary overdentures were not as successful. A number of reasons are offered, including that the patients selected had poor quality bone; short implants (7 mm) were used; only 2 implants were used; and overdenture design made cleaning the implants difficult. Because the overdenture can be an excellent functional and esthetic restoration at a relatively low cost for patients with atrophic ridges, the design and protocol for a successful maxillary overdenture is eagerly awaited. Most probably the format will include wider implants, more than 2 implants, and bone

TABLE 2.—Effect of Bone Quality on Implant Survival

	Maxilla[†]		Mandible[‡]	
Bone quality*	No. inserted	No. failed	No. inserted	No. failed
Types 1–3	87	6	366	10
Type 4	30	15	27	1

* Bone types 1 to 4 according to Lekholm and Zarb.
† Difference is significant (P < .001 using chi-square analysis.
‡ No significance could be found using chi-square analysis.
(Courtesy of Johns RB, Jemt T, Heath MR, et al: *Int J Oral Maxillofac Implants* 7:513–522, 1992.)

grafting to permit the placement of longer implants.—S.M. Roser, D.M.D., M.D.

A Retrospective Study of Osseointegrated Skin-Penetrating Titanium Fixtures Used for Retaining Facial Prostheses

Jacobsson M, Tjellström A, Fine L, Andersson H (Univ of Göteborg, Sweden; Univ of Chicago)
Int J Oral Maxillofac Implants 7:523–528, 1992   105-94-17-3

Background.—Many implant systems have been proposed over the decades, with reports of success that were not scientifically supported. A conference sponsored by the National Institutes of Health subsequently established minimum criteria for implant success. To address these criteria, osseointegrated skin-penetrating facial titanium implants used for anchoring facial prostheses were assessed over a 5-year period.

Methods and Findings.—Eighty-seven patients were divided into 3 groups—those with fixtures in place for less than 3 years, with fixtures in place for 3 to 5 years, and with fixtures in place for more than 5 years. Fixtures were auricular or orbital. Implant survival was 95.6% in patients with auricular implants and 67.2% in those with orbital implants. Approximately 10% had skin problems, with the remaining patients having no or minimal complications. The possibility of osseointegration occurring around an orbital defect was not as good as in the mastoid process.

Conclusions and Criteria.—In the first 6 to 9 months after implant fixture placement in the mastoid process, the risk of implant loss is very small. Thereafter, it is almost nonexistent. Outcomes are less predictable in the orbital region. However, it is possible to achieve osseointegration in this region, even after irradiation. The loss of 1 or more implants in this area should not deter another attempt in 9 to 12 months. There is a small risk of late implant loss in the orbital region, even after more than 5 years.

Success criteria for craniofacial implants were proposed. When clinically tested, individual unattached implants should be immobile. In more than 95% of all observations, soft-tissue reactions around skin-penetrating abutments should be of type 0 or 1. There should be no persistent and/or irreversible signs and symptoms associated with individual implant performance. The minimum criterion for success should be success rates of 95% in the mastoid process and 90% in the orbital region in nonirradiated bone tissue at 5 years.

▶ The article represents the 5-year retrospective study of extraoral titanium implants. Two of the investigators, Jacobsson and Tjellström, are considered pioneers in the use of extraoral Brånemark implants. Their excellent results of the mastoid implants mean that patients may avoid the multiple surgeons and a usually less-than-desired outcome of ear reconstruction. The less favorable results of the orbital implants are not as encouraging. Preimplant hyperbaric oxygen therapy (HBO) may improve the success rate in irradiated bone, which is the common situation after removal of an eye during tumor removal. Fortunately, similar to the intraoral situation, implant failure did not result in osteomyelitis, and implants could be replaced in sites after bone healing has occurred. Skin irritation around the implants was the most common complication, which could be significantly lessened by spacing the implants as far from each other as possible.—S.M. Roser, D.M.D., M.D.

Osseointegrated Implant Rehabilitation of the Previously Irradiated Mandible: Results of a Limited Trial at 3 to 7 Years
Taylor TD, Worthington P (Univ of Connecticut School of Dental Medicine, Farmington; Univ of Washington, Seattle)
J Prosthet Dent 69:60–69, 1993   105-94-17–4

Background.—There has been much discussion and experimentation on the use of osseointegrated dental implants in patients with a history of previous radiation to the jaws. One experience with a limited number of patients was presented.

Methods and Outcomes.—Twenty-one Brånemark implants were placed in previously irradiated mandibles of 4 patients (table). All patients had been counseled intensively as to the risks of surgery; all accepted the risks. To date, no implants have been lost. The implants have been functioning in place from 3 to 7 years. All appear stable clinically and radiographically. Perioperative hyperbaric oxygen treatment appeared to be beneficial.

Conclusion.—The outcomes in these 4 cases were encouraging. Osseointegrated dental implants can be successfully placed in patients with a history of tumoricidal doses of radiation to the mandible. Nevertheless, extreme caution is needed in considering the elective placement of osseointegrated implants in previously irradiated sites. The risks of morbidity associated from unsuccessful implantation are real and have yet to

Data Regarding Patient History and Treatment

	Patient 1	Patient 2	Patient 3	Patient 4
Original tumor	SCC floor of mouth (had had two primaries)	SCC floor of mouth nodes in left neck	SCC anterior floor of mouth	Mucoepidermoid carcinoma floor of mouth and mandible (right)
Surgical treatment	1973 Rim resection mandible	1985 Partial glossectomy, floor of mouth resection, left neck dissection, rim resection mandible	1984 Rim resection mandible, local excision 1985 (recurrence) Excision floor of mouth, bilateral supraosohyoid dissection, repair with nasolabial flaps	1986 Excision floor of mouth (right) hemimandibulectomy, partial parotidectomy (right) neck dissection
Radiation treatment	1973 Intraoral cone 6000 cGy (mandible not involved) 1978 6020 cGy external beam; entire mandible	1985 6500 cGy to entire mandible	1986 5950 cGy to entire mandible	1986 6480 cGy to entire mandible

(continued)

Table (continued)

HBO	No	Yes	Yes	Yes
Age at implantation	61	60	50	59
Phase 1 date	6-13-85	3-21-88	6-6-88	7-10-89
Implants placed (number)	6	4	5	6 (2 in bone graft)
Implants lost (number)	0	0	0	0
Implants "put to sleep"	0	0	0	2
Delay from radiation to implantation	7 Years	2 Years 3 months	2 Years 2 months	2 Years
Delay from phase 1 to phase 2	5 Months	6 Months	6 Months	6 Months
Present clinical oral status	Excellent orally. Recent third primary in base of tongue treated with further radiation and chemotherapy.	Good. Needs help with oral hygiene.	Good. Has had intermittent soft tissue inflammation on occasion, resolving with local measures.	Good

Abbreviation: SCC, squamous cell carcinoma.
(Courtesy of Taylor TD, Worthington P: J Prosthet Dent 69:60–69, 1993.)

be documented. Perioperative hyperbaric oxygen therapy should be included in the treatment protocol.

▶ The patients who derive the maximum benefit from implant-supported prostheses are those who have no other alternatives. These include patients with defects of the head and neck acquired as the result of ablative surgery for malignancy. The lack of teeth in many of these patients—complicated by the effects of tumoricidal doses of radiation, which includes radiation caries and dry mouth—makes these patients poor candidates for conventional restorative/prosthetic dentistry. The very positive results from this study should encourage all of us to pursue the option of implant-supported prostheses for our own patients. However, the numbers are small and follow-up is limited. Because the authors recommend perioperative hyperbaric oxygen therapy (HBO) as part of the treatment protocol, these patients should be referred to centers with HBO capabilities.—S.M. Roser, D.M.D., M.D.

The Effect of Aging on the Healing of Hydroxylapatite Implants
Tatsuo S, Kohsuke O, Kanako S, Ken-Ichi M (Showa Univ, Tokyo)
J Oral Maxillofac Surg 51:51–56, 1993   105-94-17-5

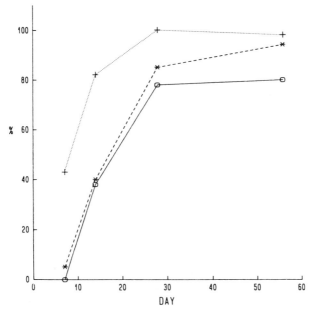

Fig 17–1.—Graph showing the mean BCSR score at each time point for the young (*plus*), adult (*asterisk*), and old (*circle*) groups. (Courtesy of Tatsuo S, Kohsuke O, Kanako S, et al: *J Oral Maxillofac Surg* 51:51–56, 1993.)

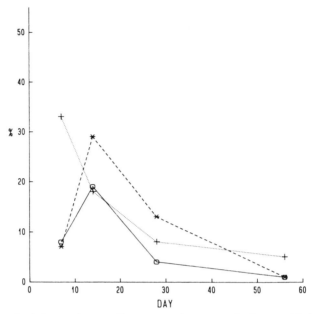

Fig 17–2.—Graph showing the mean tVsp score at each time point for the young (*plus*), adult (*asterisk*), and old (*circle*) groups. (Courtesy of Tatsuo S, Kohsuke O, Kanako S, et al: *J Oral Maxillofac Surg* 51:51-56, 1993.)

Purpose.—Hydroxyapatite (HA), used as bone implant material in a variety of situations, is especially indicated in older people. Given the bone changes that occur with advancing age, it is possible that the healing process after HA placement will be retarded as well. The potential effects of aging on the healing process after placement of HA implants into bone were investigated in rats.

Methods.—Experiments were conducted in 3 groups of Wistar rats: a young group aged 6 weeks, an adult group aged 12 weeks, and an old group aged 2 years. Each animal received 2 tibial HA implants. At intervals up to 56 days after implantation, the animals were killed for histologic examination of the healing process. A computer-based image analyzer was used to measure the percentage of HA-bone contact in the trabecular bone and medullary cavity.

Results.—The young animals had peak trabecular bone specific volume (tVsp) about 7 days after implantation. They showed rapid increase in bone contacting surface ratio (BCSR) with most of the implant surface being covered with new bone by 14 days (Figs 17-1 and 17-2). The young rats showed no fibrous tissue between the implant surface and new bone by 28 days. In the old group, as in the adult group, tVsp peaked at 14 days, though it was 10% lower in the old group. Bone contacting surface ratio progressed about equally in the adult and old group, but the old group had a BCSR of only about 80% by 56 days.

Conclusion.—Hydroxyapatite implantation in young people is followed by active formation of new bone, with quicker HA-bone contact than in adults. Older people, however, will have less HA-bone contact than adults because of their declining bone-forming capacity. Thus, aging may interfere with the achievement of good HA-bone contact.

▶ The population to receive implants initially consisted of older, totally edentulous patients. Excellent results were observed, and because of the lack of significant morbidity, old age has not been a contraindication to implant placement. However, it is well established that age results in significant differences in bone metabolism. This is seen as delayed healing of fractures of the atrophic edentulous mandible in the older individual. This study chose to look at HA implants in the older animal. As expected, less bone was found in contact with the HA implant in the older animals than in younger controls. These results cannot be extrapolated to humans, but they should make us stop and ask questions about the implant protocol for the older patient. We use the same protocol for young and old. Should it be the same?—S.M. Roser, D.M.D., M.D.

The Regenerative Potential of Plaque-Induced Peri-Implant Bone Defects Treated by a Submerged Membrane Technique: An Experimental Study

Jovanovic SA, Kenney EB, Carranza FA Jr, Donath K (Univ of California, Los Angeles: Univ of Hamburg, Germany)
Int J Oral Maxillofac Implants 8:13–18, 1993   105-94-17–6

Objective.—Of the possible complications of osseointegrated tooth implants, progressive bone loss around the implants is of special concern. In treating an implant that is failing in this way, the goals are to arrest progression of the disease process, regenerate lost bone tissue, and restore bone support for the implant. A preliminary study in dogs assessed the possibility of new bone formation on previously contaminated implants.

Methods.—After placement of dental implants into the mandibles of beagles, gross plaque was allowed to accumulate around the implants for 3 months, resulting in circumferential bone defects around the implants. At that time, all implants were treated by removal of granulation tissue, preparation of the implant surface, and placement of an expanded polytetrafluoroethylene membrane over each implant. Perforations were made into the cancellous bone before flap closure to cover the implants. Control implants were treated in the same way, except that no membrane was placed.

Results.—The initial bone defects were greater around hydroxyapatite than titanium implants. The bone defects showed signs of closure after an uneventful period of submerged healing. On histologic examination after 2 months of healing, large amounts of rapidly formed lamellar bone were noted beneath the membrane, whereas control sites in which no membrane had been placed showed little or no bone formation. In some previously contaminated implant surfaces, there was evidence of re-osseointegration.

Conclusion.—Results of this animal experiment suggest that a submerged-membrane technique can be a useful method of treating plaque-induced bone defects around osseointegrated dental implants. There is significant bone regeneration and some new, direct bone-to-implant contact. Surface preparation is an important aspect of this form of treatment.

▶ This paper represents one of many reports of experimental and clinical methods for salvaging osseointegrated implants that have begun to fail after being restored. Most commonly, late failure occurs when bone resorption at the coronal aspect of the implant weakens the support for the implant and mechanical forces loosen the implant from the remainder of the bone support. Plaque-induced inflammation around an implant, particularly a hydroxyapatite-coated implant, can cause such coronal bone loss. This animal study reports on the salvage of implants that have lost coronal bone. There are several important points: (1) laboratory animals are different than humans and these results may not be transferable; (2) preparation of the exposed surface of the implant, using a technique that includes an air-powder abrasive system and a solution of citric acid to detoxify endotoxin-contaminated implant surfaces, appears to be critical to permitting bone to once again come into intimate contact with the implant; and (3) as offered in this paper, using guided tissue regeneration with a submerged membrane enhances the process of bone growing in contact with the implant.—S.M. Roser, D.M.D., M.D.

Treatment of Ligature-Induced Peri-Implantitis Using Guided Tissue Regeneration: A Clinical and Histologic Study in the Beagle Dog
Grunder U, Hürzeler MB, Schüpbach P, Strub JR (Univ of Zurich, Switzerland; Albert-Ludwigs-Univ, Freiburg, Germany)
Int J Oral Maxillofac Implants 8:282–293, 1993   105-94-17-7

Background.—Endosseous oral implants are increasingly used as abutments for fixed or removable prostheses. Their long-term outlook is excellent, but implant threads occasionally are exposed by bacterial peri-implant destruction, a condition referred to as "peri-implantitis." The clinical and histologic findings closely resemble those of periodontitis.

Study Design.—The value of guided tissue regeneration (GTR) around submerged and nonsubmerged implants was examined as a treatment for ligature-induced peri-implantitis in beagle dogs. Titanium implants were placed in the premolar regions of the mandible in each of 10 dogs. Cotton floss ligatures were placed around the implant necks, and oral hygiene was avoided for 5 months. In 5 dogs with submerged implants, the abutments were removed and a polytetrafluoroethylene (PTFE) barrier

TABLE 1.—New Bone Formation

Study groups	Mean ± SE	Range
Submerged		
Control (n = 5)	0.3 ± 0.2	−1.0 to 2.1
Test (n = 5)	−0.1 ± 0.1	−0.7 to 1.0
Nonsubmerged		
Control (n = 5)	0.2 ± 0.1	−1.2 to 0.9
Test (n = 5)	−0.1 ± 0.2	−1.7 to 1.0

Note: No significant differences found.
(Courtesy of Grunder U, Hürzeler MB, Schüpbach P, et al: *Int J Oral Maxillofac Implants* 8:282-293, 1993.)

was placed over the implants and their adjoining bony defects. The 5 dogs with nonsubmerged implants underwent flap surgery without removal of the abutments. A PTFE barrier was placed around the abutment and adjacent defect at test sites.

Observations.—There were no significant clinical or histologic differences between experimental and control sites in dogs with submerged or nonsubmerged implants. Histomorphometric studies indicated no significant differences in new bone formation (Table 1), but significantly more regenerated connective tissue was present in GTR animals than in controls (Table 2).

Discussion.—Use of GTR was not an effective approach in this canine model of ligature-induced peri-implantitis. The finding that epithelial cells are tightly attached to the implant surface in the area between the

TABLE 2.—New Connective Tissue Formation

Study group	Mean ± SE	Range
Submerged		
Control (n = 5)	1.3 ± 0.2	0 to 3.5
Test (n = 5)	1.9 ± 0.2	0.9 to 3.6
Nonsubmerged		
Control (n = 5)	1.0 ± 0.1	0.2 to 1.8
Test (n = 5)	1.3 ± 0.1	0.7 to 1.9

* P > .01.
NS, no significant difference.
(Courtesy of Grunder U, Hürzeler MB, Schüpbach P, et al: *Int J Oral Maxillofac Implants* 8:282-293, 1993.)

sulcus epithelium and connective tissue suggests a "sealant" effect, but its clinical significance is uncertain.

▶ The findings of this study are important to recognize because the need to salvage implants around which bone has resorbed is becoming a more common situation. Decontamination of implant surface in this study was done using an air-flow powder technique, which is very effective in removing endotoxin from the titanium surfaces. However, cleaning the surface in this way may leave the implant with a different surface energy level, one that is less favorable to bone. Other reasons for failure include the difficulty in general to induce bone to regenerate after horizontal bone loss and premature membrane exposure that could lead to recurrence of inflammation around the implant. Further investigations need to be undertaken now before more implants are unnecessarily lost.—S.M. Roser, D.M.D., M.D.

18 Temporomandibular Disorders

Introduction

This year has seen considerable upheaval in the management of disorders of the TMJ. The Food and Drug Administration has withdrawn approval of all alloplastic materials designed for use in the TMJ that do not meet new and more stringent testing requirements. In reaction to this, many surgeons have voluntarily stopped using all alloplastic materials in joint reconstructive surgery. Three articles in this section deal with this issue. Additionally, the somewhat dismal outcome of attempts at reconstruction after failure of reconstruction with Teflon-Proplast implants is presented. A series of articles reporting on an international consensus conference offer guidelines for surgical management and evaluation of outcome. Acceptance of these guidelines should help surgeons share information that should help to avoid problems such as the failure to adequately test the Teflon-Proplast implant before its introduction for clinical use. One of the articles from the conference discusses the pathology of TMJ osteoarthritis and internal derangement. The authors offer the concept that osteoarthritis can occur independently of internal derangement, and internal derangement may be the result of or the cause of osteoarthritis. If true, position of the disk becomes much less of a factor in the management of temporomandibular disorder.

The effectiveness of an injection of sodium hyaluronate into a painful joint and the success of a modified condylotomy procedure also add new information regarding the etiology and management of joint symptoms. Arthroscopic surgery continues to be the most common surgical treatment to the joint. The effectiveness of arthroscopic procedures remains high. Continued efforts need to be directed toward understanding the pathogenesis of disorders of the TMJ.

Steven M. Roser, D.M.D., M.D.

Outcome of Surgical Treatment With Alloplasty

Multicenter Evaluation of Temporomandibular Joint Proplast-Teflon Disk Implant
Spagnoli D, Kent JN (Charlotte, NC; Louisiana State Univ, New Orleans)
Oral Surg Oral Med Oral Pathol 74:411–421, 1992   105-94-18-1

TABLE 1.—Patient Profile

	Data	Unilateral joints	Bilateral joints
Patients (No.)	465		
M (%)	4		
F (%)	96		
No. of joints (%)	680	188 (27.6)	492 (72.4)
In place	584 (85.9)	172 (29.4)	412 (70.6)
Removed	96 (14.1)	16 (16.6)	80 (83.4)
Incidence (%) of removal		(8.5)	(16.2)
Follow-up range (mo)	6-76		
Weighted average follow-up (mo)			
All patients	31.9		
In place implants	33		
Removed implants	20		

(Courtesy of Spagnoli D, Kent JN: Oral Surg Oral Med Oral Pathol 74:411-421, 1992.)

Introduction.—In 1986, disk replacement implants made of Proplast I and II laminated to Teflon were reported to fail in both patients and animals. Joint load and wear debris led to progressive macrophage and giant cell reaction and then to pain, bone resorption, and malocclusion. The implants were withdrawn from the market in 1988. The success and failure incidence of these implants is summarized, and recommendations for follow-up, removal, and repair surgery are made.

Patients.—The retrospective, multicenter study included 680 TMJs in 465 patients who received Proplast II Teflon interpositional implants

TABLE 2.—Patient Status of In-Place PTIPI (*n* = 584)

	Asymptomatic 540 (92.4%)	Symptomatic* 44 (7.6%)
No condylar or occlusal change	316 (58.5%)	19 (43.3%)
Condylar changes but no occlusal changes	185 (34.2%)	19 (43.3%)
Condylar and occlusal changes	39 (7.3%)	6 (13.4%)
Total	540 (100%)	44 (100)

Abbreviation: PTIPI, Proplast II-Teflon interpositional implant.
* Pain and decreased range of motion.
(Courtesy of Spagnoli D, Kent JN: *Oral Surg Oral Med Oral Pathol* 74:411–421, 1992.)

placed after meniscectomy (Table 1). The patients were followed for 6–76 months. At an average weighted follow-up of 32 months, 584 of the implants were still in place. Ninety-two percent of them were asymptomatic, but 224 asymptomatic and 25 symptomatic joints showed evidence of condylar resorption. Forty-five of these joints showed malocclusion (Table 2).

Findings.—Pain was the most common reason for the 96 implant removals (Table 3). Forty-four percent of the removed implants showed wear at the Teflon fluorinated ethylene propylene surface or through the Teflon into the Proplast; other findings included implant fracture, dis-

TABLE 3.—Reasons for PTIPI Removal
($n = 96$)

Pain	77 (80.2%)
Condylar resorption	64 (66.6%)
Malocclusion	38 (39.6%)
Hypomobility	34 (35.4%)
Trauma	14 (14.6%)
Mobility/displacement	11 (11.5%)
Legal	9 (9.4%)
Infection	3 (3.1%)

Abbreviation: PTIPI, Proplast II-Teflon interpositional implant.
(Courtesy of Spagnoli D, Kent JN: *Oral Surg Oral Med Oral Pathol* 74:411–421, 1992.)

TABLE 4.—Surgical Findings Reported at PTIPI
Removal ($n = 96$)

No wear	30 (31.3%)
Teflon® Wear only	4 (4.2%)
Wear through Teflon into Proplast	38 (39.6%)
Fractured	14 (14.6%)
Displaced	10 (10.4%)
Loose	9 (9.4%)
Buckled	3 (3.1%)
Encapsulated inferior surface	59 (61.5%)
Encapsulated superior surface	22 (21.8%)
Condylar resorption	44 (45.8%)
Fossa/eminence resorption	31 (32.3%)
Rough irregular condyle	30 (31.3%)
Smooth cortical condyle	28 (29.2%)
Granulomatous tissue	26 (27.1%)

Abbreviation: PTIPI, Proplast II-Teflon interpositional implant.
(Courtesy of Spagnoli D, Kent JN: *Oral Surg Oral Med Oral Pathol* 74:411–421, 1992.)

TABLE 5.—Condylar Resorption
Observed at PTIPI Removal ($n = 44$)

Surgical findings	%
Wear	72.7
Granuloma	45.4
Fossa resorption	50.0
Rough condyle	54.5

Abbreviation: PTIPI, Proplast II-Teflon interpositional implant.
(Courtesy of Spagnoli D, Kent JN: *Oral Surg Oral Med Oral Pathol* 74:411–421, 1992.)

TABLE 6.—Granuloma Observed at PTIPI
Removal (*n* = 26)

Surgical findings	%
Wear	76.9
Displaced IPI	38.4
Condylar resorption	76.9
Rough condyle	69.2

Abbreviation: PTIPI, Proplast II-Teflon interpositional implant.
(Courtesy of Spagnoli D, Kent JN: *Oral Surg Oral Med Oral Pathol* 74:411–421, 1992.)

placement, loosening, and buckling (Table 4). When condylar resorption was present, nearly three fourths of the implants showed wear (Table 5). In the 26 joints with granulomas, more than three fourths were associated with worn implants (Table 6). Assuming that condylar resorption suggests the presence of a worn implant, 54% of the implants can be expected to fail. The reported annual failure rates range from 3%, reported by the manufacturer, to an average of 18% reported by individual clinicians. In vivo service life appears to be only 3 years, and there have been no reports of follow-up beyond 5 years.

Conclusion.—Yearly imaging studies are recommended for asymptomatic patients with Proplast-Teflon disk implants still in place. For symptomatic patients, evaluation should be performed 2 or 3 times a year. Patients in whom occlusal changes or changes in the condyle or fossa articular bone develop beyond the expected remodeling time should have the implants removed. Early, aggressive postoperative physical therapy may be contraindicated.

Long-Term Results on VK Partial and Total Temporomandibular Joint Systems
Kent JN, Block MS, Halpern J, Fontenot MG (Louisiana State Univ, New Orleans)
J Long Term Effects Med Implants 3:29–40, 1993   105-94-18–2

Background.—Two total TMJ systems, the VK I and II, have been used in the past decade to reconstruct the TMJ. The long-term results of VK partial and total TMJ systems were investigated.

VK System Evaluation (VK I Placed 1982–1986; VK II Placed 1986–1990)

Prosthesis	Years followed	No. entering interval	Failures	Lost to follow-up	For evaluation	Interval success rate (%)	Cumulative success rate (%)
VK I Partial	10	42	36	1	41	14.34	7.84
VK II Partial	6	6	0	0	6	100	100
VK I Total	10	96	58	11	85	39.68	19.83
VK II Total	6	118	21	2	116	82.2	79.3

(Courtesy of Kent JN, Block MS, Halpern J, et al: *J Long Term Effects Med Implants* 3:29–40, 1993.)

Methods and Findings.—Two hundred sixty-two procedures done during a 10-year period were reviewed. The VK I total joint was used between 1982 and 1986, and the VK II was used from 1986 to 1990. The cumulative success rate with the VK I was 44% at 6 years and 20% at 10 years. The cumulative success rate of the VK II at 6 years was 80%. The most common reason for failure was material wear of the Teflon fluorinated ethylene propylene surface of the VK I fossa. No material failures occurred with the VK II. Clinical success parameters for both prostheses were significantly improved when no previous surgery had been done before prosthetic total joint placement. In patients with a history of multiple procedures, rib grafts were not helpful after removal of total joint prostheses (table).

Conclusion.—Total TMJ prostheses must be reserved for patients in whom alternative surgery fails or when no other procedure is indicated. Patients with total TMJ prostheses should be closely monitored by clinical assessment and imaging.

▶ The publication of these 2 articles immediately preceded the recommendation that all Proplast-Teflon disk implants and VK I partial and complete joint replacements be removed. The crux of the matter is that the Teflon surface of the implant deteriorates as the result of what appears to be normal forces found in the TMJ. The deteriorated particles of Teflon produce a foreign body response that may or may not be symptomatic, but in all cases results in a destructive process of the joint structures. Polyethylene, the surface used in the VK II system, is thought to be able to resist the usual range of forces applied during TMJ function. However, the Food and Drug Administration has required all manufacturers of TMJ prostheses to submit more testing before giving even currently used prostheses approval for use. The authors discuss 2 of their concerns about TMJ surgery. The first is that there is very little reliable long-term data available regarding any technique of joint reconstruction, including rib grafts. Second, without this data, there can be no basis to recommend one reconstruction technique over another for patients from whom deteriorating alloplastic material must be removed. We indeed find ourselves in a dilemma as does this very unfortunate group of patients. For more insight into this area, the reader is encouraged to read the complete articles.—S.M. Roser, D.M.D., M.D.

Treatment Outcomes for Temporomandibular Joint Reconstruction After Proplast-Teflon Implant Failure
Henry CH, Wolford LM (Baylor Univ Med Ctr, Dallas)
J Oral Maxillofac Surg 51:352–358, 1993   105-94-18–3

Introduction.—It has proved difficult to treat complications developing when a Proplast-Teflon (PT) interpositional TMJ implant fails. Temporary and permanent alloplastic materials have been used interpositionally in the TMJ. Use of a PT implant may initially relieve symptoms and provide acceptable function, but many recipients later have changes in the mandibular condyle, severe pain, and malocclusion.

Patients and Methods.—The sequelae of PT implants were examined in 107 patients receiving implants in 163 joints. The PT implant was in place for 5 years on average, and patients were followed up for an average of 7.5 years.

Findings.—Only 12% of operated joints were free of significant bony changes on radiographic assessment. Of 45 patients with PT implants still in place, 36% have pain requiring medication. One fourth of these patients have had anterior open bite and malocclusion develop, and 9% have limited vertical opening.

Management and Outcome.—Five autologous tissues and total joint prostheses were used for TMJ reconstruction after failure of the PT implant. Temporalis fascia/muscle grafts were successful in only 13% of cases, but when combined with sagittal split ramus osteotomy, the success rate rose to 31%. Dermal grafts succeeded in only 1 of 9 cases, whereas conchal cartilage grafting was successful in 25% of attempts. The success rate for costochondral grafts was 12%, and for sternoclavicular grafts, 21%. Failures were most often the result of fibrous or bony ankylosis. When total joint prostheses were used in 26 patients, 88% gained functional and occlusal stability and nearly half the patients had a good pain response. The average interincisal opening was 33 mm after 2 years.

Conclusion.—Fibrous or bony ankylosis is the most common cause of failure of autologous tissues after placement of a PT implant. Reconstruction with a total joint prostheseis may be the only predictable effective measure in these patients, although longer follow-up is needed.

▶ The American Association of Oral and Maxillofacial Surgeons recommends that all Proplast-Teflon interpositional TMJ implants be removed even for those patients who are asymptomatic. They believe it is a matter of time before all implants break down and produce a foreign body giant cell reaction with destruction of the condyle and glenoid fossa. This article discusses the difficulty encountered removing the implant that has deteriorated and offers recommendations on how to reconstruct the TMJ after removal of the implant. The authors recommend using a total joint replacement technique and report a higher success using an alloplastic total joint than when autologous material is used. The technique of total joint prosthesis as described is technically demanding, and many believe it should be reserved for those patients who have failed to improve after removal of the implant and reconstruction with autologous material such as a temporalis muscle flap. Unfortunately, the outcome of these techniques is not always successful.—S.M. Roser, D.M.D., M.D.

Surgical Management

The Opinions of 100 International Experts on Temporomandibular Joint Surgery: A Postal Questionnaire
Goss AN (Univ of Adelaide, Australia)
Int J Oral Maxillofac Surg 22:66–70, 1993   105-94-18–4

Objective and Methods.—Results of a questionnaire sent to a representative group of oral and maxillofacial surgeons considered to be leaders in the field of TMJ surgery are reported. The questionnaire covered current areas of controversy related to TMJ surgery. One hundred international experts were selected from recommendations by their colleagues in the field. A second mailing was sent to nonrespondents after 3 months.

Results.—The overall response rate was 77%. Questions dealt with definitions, diagnosis, and broad treatment principles. There was generally strong support for the 5-stage concept of internal derangements (Fig 18-1); other variations or additions were proposed by 13% of respondents. Apart from some form of simple radiograph, no single investigational technique was predominant (Table 1). The responses were varied regarding the surgeon's performance of nonsurgical treatment (Table 2). On the question of nonsurgical treatment, only reassurance and splints to disengage the occlusion received more than 50% support (Table 3). Few respondents believed that a trial of nonsurgical treatment should exceed 6 months (Table 4). Only 30% of surgeons would operate in the early stage of internal derangement; operative treatment was considered appropriate in all other stages by 95% to 100% of respondents. The choice of interventional procedure varied from one country to another. Surgeons' opinions on the appropriateness of criteria for success varied (Table 5), as did their assessment of their own success (Table 6). Complications reported with arthroscopy (Table 7) and arthrotomy (Table 8) were broadly similar. Most surgeons used both approaches and followed patients for at least 1 year (Table 9).

Conclusion.—International experts on TMJ surgery showed a considerable degree of consensus in many areas. Techniques of surgery for particular stages of internal derangements and osteoarthrosis and the mea-

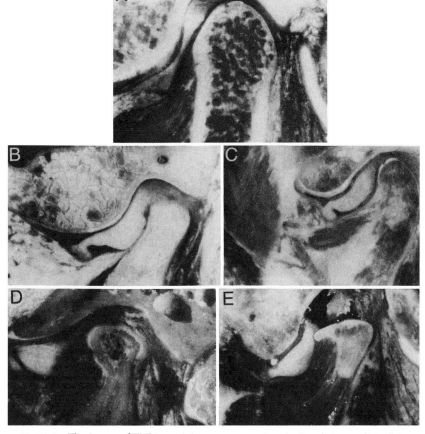

Fig 18–1.—The 5 stages of TMJ internal derangement are: **A,** early; **B,** early intermediate; **C,** intermediate; **D,** intermediate/late; and **E,** late. (Courtesy of Goss AN: *Int J Oral Maxillofac Surg* 22:66–70, 1993.)

TABLE 1.—Investigational Techniques

Technique	Always	Usually	Occasionally	Never	Not available
Transcranial radiograph	35	12	26	26	1
Transpharyngeal radiograph	15	5	25	53	2
Tomogram	22	32	39	6	1
Panorex (OPG)	67	18	12	3	–
Arthrogram	10	33	42	15	–
CT scan	3	10	74	13	–
MRI	7	25	58	5	5
Diagnostic arthroscopy	3	17	51	15	14

(Courtesy of Goss AN: *Int J Oral Maxillofac Surg* 22:66–70, 1993.)

TABLE 2.—Nonsurgical Treatment

Do you	Usually	Sometimes	Never
Do it yourself	35	39	26
Accept what the referring dentist has done	13	74	13
Work with a prosthodontist or other specialist	44	41	15

(Courtesy of Goss AN: *Int J Oral Maxillofac Surg* 22:66–70, 1993.)

TABLE 3.—Use of or Belief in Appropriateness of Various Nonsurgical Treatments

Treatment	Usually	Sometimes	Never
Reassurance	64	32	4
Jaw exercises	40	53	7
Splints			
• to increase vertical dimension	37	53	10
• to disengage occlusal guidance	51	38	11
• anterior repositioning splint	16	57	27
Permanent occlusal alteration by			
• grinding	3	67	30
• crowns	5	63	32
• orthodontics	12	75	13
• orthognathic surgery	5	80	15

(Courtesy of Goss AN: *Int J Oral Maxillofac Surg* 22:66–70, 1993.)

TABLE 4.—Minimum Time for Trying
Nonsurgical Treatment Before
Considering Surgery

1 month	9
2 months	34
6 months	51
12 months	5
more than 12 months	1

(Courtesy of Goss AN: *Int J Oral Maxillofac Surg* 22:66–70, 1993.)

TABLE 5.—Acceptance of Various Criteria for Success of Surgery

Criterion	Yes	No
Pain absent or so mild that patient not concerned	100	–
Range of motion greater than 35 mm interincisal and 6 mm lateral and protrusive	90	10
Absence of joint sounds	38	62
Regular diet which, at worst, avoids tough or hard foods – patient minimally inconvenienced by diet	91	9
Return of normal imaging appearance	32	68
Absence of significant complications	97	3
Absence of symptoms for at least 2 years	78	22

(Courtesy of Goss AN: *Int J Oral Maxillofac Surg* 22:66–70, 1993.)

surement of treatment outcome are topics requiring additional consideration.

▶ Expert surgeons were questioned in preparation for the Second International Consensus Conference on Temporomandibular Joint Surgery, which was held in April 1992. The experts were asked questions about internal derangement and the management of symptomatic patients. Favored surgical management approaches differed by region, and a broad range of success or failure was reported. The majority of surgeons did not advocate early surgical intervention. This is good, because the pathogenesis of inflammatory TMJ disease and its sequelae, osteoarthrosis, has not been established, and early intervention might be harmful. It is worthy to note that this conference occurred before the U.S. Congress publicly investigated the role of the Teflon-Proplast interpositional implants. It would be interesting to undertake a similar survey today. My impression is that the results would show a much lower percentage of those in favor of early surgical intervention, the number of arthroscopic procedures would be greater, and the success rate would still be reported at about 80%. As the authors state in the paper, further investigation is needed.—S.M. Roser, D.M.D., M.D.

TABLE 6.—Estimate of Success of Surgery for Internal Derangement/Osteoarthrosis

Symptom	0–10%	11–20%	21–30%	31–40%	41–50%	51–60%	61–70%	71–80%	81–90%	91–100%
Pain	14	1	–	1	–	1	3	10	29	41
Locking	35	3	–	1	–	1	–	5	12	43
Clicking	10	1	4	–	5	3	14	9	20	34
Limitation of opening	16	–	1	–	1	4	1	13	26	38

Response in percentage.
(Courtesy of Goss AN: *Int J Oral Maxillofac Surg* 22:66–70, 1993.)

TABLE 7.—Complications With Arthroscopy

	0%	0–5%	6–10%	11–20%	20 + specify
Intraoperative					
Persistent bleeding	58	32	8	1	1
Iatrogenic damage	46	46	2	3	3
Postoperative					
Persistent pain	15	36	29	13	7
Facial weakness (temporary)	11	61	21	7	–
Facial weakness (permanent)	72	27	1	–	–
Infection	62	38	–	–	–
Deafness	94	6	–	–	–
Unaesthetic scar	66	33	–	1	–

(Courtesy of Goss AN: *Int J Oral Maxillofac Surg* 22:66–70, 1993.)

TABLE 8.—Complications With Arthrotomy

	0%	0–5%	6–10%	11–20%	20 + specify
Intraoperative					
Persistent bleeding	69	25	6	–	–
Iatrogenic damage	38	53	6	–	3
Postoperative					
Persistent pain	25	36	25	8	6
Facial weakness (temporary)	39	56	5	–	–
Facial weakness (permanent)	97	3	–	–	–
Infection	89	11	–	–	–
Deafness	92	8	–	–	–
Unaesthetic scar	94	6	–	1	–

(Courtesy of Goss AN: *Int J Oral Maxillofac Surg* 22:66–70, 1993.)

TABLE 9.—Personal Experience

Surgical approach					
Only use arthrotomy	29				
Only use arthroscopy	2				
Use both approaches	69				
	0–2	3–5	6–10	11–20	20+ specify
Number of new TMJ patients seen per week	8	27	33	27	5
Number of TMJ cases treated surgically per month	42	33	18	7	–

My usual follow-up

0–3 mth	4–6 mth	7–12 mth	1–2 yrs	2 yrs+
8	3	21	30	38

Years experience performing TMJ surgery

1–2 yrs	6–10 yrs	11–20 yrs	20 yrs+
1	39	42	18

(Courtesy of Goss AN: *Int J Oral Maxillofac Surg* 22:66–70, 1993.)

Pathology of Temporomandibular Joint Internal Derangement and Osteoarthrosis

de Bont LGM, Stegenga B (Univ Hosp Groningen, The Netherlands)
Int J Oral Maxillofac Surg 22:71–74, 1993   105-94-18-5

Introduction.—Although there is a strong relationship between TMJ osteoarthrosis (OA) and internal derangement (ID) of the joint, OA may develop without disk displacement. Relevant aspects of normal physiology and degeneration of the TMJ and the relationship between OA and ID are discussed. A general classification of temporomandibular disorders is proposed (table).

Normal Physiology.—The basic elements in a synovial joint are articular cartilage, the synovial membrane, and synovial fluid. Unlike most other synovial joints, the TMJ has fibrocartilage instead of hyaline cartilage. Joint lubrication and nutrition depend upon synovial fluid covering the articular surface. During normal functioning of the TMJ, the external pressure from loading is in equilibrium with the internal cartilage pressure.

TMJ Pathology.—The pathologic state in the TMJ seems to be the same as in other synovial joints. An insult, whether mechanical, chemical, or inflammatory, can result in cartilage degeneration. In OA, all synovial joint components are affected including the subchondral bone, the synovial lining cells, the synovial fluid, and the capsular ligaments. Degenerative changes of OA in the TMJ are clearly present in the deeper layers of

Classification of Temporomandibular Disorders

(continued)

Articular disorders

1. Noninflammatory chondro-osteoarthropathies

Chondromalacia

Internal derangement

reducing disk displacement (I–II)[a]

permanent disk displacement

acute/subacute (III)[a]

chronic (IV and V)[a]

residual osteoarthrosis (V)[a]

Osteoarthrosis and internal derangement

Mechanical derangements

Internal derangements

osteochondritis dissecans

disk displacement

[anterior, posterior, medial, lateral, or combinations]

Condyle-eminence mobility disturbances

subluxation

luxation

hypermobility syndromes

capsular fibrosis (contracture)

ankylosis [fibrous, bony]

Direct results from traumatic injury

fracture [intracapsular, collum]

laceration/rupture attachments

Neoplasm

Pseudotumors

[e.g. chondromatosis]

Benign

[e.g. chondroma, osteoma]

Malignant

[primary, metastatic]

III. Arthritides

Primary

Rheumatoid arthritis

rheumatoid arthritis

[active/inactive]

juvenile rheumatoid arthritis

Other arthritides

seronegative polyarthritis

ankylosing spondylitis

psoriatic arthritis

infectious arthritis

[bacterial, viral, fungal]

Reiter's syndrome

Secondary

Synovitis

traumatic arthritis

osteoarthritis

[osteoarthrosis and synovitis]

Capsulitis

V. Miscellaneous articular disorders

Nonarticular disorders

I. Muscle disorders

Myofascial pain

Regional

Generalized (fibromyalgia)

Muscle fibrosis

Contracture

Chronic muscle strain

Bruxism

Muscle inflammation

Tenomyositis

Infection

Motor-function disorders

Orofacial dyskinesia

Cramp/spasm

Miscellaneous muscle disorders

Degenerative [dystrophy]

Myasthenia

Myotonia

Neoplasm

II. Growth disorders

Table (*continued*)

Bone and cartilage disorders with articular manifestations
Avascular necrosis
Miscellaneous
[osteomalacia, osteoporosis]

II. Growth disorders

Nonmeoplastic
Developmental
hypoplasia
hyperplasia
dysplasia
Acquired
condylolysis
(post-)juvenile osteoarthrosis or rheumatoid arthritis

(capsular) sprain
adhesive capsulitis
Crystal-induced arthropathy
hyperuricemia
calcium pyrophosphate
dihydrate deposition
hydroxyapatite deposition

IV. Diffuse connective-tissue disorders

Systemic lupus erythematosus
Mixed connective-tissue disease
Polymyositis
Scleroderma
Sjögren's syndrome
Rheumatic fever
Polymyalgia rheumatica
Arteritis temporalis

Eagle's syndrome
Coronoid impingement
syndrome
Neoplasm

III. Miscellaneous nonarticular disorders

[a] **I, II, III, IV,** and **V,** refer to Wilkes' staging.
(Courtesy of de Bont LGM, Stegenga B: *Int J Oral Maxillofac Surg* 22:71-74, 1993.)

tissue, but not detectable on inspection of joint structures during arthroscopy or open-joint surgery.

Disk Displacement.—It is uncertain whether disk displacement is a cause or a sign of TMJ OA. There is a sequence of events, however, that explains the relationship between OA and ID. Cartilage breakdown in OA affects the sliding properties of the joint surfaces. The deterioration of synovial fluid in OA results in friction and adhesive wear, impairing the movement of the disk. Repetitive stretching of disk attachments may permit disk displacement. An autopsy study of elderly patients indicates that displacement of the articular disk is a sign of TMJ OA rather than its cause.

Conclusion.—Primary OA with disk displacement can be distinguished from primary OA without disk displacement. Secondary OA is the result of other joint disorders such as rheumatoid arthritis and avascular necrosis. In the classification proposed by the authors, TMJ OA and ID represent a substantial portion of temporomandibular disorders. Although they appear to be strongly related, TMJ OA and ID may be mutually independent.

▶ This article is an example of the type of work that will lead to a better understanding of inflammatory TMJ disease. The authors make some key statements. First, although the etiology is unknown, OA of the TMJ can occur as a primary process leading to joint symptoms and dysfunction not unlike other constantly used synovial joints in the body. Secondary OA also can occur as the result of disk displacement, internal derangement, or joint hypermobility. Two independent processes can produce identical clinical findings. Knowing what is primary would greatly assist in early treatment planning. The proposed classification of TMJ disorders is useful.—S.M. Roser, D.M.D., M.D.

Surgery for TMJ Internal Derangement: Evaluation of Treatment Outcome and Criteria for Success
Holmlund AB (Karolinska Inst, Huddinge, Sweden)
Int J Oral Maxillofac Surg 22:75–77, 1993   105-94-18–6

Background.—Most follow-up studies of patients undergoing surgery for TMJ internal derangement are flawed methodologically. The literature on treatment evaluation and methods for assessment was reviewed, and recommendations for TMJ surgery were given.

Discussion.—Because the etiopathogenesis of TMJ internal derangement is still unclear, it is not possible to eliminate the disease. The least treatment that benefits the patient is the best in TMJ cases. Nonsurgical management should always precede surgery. The goals of TMJ derangement management are to arrest the disease or eliminate disturbing manifestations, improve mandibular function, and alleviate pain. Properly conducted follow-up studies of patients treated for TMJ derangement should include the goals of treatment, prospective design, inclusion and exclusion criteria, proper evaluation methods, defined outcome criteria, a long follow-up, minimal dropout, and appropriate statistical analysis. Randomized clinical trials are the best for assessing treatment. For TMJ surgery, success criteria have been proposed: absent or mild pain; range of motion greater than 35 mm for vertical and greater than 6 mm for protrusive and lateral excursions; regular diet that, at worst, avoids tough or hard foods; unimportant radiographic changes in the joint, unless destructive changes are severe; and absence of significant complications. Recommendations for follow-up include prospective preoperative and postoperative recordings; standard methods for clinical assessment; follow-up of at least 1 year for arthroscopic surgery, disk repositioning, and diskectomy without implants; follow-up of at least 3 years for diskectomy with implants and arthroplasty; American Association of Oral and Maxillofacial Surgeons outcome criteria.

Conclusion.—Previous follow-up studies of TMJ surgery are retrospective and do not specify inclusion and exclusion criteria, assessment methods, and other important information. Randomized clinical trials are needed to assess the value of surgery for TMJ internal derangement.

▶ For those interested in reading the literature on the topic of TMJ disorders, the challenge is formidable. This article offers the serious reader a set of criteria to evaluate the articles written on the surgical management of TMJ disorders. This is important because almost every new technique offered is reported by the authors to enjoy an 80% success rate. These are not modifications of a basic technique, but quite different approaches. It seems that surgical treatment, regardless of what is done, is reported to have an 80% success rate. Lack of consistent criteria for evaluating outcome of surgical treatment is one of the primary reasons this happens. By keeping the recommendations made in this article in mind, the reader should be able to more critically evaluate the surgical TMJ disorder literature.—S.M. Roser, D.M.D., M.D.

Toward an International Consensus on Temporomandibular Joint Surgery: Report of the Second International Consensus Meeting, April 1992, Buenos Aires, Argentina
Goss AN (Univ of Adelaide, Australia)
Int J Oral Maxillofac Surg 22:78–81, 1993   105-94-18–7

Background.—Although surgery undoubtedly has a place in the management of TMJ disorders, the rationale, indications, and contraindications for it and preferred techniques are debated. The International Association of Oral and Maxillofacial Surgeons (IAOMS) recently held a consensus meeting in an attempt to settle this controversy.

Definitions.—It was agreed that internal derangement is "a localized mechanical fault in the joint which interferes with its smooth action."

Osteoarthritis was defined as a noninflammatory condition of a movable joint, characterized by articular connective tissue deterioration and abrasion and new bone formation at the articular surfaces.

Diagnosis.—It was agreed that distinguishing intra-articular joint problems from the many other causes of facial pain and jaw dysfunction is essential. A range of imaging modalities can be used to determine the morphologic state of the joint. Typically, a demonstration by imaging of derangement or pathologic conditions amenable to surgery is required for surgery.

Indications.—Three general indications were agreed on. A surgical candidate would usually meet all 3. First, appropriate nonsurgical treatment should have proved unsuccessful. Second, the patient has requested additional treatment, including surgery, if needed. Third, there are no medical or psychological contraindications to surgery. Consensus was also reached on indications for several specific surgical procedures.

Summary.—Surgery of the TMJ should be aimed at conserving existing joint tissues consistent with the degree of disorder. Arthroscopy should be considered in the early stages of the disorder. Arthrotomy should be aimed at restoring normal function and structure, if possible. Long-term outcome criteria for all surgical procedures need to be developed.

▶ This article is a summary of key issues discussed at a consensus conference on the management of TMJ disorders held in 1992 and attended by surgeons from all over the world. The meeting was not intended to bring together all interested parties in TMJ disorder but to try to develop consensus in the surgical arena on definitions, pathogenesis of disease, and how to evaluate surgical outcome. Current thinking on joint physiology and pathophysiology played a prominent role in the outcome of the conference. One can only speculate about where we would be in the management of TMJ disorder/facial pain if there was universal agreement on definitions and well-understood criteria to measure treatment outcome. For sure, millions of health care dollars now going to pay for unproved treatment for TMJ disorder could be saved or be used to support more appropriate treatments.—S.M. Roser, D.M.D., M.D.

Efficacy of Temporomandibular Joint Arthroscopy: A Retrospective Study
Mosby EL (Univ of Missouri Schools of Dentistry and Medicine, Kansas City)
J Oral Maxillofac Surg 51:17–21, 1993   105-94-18-8

Introduction.—The outcome of arthroscopic surgery on the TMJ was reviewed in 109 patients, 87 women and 22 men, who had a total of 150 TMJ arthroscopies, most often after nonoperative measures had failed to relieve symptoms. Forty-one patients had bilateral procedures. In 10 cases, manipulation was carried out to increase the range of motion before arthroscopy.

Findings.—Before arthroscopy, 47% of patients had an interincisal opening less than 35 mm, and postoperatively 75% had an opening more than 40 mm. Both lateral and protrusive excursions increased postoperatively. Pain was substantially reduced in about three fourths of patients 1–5 years after the procedure. Headaches persisted in half of the 90 patients affected. Muscle tenderness was nearly always less severe after arthroscopic surgery.

Discussion.—Arthroscopy of the TMJ consistently reduces pain and enhances function to a manageable level. Noises representing internal derangement of the TMJ do not preclude a functional occlusion and a normal or functional range of motion.

▶ Early reports in the mid-1980s told of the success of TMJ arthroscopic procedures in reducing or eliminating signs and symptoms associated with a variety of TMJ disorders. However, these were criticized because of the lack of adequate clinical studies. This moderate-sized clinical retrospective study supports the effectiveness of arthroscopic lysis of adhesions and lavage of the joint space. Although it is hard to argue with well-documented clinical success, we should not forget what is necessary to validate treatment modalities for TMJ disorders. The best studies are those that are prospective and include inclusion and exclusion criteria, standard assessment methods for pain, mandibular function, hard tissue changes, and disk position and form; they also follow the patients for at least a 3-year period. Studies such as this one are important and give us some comfort while we await the prospective trials. One hopes that someone is doing them.—S.M. Roser, D.M.D., M.D.

Modified Condylotomy for Treatment of the Painful Temporomandibular Joint With a Reducing Disc

Hall HD, Nickerson JW, McKenna SJ (Vanderbilt Univ, Nashville, Tenn)
J Oral Maxillofac Surg 51:133–142, 1993   105-94-18–9

Introduction.—The modified condylotomy has several advantages compared with the original condylotomy and other surgical and nonsurgical disk-preserving treatments for painful temporomandibular joint. It is performed to eliminate pain and dysfunction, to reverse the disease process, and to prevent progression by reestablishing a normal disk/condyl relationship. The chief contraindication is the inability to control the occlusion well. The procedure is also contraindicated in a patient with poor intercuspation.

Method.—Data on the results of the modified condylotomy were derived from 2 published reports and personal experience of more than 400 cases.

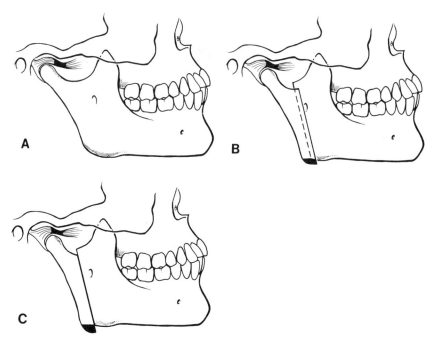

Fig 18–2.—Condylar and disk position before and after modified condylotomy. **A,** mandible with an anteriorly displaced disk that reduces. **B,** lateral overlap of the proximal segment with anterior and inferior displacement of the condyle to a position beneath the disk. **C,** butt joint formed after removal of bone from the anterior edge of the proximal segment. Same movement of condyle occurs as in **B.** (Courtesy of Hall HD, Nickerson, JW, McKenna SJ: *J Oral Maxillofac Surg* 51:133–142, 1993.)

Modified Condylotomy.—In a modified condylotomy, the bone cut differs from the intraoral vertical ramus osteotomy (Figs 18-2 and 18-3) technique, and the inferior 50% to 60% of the medial pterygoid muscle is detached from the proximal segment to permit "sag" or anterior and inferior displacement of the condyle with an increase in joint space (Fig 18-4 and 18-5). Maxillomandibular fixation is maintained for 3 to 6 weeks. The critical components of the operation are the placement of the osteotomy and the amount of muscle retained on the proximal segment.

Discussion.—Condylar morphology changes after condylotomy. New bone formation can be seen radiographically on the posterior and superior aspects of the condyle in 90% of cases (Fig 18-6). A less common finding is a deformed condyle, possibly representing regressive modeling. Morbidity from the procedure is significantly less than after arthrotomy, and the more frequent relief of pain and shorter rehabilitation time favor modified condylotomy. The procedure also appears to reverse and prevent progression of internal derangement. The modified condylot-

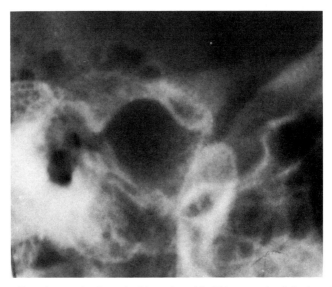

Fig 18–3.—Transpharyngeal radiograph of luxated condyle. This occurred early in the series, before the need to make a vertical cut, as shown in **Figure 18–2,** became evident. (Courtesy of Hall HD, Nickerson JW, McKenna SJ: *J Oral Maxillofac Surg* 51:133–142, 1993.)

omy produces good results and avoids some of the problems associated with the original procedure.

▶ The condylotomy procedure for relief of TMJ pain and dysfunction has been around for a long time. It has its champions, including the authors of

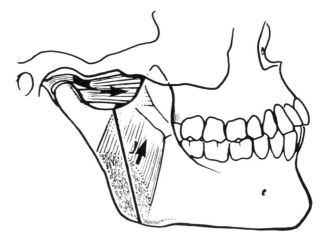

Fig 18–4.—Drawing shows direction of pull of medial and lateral pterygoid muscles. Note the extent of medial pterygoid attachment to mandible. (Courtesy of Hall HD, Nickerson JW, McKenna SJ: *J Oral Maxillofac Surg* 51:133–142, 1993.)

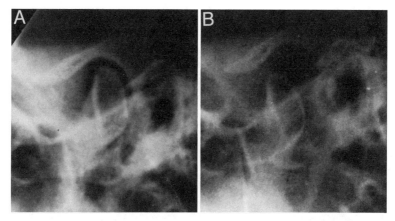

Fig 18–5.—Transcranial radiographs of condylar position before and after modified condylotomy. **A,** position of condyle in the glenoid fossa before modified condylotomy. **B,** position after modified condylotomy. Note the moderate anterior and inferior displacement of the condyle, with a slight increase in joint space. (Courtesy of Hall HD, Nickerson JW, McKenna SJ: *J Oral Maxillofac Surg* 51:133–142, 1993.)

this article. The report suffers from some of the same problems as does much of the surgical treatment literature, including being a retrospective study and lacking standardized criteria to evaluate the outcome. However, the results are important because of the consistent reduction in pain and dysfunction that results from the procedure. What happens in the procedure is that an anteriorly displaced reducing disk assumes a more normal disk-condyle relationship. The disk-condyle-fossa relationship is changed, with a significant opening of the space between the condyle and the fossa. The condyles appear to remodel over time. The postoperative sequence of events and the improvements in symptoms and function should be used as a model to test the current theories of the pathogenesis of osteoarthritis that involves disk displacement. The article also raises the issue of the impact of disk displacement on the growing mandible. Is it possible that many of the mandibular asymmetries that are accompanied by a small deformed condyle on one side and no history of trauma are the result of a disk displacement at an early age that may have been minimally symptomatic? This needs further investigation.—S.M. Roser, D.M.D., M.D.

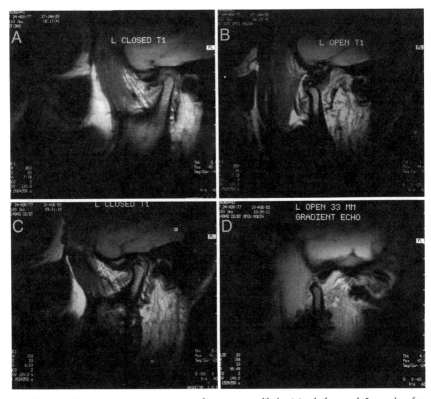

Fig 18–6.—Magnetic resonance imaging of temperomandibular joint before and 5 months after modified condylotomy in a 14-year-old girl. **A,** anteriorly displaced disk before operation. Disk is slightly folded, and there is a defect in the cortex on the anterior superior surface of the condyle (mouth closed). **B,** reduction of the disk during opening of the mouth before operation. **C,** reversal of the internal derangement 5 months after condylotomy. The posterior band of the disk has moved posteriorly and superiorly in the fossa to the 12-o'clock position, and the disk is no longer folded. The "double contour" on the posterior and superior aspects of the condyle represents new bone growth (mouth closed). **D,** translation of the disk with the condyle during opening of the mouth 5 months after surgery. Disk is fully reduced. (Courtesy of Hall HD, Nickerson JW, McKenna SJ: *J Oral Macillofac Surg* 51:133–142, 1993.)

Use of Sodium Hyaluronate in Treating Temporomandibular Joint Disorders: A Randomized, Double-Blind, Placebo-Controlled Clinical Trial

Bertolami CN, Gay T, Clark GT, Rendell J, Shetty V, Liu C, Swann DA (Univ of California, Los Angeles; Univ of Connecticut, Farmington; MedChem Products, Woburn, Mass)
J Oral Maxillofac Surg 51:232–242, 1993   105-94-18–10

Introduction.—A trial was designed to determine whether intra-articular administration of sodium hyaluronate will improve joint function and combat pain in patients with severe TMJ disorders. Hyaluronate is a soft tissue lubricant that hopefully can provide a conservative yet effective alternative to current, less successful measures.

Treatment.—A total of 121 patients with degenerative joint disease, reducing displaced disk, or nonreducing displaced disk who had failed to respond to other nonoperative measures and had evidence of severe dysfunction received an injection of either 1% sodium hyaluronate in saline or physiologic saline alone into the upper joint space on one side.

Results.—No significant difference in outcome was evident between patients with degenerative changes who received hyaluronate and those given placebo treatment. Hyaluronate-treated patients with a reducing displaced disk exhibited improvement in the Helkimo index, visual analogue scales, and joint noise during the 6-month study period. Nearly one third of placebo recipients and only 3% of patients who were given active treatment relapsed. Too few patients with a nonreducing displaced disk were followed to assess the efficacy of hyaluronate.

Discussion.—The mechanism by which hyaluronate injection relieves symptoms of reducing displaced disk is unclear, but it may be a purely mechanical effect of this soft tissue lubricant. Experience with hyaluronate in animals and in human joints other than the TMJ has been relatively favorable. Benefit persists beyond the time that hyaluronate remains present in the joint, possibly because it is bound to hyaluronate receptors on the cell surface.

▶ Because of the unexplained successes and failures, some of them disasters, of treatments for TMJ disorders, it is time that efforts are redirected to understanding disease pathogenesis. Treatment modalities should be rationalized and based on physiologic principles. The use of sodium hyaluronate is based on just such principles. In this very well-designed study, the authors found that 1 injection of sodium hyaluronate into symptomatic joints with displaced reducing disks resulted in a reduction of symptoms that lasted up to 6 months. The authors postulated that sodium hyaluronate, which acts as a joint lubricant, interrupted a destructive cycle caused by friction between inflamed articular surfaces, thus permitting healing of these surfaces. According to the authors, reduction of inflammation and healing is what accounts for the long-term reduction in symptoms, which occurred far beyond the time the injected hyaluronate had been cleared from the joint. The use of sodium hyaluronate in treatment protocols for TMJ disorders awaits confirmation by others, but these results should stimulate clinical researchers to continue to explore the exciting concept offered by the authors.—S.M. Roser, D.M.D., M.D.

19 Maxillofacial Trauma and Reconstruction

Introduction

Rigid fixation has revolutionized the treatment of maxillofacial trauma. Although rigid fixation techniques are associated with a higher incidence of complications, the benefits of recovery without maxillomandibular fixation outweigh the risks. Because of the relatively high cost of plates, the cost effectiveness of rigid fixation can be debated. Opinions differ about what to do with teeth in the line of fracture. Some advocate removal of all teeth in fracture lines, but others leave in all but those teeth that are themselves fractured. An article in this chapter discusses the high incidence of nonvitality of retained teeth in and adjacent to fracture lines of mandibular fractures repaired with rigid fixation. Other articles include an interesting discussion on the changing trend in management of facial fractures in children during the past 5 years, a follow-up study on biodegradable plates that indicates that more work needs to be done in this area, and a treatment protocol for avulsed teeth that appears to significantly enhance their survival.

The mandible can be successfully reconstructed after resection for cancer with rigid reconstruction plates without bone grafts, although esthetics and function are compromised. Vascularized bone grafts stabilized by rigid reconstruction plates are reported to be successful, particularly in situations of symphyseal reconstruction and irradiated tissue sites, both previously thought to be almost impossible reconstruction challenges. Immediate or delayed implants can be used with vascularized bone grafts, permitting complete rehabilitation of the patient.

Steven M. Roser, D.M.D., M.D.

Maxillofacial Trauma

The Functional Case for Miniplates in Maxillofacial Surgery

Hayter JP, Cawood JI (Chester Royal Infirmary, England)
Int J Oral Maxillofac Surg 22:91–96, 1993   105-94-19-1

Introduction.—Intermaxillary fixation (IMF) has been the traditional means of achieving healing in fractures of the facial skeleton. Osteosynthesis, originally developed for orthopedic practice, is now applied in

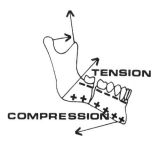

Fig 19–1.—Tension and compression forces in fractured mandible. (From Hayter JP, Cawood JI: *Int J Oral Maxillofac Surg* 22:91-96, 1993. Courtesy of the editor of *Br J Oral Maxillofac Surg.*)

the maxillofacial region to achieve early recovery of function. The functional advantages of osteosynthesis over IMF are discussed.

Compression Plates.—Rigid internal fixation by compression bone plates, developed for the treatment of long bone fractures, has been difficult to apply in maxillofacial surgery. A miniplate technique, using malleable plates inserted intraorally, overcomes these difficulties. The theory behind small-plate osteosynthesis in the treatment of mandibular fractures is based upon the forces of tension and compression produced by jaw function (Fig 19–1). Plate thickness can be minimized by placing the plates at the most biomechanically favorable site to neutralize the tension forces causing fracture distraction (Fig 19–2).

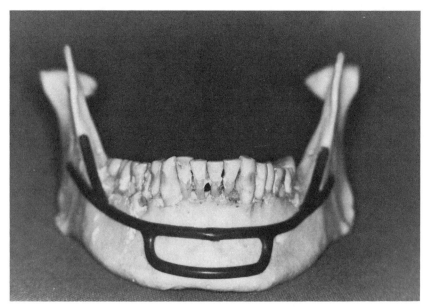

Fig 19–2.—Ideal sites for miniplate osteosynthesis in mandible. (Courtesy of Hayter JP, Cawood JI: *Int J Oral Maxillofac Surg* 22:91-96, 1993.)

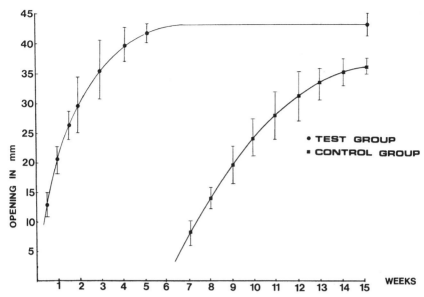

Fig 19–3.—Differences in jaw opening after treatment of fractured mandible. Test group treated by miniplate osteosynthesis (*circles*); control group treated by IMF (*squares*). (From Hayter JP, Cawood JI: *Int J Oral Maxillofac Surg* 22:91–96, 1993. Courtesy of the editor of *Br J Oral Maxillofac Surg.*)

Results of the Two Methods.—A prospective study comparing IMF and miniplate osteosynthesis revealed significant differences in the recovery of normal mouth opening (Fig 19–3). Improvements in the patient's ability to eat means that the extent and duration of weight loss is

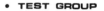
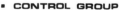

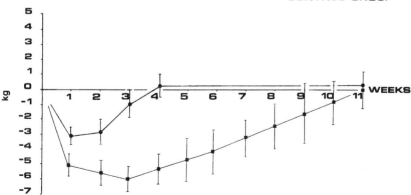

Fig 19–4.—Weight changes after treatment of fractured mandible. Test group treated miniplate osteosynthesis (*circles*); control group treated by IMF (*squares*). (From Hayter JP, Cawood JI: *Int J Oral Maxillofac Surg* 22:91–96, 1993. Courtesy of the editor of *Br J Oral Maxillofac Surg.*)

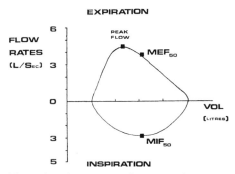

Fig 19–5.—A normal flow-volume loop. MIF$_{50}$ and MEF$_{50}$ are the mean inspiratory and expiratory flow rates, respectively, when the lung volume is the residual volume plus 50% of vital capacity. (Courtesy of Hayter JP, Cawood JI: *Int J Oral Maxillofac Surg* 22:91–96, 1993.)

reduced with miniplate treatment (Fig 19-4). Intermaxillary fixation causes a significant degree of airway obstruction, resulting in a significant decrease in all dynamic respiratory values (Figs 19-5 and 19-6). These effects on pulmonary function can cause serious complications in the previously healthy patient and endanger those with preexisting chronic obstructive airways disease or asthma.

Conclusion.—Miniplate osteosynthesis is applicable at many sites in the facial skeleton (Fig 19-7). As compared with IMF, miniplates offer all the advantages of improved function with few disadvantages. There is, however, a slightly higher incidence of malocclusion in patients with mandibular fractures treated by small-plate osteosynthesis. The risk to facial nerve function can be reduced through an intraoral approach during insertion of the miniplates. With the advantages of patient safety and comfort, a shorter hospital stay, and early return to work offered by miniplate osteosynthesis, IMF appears to be obsolete.

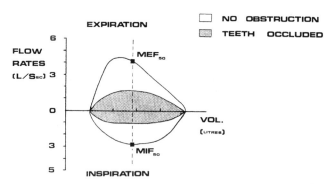

Fig 19–6.—Change of flow-volume loop after IMF. (Courtesy of Hayter JP, Cawood JI: *Int J Oral Maxillofac Surg* 22:91–96, 1993.)

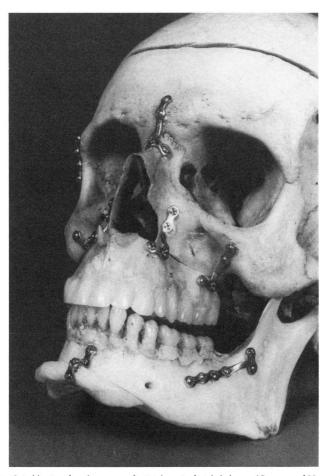

Fig 19–7.—Suitable sites for placement of miniplates in facial skeleton. (Courtesy of Hayter JP, Cawood JI: *Int J Oral Maxillofac Surg* 22:91-96, 1993.)

▶ Intermaxillary fixation for treatment of maxillary and mandibular fractures is obsolete. If this statement is surprising, further reading about miniplate osteosynthesis is necessary. Not having to wire jaws together for 4 to 6 weeks means a much more rapid recovery from trauma. For patients with multiple injuries, the return to a more normal oral intake will impact in a very positive way on the healing of other injuries. Comparing the final outcome of either method demonstrates far less difference, with a higher complication rate seen in patients who are plated. These include a higher incidence of post-repair malocclusion and sensory disturbances, and as demonstrated in Abstract 105-94-19-2, in nonvitality in teeth near the fracture. Thus, fracture plating is a technique-sensitive procedure, and the principles and techniques must be thoroughly understood by all those who use them.—S.M. Roser, D.M.D., M.D.

The Fate of Teeth in Mandibular Fracture Lines: A Clinical and Radiographic Follow-Up Study

Kamboozia AH, Punnia-Moorthy A (Univ of Sydney, Australia)
Int J Oral Maxillofac Surg 22:97–101, 1993   105-94-19-2

Introduction.—No definite guidelines have been established for the management of teeth in mandibular fracture lines. Previous recommendations to extract involved teeth assumed that communication of the fracture to the oral cavity via periodontal space fostered infection. More recent studies suggest that vital teeth can be preserved when antibiotics are used prophylactically. This study of teeth in the line of mandibular fractures compares the morbidity of teeth treated with plates with those treated with interdental wiring.

Methods.—Forty patients with mandibular fractures involving completely erupted permanent teeth took part in the study. Fractures involving the lower third molars were excluded, because most third molars were removed for technical and clinical reasons when plating was undertaken. Four fracture types were identified (Fig 19–8), and the degree of fracture displacement was classified as hairline, minimal, or gross. Affected teeth were examined clinically and with periapical radiographs. Pulpal response was measured with an electric pulp tester. The follow-up ranged from 1 to 4 years.

Results.—Most of the mandibular fractures (90%) occurred in males; assault was the main cause (90%). The most common site of fracture was the mandibular canine region (Fig 19–9). Thirty-four teeth (20 patients) were plated, and 29 teeth (20 patients) were treated with wiring. Patients

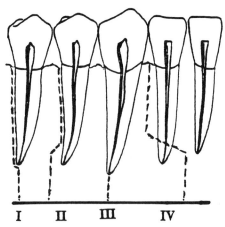

I   II   III   IV

Fig 19–8.—Fracture types based on relationship of fracture line to periodontium. (Courtesy of Kamboozia AH, Punnia-Moorthy A: *Int J Oral Maxillofac Surg* 22:97–101, 1993.)

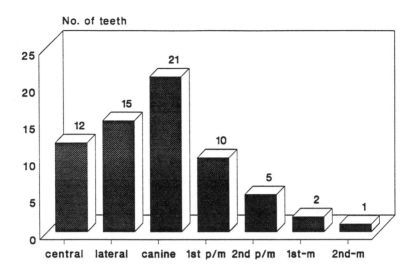

n=66

Fig 19–9.—Distribution of teeth in line of fractures. (Courtesy of Kamboozia AH, Punnia-Moorthy A: *Int J Oral Maxillofac Surg* 22:97–101, 1993.)

in the plated group had more nonvital teeth (68%) than did the wired group patients (41%) (Fig 19–10). There was also a higher incidence of nonvital involved adjacent teeth in the plated group patients (Fig 19–11). The frequency of tooth vitality was closely related to the degree of frac-

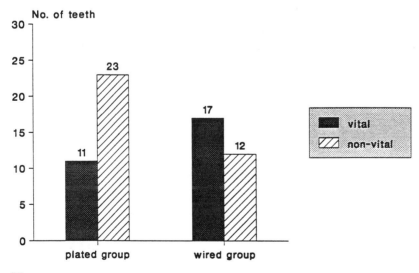

n=63

Fig 19–10.—Incidence of vitality/nonvitality of teeth in fracture lines in plated and wired patients. (Courtesy of Kamboozia AH, Punnia-Moorthy A: *Int J Oral Maxillofac Surg* 22:97–101, 1993.)

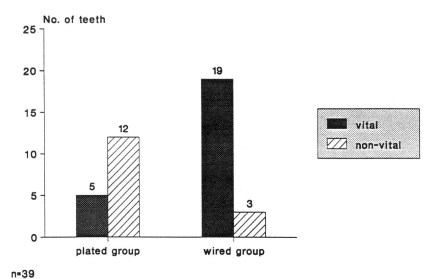

Fig 19–11.—Incidence of vitality/nonvitality of involved adjacent teeth in plated and wired patients. (Courtesy of Kamboozia AH, Punnia-Moorthy A: *Int J Oral Maxillofac Surg* 22:97–101, 1993.)

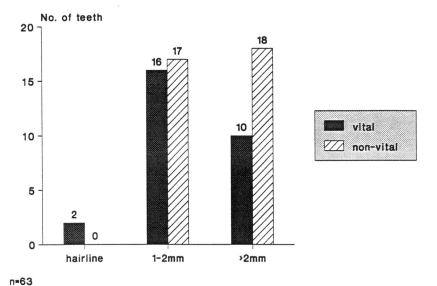

Fig 19–12.—Relationship of tooth vitality/nonvitality to degree of fracture displacement. (Courtesy of Kamboozia, AH, Punnia-Moorthy A: *Int J Oral Maxillofac Surg* 22:97–101, 1993.)

TABLE 1.—Fracture Displacement and Complications of Involved Teeth

Degree of displacement	plated group (n_1=34)			wired group (n_2=29)			Total
	vital	non-vital (no apical lesion)	non-vital (with apical lesion)	vital	non-vital (no apical lesion)	non-vital (with apical lesion)	
hair line	0	0	0	2	0	0	2
minimal	3	5	7	13	3	2	33
gross	8	3	8	2	5	2	28
Total	11	8	15	17	8	4	63

(Courtesy of Kamboozia AH, Punnia-Moorthy A: *Int J Oral Maxillofac Surg* 22:97–101, 1993.)

ture displacement (Fig 19–12 and Table 1). In the most common type of fracture line, type I, 65% of teeth were nonvital (Fig 19–13 and Table 2).

Conclusion.—There was a significant increase in nonvitality of teeth, both in the line and adjacent to the fractures of the mandible, when plate treatment rather than interdental wiring was used. The increase in tooth nonvitality with plating can be attributed to the open nature of the

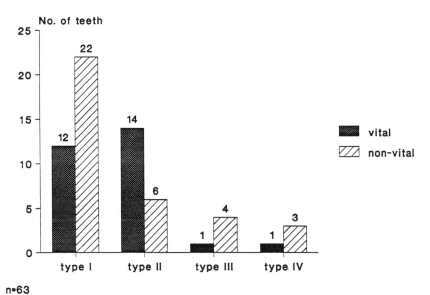

n=63

Fig 19–13.—Relationship of tooth vitality/nonvitality to type of fracture line in relation to involved tooth. (Courtesy of Kamboozia AH, Punnia-Moorthy A: *Int J Oral Maxillofac Surg* 22:97–101, 1993.)

TABLE 2.—Fracture Types and Complications of Involved Teeth

Type of fractures	plated group (n₁=34)			wired group (n₂=29)			Total
	vital	non-vital (no apical lesion)	non-vital (with apical lesion)	vital	non-vital (no apical lesion)	non-vital (with apical lesion)	
I	4	5	11	8	3	3	34
II	7	1	1	8	3	0	20
III	0	1	2	1	0	1	5
IV	0	1	1	0	2	0	4
Total	11	8	15	17	8	4	63

(Courtesy of Kamboozia AH, Punnia-Moorthy A: Int J Oral Maxillofac Surg 22:97–101, 1993.)

procedure and the degree of manipulation of fragments required. Unless there is an absolute indication for removal, the authors recommend retention of teeth associated with fracture lines. Patients should be followed for at least 1 year to determine if endodontic treatment is needed.

▶ The unexpected but not surprising finding is the lack of vitality in a significant number of teeth in or adjacent to a plated mandibular fracture site. This is compared with teeth in the line of fracture treated in a closed manner using arch bars and intermaxillary fixation. The disruption of blood supply by the open procedure necessary to successfully plate a fracture is implicated by the authors. Most of the nonvital teeth were asymptomatic during the 1–4 years of the study. Thus, these teeth must be followed on a regular basis throughout the patient's lifetime.—S.M. Roser, D.M.D., M.D.

Diagnosis and Treatment of Fractures of the Facial Bones in Children 1943–1993
Kaban LB (Univ of California, San Francisco)
J Oral Maxillofac Surg 51:722–729, 1993   105-94-19-3

Background.—Since 1943, significant advances have been made in pediatric airway management, metabolic management of pediatric patients, pediatric anesthesia, antibiotic therapy, and surgical techniques for the management of facial fractures. There is also a better understanding of the etiology, incidence, and prevention of these fractures. Current concepts of diagnosing and managing pediatric facial fractures were reviewed.

Incidence, Etiology, and Prevention.—The incidence of facial fractures is lower in children than in adults, with children younger than age 12 years accounting for 1.5% to 8% of all facial fractures treated in trauma centers. Mandibular fractures are the most common; the midface is relatively protected in children because it is retruded relative to the calvaria. The most common cause of pediatric facial fractures is a fall from a bicycle, steps, or climbing apparatus, although more fractures are occurring in motor vehicle accidents. Other vehicles, such as dirt bikes and offroad vehicles, are also an increasingly important cause. Child abuse must also be considered in the differential diagnosis.

Diagnosis and Management.—Computed tomography is now the standard imaging technique used for pediatric trauma victims. In terms of management, maintenance of normal fluid and electrolyte balance is a critical consideration. Airway management is another important issue, although fiberoptic laryngoscopy has decreased the need for tracheotomy.

For mandibular fractures in children with deciduous dentition, closed reduction and immobilization, either with splints or with splints and maxillomandibular fixation, remain the standard of care. With the availability of miniplates and microplates, open reduction is no longer contraindicated. Condylar fractures are treated with analgesics and a liquid or soft diet for children without malocclusion or a short period of immobilization for those with pain and malocclusion. Midface fractures are approached via a coronal incision and craniofacial dissection. Supplementary incisions can avoid the need for external fixators and maxillomandibular fixation. For all facial fractures, healing is generally better in children than in adults. Questions remain about the significant problem of infection and the effects of rigid internal fixation on the growing facial skeleton.

Summary.—Although many major advances have been made, the fundamentals of diagnosis and management of pediatric facial fractures have changed little since 1943 and probably since the work of Kazanjian in World War I. Significant advances have been made since the development of craniofacial techniques. Further progress in the biology of bone healing will surely mark the next 50 years.

▶ This is an important review article to be read by those practitioners who provide care to children. The etiology and incidence of facial fractures have changed during the last 50 years. Rigid fixation and plates and screws are often used to repair mandibular and midface fractures, shortening the postoperative recovery time, mostly by minimizing or eliminating maxillomandibular fixation and, in some cases, enhancing the esthetic and functional results. The short-term results are in and they are good; the long-term effects of rigidly fixing the growing bones of children remain to be determined.—S.M. Roser, D.M.D., M.D.

Foreign Body Reactions to Resorbable Poly(L-Lactide) Bone Plates and Screws Used for the Fixation of Unstable Zygomatic Fractures

Bergsma EJ, Rozema FR, Bos RRM, de Bruijn WC (Univ Hosp, Groningen, The Netherlands)

J Oral Maxillofac Surg 51:666–670, 1993   105-94-19-4

Background.—Although metallic bone plates and screws provide a reliable method of internal fracture fixation, they also carry several disadvantages, such as the possibility of bone atrophy from stress shielding by the rigid bone plates and screws. As an alternative, bioresorbable polymeric plates and screws gradually transduce functional stress to the bone because of resorption of the material. In a previous study, good results were obtained with the use of resorbable poly(L-lactide) (PLLA) plates

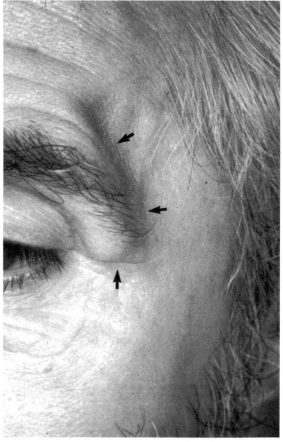

Fig 19–14.—Subcutaneous swelling (*arrows*) in the left front zygoma region. (Courtesy of Bergsma EJ, Rozema FR, Bos RRM, et al: *J Oral Maxillofac Surg* 51:666–670, 1993.)

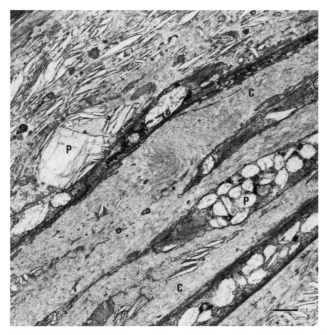

Fig 19–15.—Particles of PLLA lying between sheets of collagen fibers (C) and intracellularly in the fibrocytic cells in membrane-bound phagosomes (P). *Bar* = 1.1 μm Uranylacetate/lead citrate stain. (Courtesy of Bergsma EJ, Rozema FR, Bos RRM, et al: *J Oral Maxillofac Surg* 51:666–670. 1993.)

and screws for the fixation of unstable zygomatic fractures in 10 patients. Clinical and histologic characteristics of a late tissue reaction in 4 patients were reported.

Patients.—The patients returned 3 years postoperatively with an intermittent swelling at the implantation site. The other 5 living patients were also recalled for clinical examination at that time. The affected patients showed a mobile swelling relative to the underlying bone (Fig 19–14). The contours of the bone plates and screws were palpable. Six of the 9 patients underwent reoperation to investigate the nature of the tissue reaction.

Findings.—At surgery, remnants of degraded PLLA surrounded by a dense fibrous capsule made up a significant part of the swelling. Light microscopic analysis disclosed a foreign body reaction with no evidence of inflammation. On ultrastructural evaluation, the cytoplasm of various cells in the degraded material showed internalized, crystal-like PLLA material (Fig 19–15).

Conclusion.—Although PLLA plates and screws can allow undisturbed healing of unstable zygomatic fractures, a foreign body reaction with swelling may appear some years later. Disintegration of the material causes biomechanical alterations and increased volume of the PLLA ma-

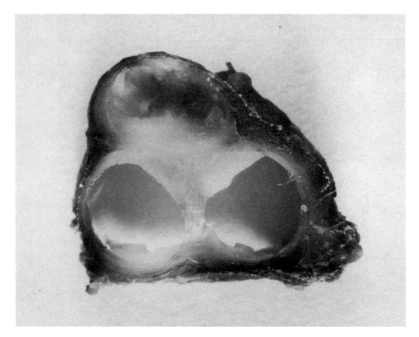

Fig 19–16.—Cross-section of one of the explanted tissue masses. The lower cavities contained the degraded PLLA bone plate. The upper cavity contained remnants of the PLLA screw head. Original magnification, ×7.5. (Courtesy of Bergsma EJ, Rozema FR, Bos RRM, et al: *J Oral Maxillofac Surg* 51:666–670, 1993.)

terial (Fig 19-16). Further use of PLLA for internal fixation should await more study of the cause of this foreign body reaction.

▶ Resorbable bone plates and screws have been eagerly awaited by surgeons and patients. In addition to removing the worry of corrosion and toxic breakdown products, resorption of the plate will eliminate the problem of stress shielding. Stress shielding is the phenomenon in which the rigid plate absorbs much of the stress placed on the bone/plate combination. The bone within the confines of the plate is shielded from stress and can become thin and osteoporotic. If the plate should fatigue and fracture, the stress-shielded bone may not be able to withstand forces placed upon it, and it will fracture itself. A resorbable plate will dissolve and allow the healed bone to develop the strength needed for its function. Great idea, but more research and development needs to be done before an acceptable resorbable plate is available.—S.M. Roser, D.M.D., M.D.

Dentoalveolar Trauma

Preserving Avulsed Teeth for Replantation
Krasner P, Person P (Temple Univ, Philadelphia; New York Univ, New York)
J Am Dent Assoc 123(12):80–88, 1992   105-94-19-5

Introduction.—Preservation of avulsed teeth relies on storage in a physiologic medium, replenishing the nutrients of the periodontal ligament (PDL) cells, protecting the root PDL cell from trauma, elimination of infection, physiologic splinting of the avulsed tooth, timely pulpal extirpation, and placement of calcium hydroxide. Although immediate replantation is generally the best treatment, it cannot always be accomplished. The success of replantation can be enhanced by using an optimum preservation medium, such as Hank's Balanced Salt Solution (HBSS).

Methods.—In a retrospective study, the effect of storage in a biological environment, as provided by the Emergency Tooth Preserving System (ETPS), on the success of tooth replantation was determined. In this system, HBSS serves as an optimum storage and transport medium, along with an apparatus for reducing trauma to the PDL cells. The dentists of 34 patients with traumatic tooth avulsion who were treated with the ETPS were surveyed.

Results.—Replantation was very successful in 85% of cases (Table 1). Time between avulsion and placement of the tooth in the ETPS ranged from 15 to 120 minutes, and total extraoral time ranged from 45 to 360

TABLE 1.—Fate of Tooth Replants at Follow-Up Intervals

Months	Very successful	Moderately successful	Unsuccessful
3	2	0	1
6	9	0	1
9	1	0	0
12	8	1	0
18	4	1	0
24-30	5	0	1
Total	29 (85.3%)	2 (5.9%)	3 (8.8%)

(Courtesy of Krasner P, Person P: *J Am Dent Assoc* 123(12):80–88, 1992.)

TABLE 2.—Fate of Tooth Replants Related to Time Between
Avulsion and Placement in the Emergency Tooth Preserving System

Minutes	Very successful	Moderately successful	Unsuccessful
15	4	0	0
30	6	1	1
45	5	1	1
60	13	0	1
120	1	0	0
Total	29 (85.3%)	2 (5.9%)	3 (8.8%)

(Courtesy of Krasner P, Person P: *J Am Dent Assoc* 123(12):80–88, 1992.)

minutes (Tables 2 and 3). There were no adverse reactions, and all dentists stated that the ETPS was a useful adjunct for replantation.

Conclusion.—Use of the ETPS increases the chances of success in the replantation of avulsed teeth. The reconstitutive nature of the HBSS and the protective characteristics of the ETPS both appear to contribute to a high success rate.

▶ The principles recommended by Andreasen for replacing traumatically avulsed teeth have guided the dental profession since the 1960s. This study

TABLE 3.—Fate of Tooth Replants Related to Total Length of Extraoral Time

Minutes	Very successful	Moderately successful	Unsuccessful	Total
0-15	0	0	0	0
16-30	0	0	0	0
31-60	9 (90%)	0	1 (10%)	10 (29.4%)
61-120	16 (88.9%)	0	2 (11.1%)	18 (52.9%)
121-240	2 (66.6%)	1 (33.4%)	0	3 (8.8%)
241-360	2 (66.6%)	1 (33.4%)	0	3 (8.8%)

(Courtesy of Krasner P, Person P: *J Am Dent Assoc* 123(12):80–88, 1992.)

used the work of Andreasen and others as a control, because the authors believed a double-blind study for avulsed teeth was not feasible. This study demonstrates that storing or even exposing an avulsed tooth to a physiological saline solution increases its survival rate after replantation. If these results are reproducible, the profession and public will have to be instructed to reach for a physiologic solution when a tooth is avulsed.—S.M. Roser, D.M.D., M.D.

Reconstruction

Rigid Reconstruction Plates for Immediate Reconstruction Following Mandibular Resection for Malignant Tumors
Lindqvist C, Söderholm A-L, Laine P, Paatsama J (Helsinki Univ)
J Oral Maxillofac Surg 50:1158–1163, 1992   105-94-19–6

Background.—Rehabilitating patients with mandibular continuity defects has always been difficult. Rigid reconstruction plates have been used for immediate reconstruction after mandibular resection for malignant tumors was reported.

Patients and Findings.—Thirty-four primary alloplastic reconstructions of segmental defects resulting from surgery for malignancies were done over 6 years. Eighty-eight percent of the tumors were staged as III or IV. During the mean follow-up of 29 months, one third of the patients died, 9 with the primary reconstruction plate in place. Plates had to be removed in 12 cases because of complications. Four of these patients re-

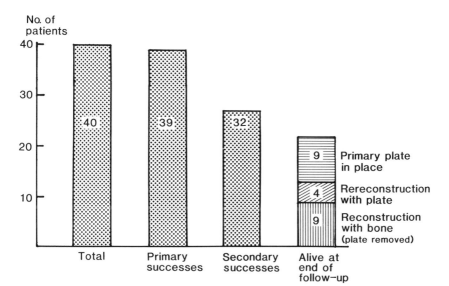

Fig 19–17.—Summary of the results of mandibular rigid plate reconstruction in 34 patients. (Courtesy of Lindqvist C, Söderholm A-L, Laine, P et al: *J Oral Maxillofac Surg* 50:1158–1163, 1992.)

ceived another plate. Nineteen of the 21 patients still alive at the end of follow-up were disease free, 10 of whom had their primary plate still in place. Four had a different plate placed because of plate fracture or screw loosening. Three patients had permanent reconstruction of the mandible with bone. In most cases, the functional and esthetic outcomes were excellent or fair (Fig 19–17).

Conclusion.—Because the recurrence rate for mandibular cancer is high, it is reasonable to question the use of an immediate, permanent, hard-tissue reconstruction with bone. The authors of the current study have adopted a policy of immediate soft-tissue reconstruction and temporary, alloplastic hard-tissue reconstruction, and their findings demonstrate that this policy is justified.

Critical Analysis of Mandibular Reconstruction Using AO Reconstruction Plates

Kim M-R, Donoff RB (Ewha Womans Univ, Seoul, Korea; Massachusetts Gen Hosp, Boston)
J Oral Maxillofac Surg 50:1152–1157, 1992   105-94-19–7

Objective.—For patients with large mandibular defects, primary internal stabilization using metal plates and delayed reconstruction using bone grafts are the most frequently recommended procedures. The AO plates are sufficiently rigid to hold the remaining mandibular stumps, avoiding the need for maxillomandibular fixation, and are easy to use; early wound dehiscence and thinning of the soft tissue coverage may cause problems, however.

Patients.—Forty-one mandibular reconstructions using AO plates were performed in 37 patients. The patients, mean age 52 years and mean follow-up 13 months, were treated in a 3-year period. Twelve cases, com-

Incidence of Revision or Plate Removal by the Location of Reconstruction			
Location	No. of Reconstructions	No. of Revisions	Revision Incidence (%)*
Group A	12	6	52.2
Group B	16	2	12.5
Group C	13	1	7.7
Total	41	9	22.2

Note: Differences between the groups are significant ($P < .02$, chi-square). Time of revision: postoperative 8.2 ± 3.7 months.
* Revision incidence was calculated by actuarial analysis considering the lost or the dead.
(Courtesy of Kim M-R, Donoff RB: *J Oral Maxillofac Surg* 50:1152–1157 1992.)

prising group A, involved reconstruction crossing the midline; 16 involved the mandibular body, group B; and 13 involved the mandibular condyle and ramus, group C.

Outcomes.—Revision surgery or plate removal was required in 22% of the cases, including 52% of group A, 13% of group B, and 8% of group C (table). Infection was the most common cause of revision. Revision was needed in 33% of cases involving combined use of an AO plate and bone grafting, compared with 17% for plate-only reconstructions. Nineteen percent of reconstructions were immediate and 27% delayed, a nonsignificant difference. Failure rate was the highest, 57%, with delayed reconstruction of the anterior mandible. One third of cases whose management included radiation required revision, compared with only 6% of nonirradiated cases. The failure rate in the radiated group was especially high—63% in irradiated patients in group A. Just 52% of group A cases had a mouth opening greater than 30 mm, compared with 69% of group B and 92% of group C. Three patients in the latter group reported mild and tolerable joint pain.

Conclusion.—Immediate mandibular reconstruction using AO plates does not appear to lead to poorer results. Most failures and complications occur in reconstruction of the anterior mandible. Radiation appears to be one of the most important factors in unfavorable results and so may be contraindicated before reconstruction. It should be borne in mind that in AO plate reconstruction with bone grafting, revision does not always mean complete reconstructive failure.

▶ These 2 articles objectively report on the outcome of mandibular reconstruction after resection for oral cancer. In total, the outcome of 75 patients was reviewed. From these articles, it appears the least successful area to be reconstructed is the anterior mandible, or symphysis, particularly in an irradiated patient. The same complication rate occurs when the reconstruction is done with a plate only or a plate and bone graft, except for a vascularized bone graft (a bone graft accompanied by the blood vessels that are anastomosed with facial blood vessels, immediately reestablishing a blood supply to the bone). Vascularized grafts stabilized with plates were very successful. However, the morbidity to the patient, including the donor site and the significant time it adds to the procedure, may outweigh the benefits of the procedure, particularly in advanced (stage IV) cancers that have a 15% to 20% 5-year survival rate. From the articles there is a sense that primary reconstruction with a plate followed by secondary bone graft reconstruction may be most appropriate for most situations. A significant benefit to the patient of a vascularized bone graft reconstruction is the early, even at the time of grafting, placement of implants. To be able to prosthetically restore these patients significantly enhances rehabilitation.—S.M. Roser, D.M.D., M.D.

20 Surgical Oral Pathology

Introduction

The diagnosis of oral cancer is a responsibility of the dental practitioner. Usually, physical examination and biopsy are the methods used. Staining techniques have been available for a long time but have not gained wide acceptance because of their lack of reliability. Using a combination of toluidine blue and Lugol's iodine appears superior to using either stain alone. Practitioners with an at-risk geriatric patient population should consider this technique. The reports of exsanguination after a routine extraction because of an undiagnosed high-flow vascular lesion are becoming fewer as a result of awareness of the problem and better diagnostic and management protocols. Included in this chapter is a discussion of a systematic approach to the management of high-flow vascular lesions of the jaws. Two articles describe the use of established diagnostic imaging techniques in areas not previously considered. The use of CT for determination of implant sites is proposed for imaging odontogenic cysts, and sonography is proposed for diagnosing salivary gland lesions. The cost effectiveness and ease of use of these techniques will ultimately determine their popularity. Also included are articles on a new topical steroid preparation for treatment of lichen planus, management of salivary gland calculi and management of neoplastic disease in patients with AIDS.

Steven M. Roser, D.M.D., M.D.

Oral Carcinoma

Toluidine Blue and Lugol's Iodine Application in the Assessment of Oral Malignant Disease and Lesions at Risk of Malignancy
Epstein JB, Scully C, Spinelli JJ (Univ of British Columbia, Vancouver, Canada; Bristol Dental School and Hosp, England)
J Oral Pathol Med 21:160–163, 1992   105-94-20–1

Background.—Early diagnosis of oral cancer is vital to reducing morbidity and improving survival. In the oral cavity, esophagus, and the cervix, toluidine blue has been found to differentiate normal from abnormal epithelium. Lugol's iodine, has also been used to differentiate abnormal from normal mucosa in the esophagus and cervix. The use of both agents simultaneously has been reported but not in the case of oral lesions.

TABLE 1.—Formulation of
Tissue Stains

Toluidine blue solution:
Toluidine blue 1 g
Acetic acid 10 cc
Absolute alcohol 4.19 cc
Distilled water 86 cc
ph adjusted to 4.5

Lugol's iodine solution
Iodine 2 g
Potassium iodide 4 g
Distilled water 100 cc

(Courtesy of Epstein JB, Scully C, Spinelli JJ:
J Oral Pathol Med 21:160-163, 1992.)

Methods.—Whether simultaneous staining with toluidine blue and Lugol's iodine could aid in the diagnosis of oral lesions at risk of malignant change in 59 patients was determined. Toluidine blue was applied, followed by counterstaining with Lugol's iodine (Tables 1 and 2). Multiple punch biopsy specimens were taken from each area of tissue change.

Findings.—There were 19 benign lesions, most commonly keratosis; 15 cases of dysplasia; and 25 carcinomas. On analysis of toluidine blue staining alone, there was 1 false negative result and 1 equivocal result. On Lugol's iodine staining, there were 3 false negative and 2 equivocal results (Table 3).

TABLE 2.—Tissue Stain Application Sequence

1. Photograph untreated lesion
2. Application of 1% acetic acid with
   Q-tip (20 s)
3. Rinse with water
4. Apply toluidine blue 1% with Q-tip
   (10–20 s)
5. Decolorize with 2% acetic acid,
   Q-tip (20–30 s)
6. Photograph
7. Apply Lugol's iodine Q-tip (10–20 s)
8. Photograph

(Courtesy of Epstein JB, Scully C, Spinelli JJ: *J Oral Pathol Med* 21:160-163, 1992.)

TABLE 3.—Histologic Diagnosis Compared With the Results of Toluidine Blue and Lugol's Iodine Applications

	Toluidine blue Histologic diagnosis			Lugol's iodine Histoligic diagnosis	
	Benign	Dysplatic/ malignant		Benign	Dysplastic/ malignant
Dye retention	+ 7	37	Dye retention	+ 3	35
	− 12	3		− 16	5

Sensitivity = 0.925 Sensitivity = 0.875
Specificity = 0.632 Specificity = 0.842
Positive predictive value = 0.841 Positive predictive value = 0.921
Negative predictive value = 0.800 Negative predictive value = 0.762

	Either tissue stain Histologic diagnosis			Both stains Histologic diagnosis	
	Benign	Dysplastic/ malignant		Benign	Dysplastic/ malignant
Dye retention	+ 8	38	Dye retention	+ 2	34
	− 11	2		− 17	6

Sensitivity = 0.950 Sensitivity = 0.850
Specificity = 0.579 Specificity = 0.895
Positive predictive value = 0.826 Positive predictive value = 0.944
Negative predictive value = 0.846 Negative predictive value = 0.739

(Courtesy of Epstein JB, Scully C, Spinelli JJ: *J Oral Pathol Med* 21:160–163, 1992.)

Conclusion.—Staining with toluidine blue and Lugol's iodine appears to be sensitive and specific in the assessment of oral dysplastic or malignant lesions. They improve demarcation of both oral squamous cell carcinoma and dysplasia and help in biopsy site selection. They should not be used as screening measures in the general population; rather, they should be used as adjuncts in high-risk patients and those with suspicious oral lesions.

▶ The use of toluidine blue staining for detection of oral carcinoma has been advocated for more than 20 years. Although toluidine blue is quite sensitive, because almost all dysplastic oral tissue will be stained, it is considered nonspecific; it stains areas of benign ulceration and inflammation. Lugol's solution, which stains only normal mucosa, is considered less sensitive and has a higher incidence of false negative results, but it is more specific and has fewer false positives than toluidine blue. The use of both agents simultaneously in the oral cavity has not previously been reported. The authors found that positive predictive value is greater when both stains are positive as compared with either stain being positive, and they recommended routinely using both agents together. They recommended that the agents be used as an adjunct to clinical judgment, assisting in delineation of the extent of erythroleukoplakic lesions, identifying areas of field cancerization, determining biopsy sites, and in follow up of patients after treatment of oral cancer. They also recommended that the agents not be used for screening measures in the general population because of the low incidence of oral malignancy and the possibility of false positive results.—S.M. Roser, D.M.D., M.D.

Neoplastic Disease in the Head and Neck of Patients With AIDS

Epstein JB, Scully C (Vancouver Gen Hosp, BC, Canada; Univ of Bristol, England)
Int J Oral Maxillofac Surg 21:219–226, 1992   105-94-20–2

Introduction.—Immunosuppressed patients, such as patients with AIDS, are at increased risk of developing malignant disease. Kaposi's sarcoma (KS) usually develops first, followed by lymphoma and, later, epithelial neoplasms. Presumably, a failure of immune surveillance mechanisms to recognize malignant cells has a major role in these malignancies.

Kaposi's Sarcoma.—Since the advent of AIDS, KS is most often seen as a manifestation of HIV infection. It is, in fact, a diagnostic criterion. The disorder involves a multifocal proliferation of endothelial cells and fibroblasts. It is not entirely clear that KS is a true neoplasm. It is not uncommonly the presenting feature of AIDS. In the head and neck region, KS often involves the nasal tip, skin folds of the neck, the auricular and preauricular areas, and periorbital regions. In the mouth, the palate is involved most frequently, followed by the gingiva. In patients with AIDS, KS is progressive, extending to lymph nodes and the viscera.

Malignant Lymphoma.—About half of HIV-related lymphomas are associated with Epstein-Barr virus. Most are immunoblastic lymphomas, but primary lymphomas of the brain also are seen. Lymphomas are becoming more frequent in this setting, and they are an increasingly common cause of death in HIV-infected persons. Intravenous drug abusers are most often affected. A majority of lesions are nonHodgkin's lymphomas of B-cell origin. Most often lymphomas present extranodally, often involving the CNS. Oral lymphomas are infrequent, seen as a rapidly growing mass in the fauces, gingiva, or elsewhere.

Squamous Cell Carcinoma.—Some oropharyngeal squamous cell cancers in patients with HIV disease harbor human papillomavirus. This cancer tends to occur in younger persons and in those lacking the usual risk factors for squamous cell carcinoma. It may present as leukoplakia or erythroplakia, with or without induration and ulceration. The most common oral sites are the posterior third of the tongue, the floor of the mouth, the tonsillar fossa, and the soft palate.

▶ This article provides a comprehensive review of malignant neoplasms that occur in the head and neck in patients with AIDS, including incidence, clinical presentation, and current therapeutic modalities. The mechanism of malignant disease formation in immunosuppressed individuals may be the result of failure of the immune system to recognize malignant cells or allowing viruses to induce sustained proliferations of specific cell populations. The take-home message for clinicians is to be alert to the possibility of tumors other than KS to occur in HIV-infected individuals. In particular, squamous cell carcinoma has been reported in this population, without the commonly identified risk factors.—A. Schreiber, D.M.D., and S.M. Roser, D.M.D., M.D.

Vascular Lesions

A Systematic Approach to Management of High-Flow Vascular Malformations of the Mandible

Larsen PE, Peterson LJ (Ohio State Univ, Columbus)
J Oral Maxillofac Surg 51:62–69, 1993   105-94-20-3

Introduction.—In the past, patients with high-flow vascular malformations of the mandible were at significant risk of exsanguination during surgery. Morbidity and mortality remain high. The primary reason for this is failure to properly diagnose and assess these lesions before surgery. A systematic approach to the diagnosis and treatment of these malformations was outlined.

Classification.—Unlike true hemangiomas, vascular malformations are commonly intraosseous, do not regress with age, and are often associated with life-threatening bleeding. They may be capillary, lymphatic, venous, arterial, or combinations of these, with the latter 2 types causing

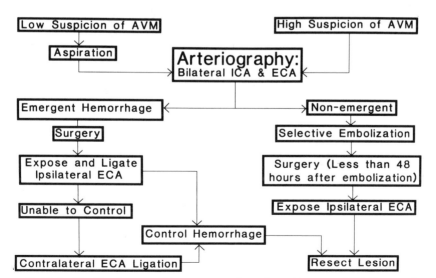

Fig 20–1.—Algorithm for sequential management of a patient with suspected high-flow vascular malformation. (Courtesy of Larsen PE, Peterson LJ: *J Oral Maxillofac Surg* 51:62–69, 1993.)

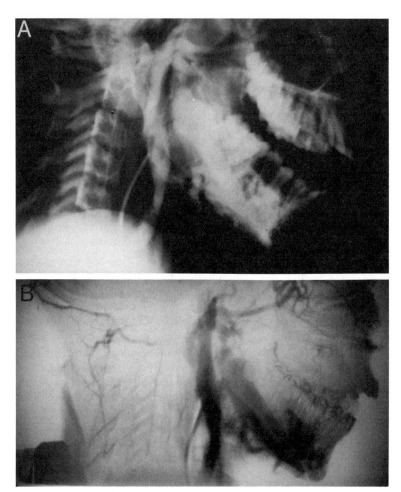

Fig 20–2.—A, arteriogram of the right common, external and internal carotid arterial system shows evidence of a large vascular malformation of the right mandibular body. **B,** substraction techniques allow the extent of the lesion to be more clearly delineated and also allow better visualization of the venous drainage, which is not clearly seen on the presubtraction radiographs. (Courtesy of Larsen PE, Peterson LJ: *J Oral Maxillofac Surg* 51:62–69, 1993.)

the most severe hemorrhage and morbidity. In most vascular malformations, the lower pressure of the large central channel drives the development of feeder vessels around it. Because of the lower pressure within the vessels of the malformation blockage of flow in the proximal part of any feeder without concomitantly blocking flow within the malformation itself results in the development of increased flow in the collateral circulation and subsequently recruitment of new supplying vessels. Therefore, if treatment does not address the central channel of the lesion, collateral circulation will increase—thus the failure of ligation of the ipsilateral and

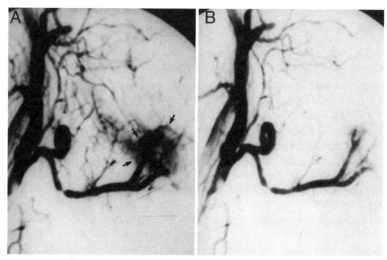

Fig 20–3.—Embolization treatment resulted in significantly decreased flow through the lesion. The radiologist wanted to perform another arteriogram on the patient 7 days after the first embolization and re-treat any problem areas. In the 7 days after the first embolization, flow to the lesion was somewhat reestablished (*arrows*) through feeders from the lingual artery. *B*, re-treatment of the lesion at the time of the repeated arteriogram reduced flow to the lesion, with surgery following within 24 hours. (Courtesy of Larsen PE, Peterson LJ: *J Oral Maxillofac Surg* 51:62-69, 1993.)

even bilateral external carotid arteries to control flow to the lesion. Collateral supply can come from the internal carotid artery, the contralateral external carotid, or the vertebral basilar system.

Diagnosis and Preparation.—A systematic approach to treatment can avoid morbidity (Fig 20-1). Diagnosis includes arteriography with de-

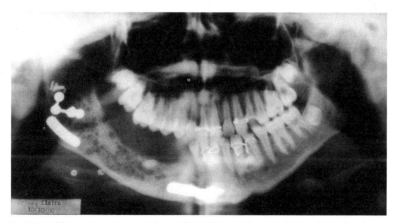

Fig 20–4.—The autogenous tray and cancellous iliac crest bone graft have been placed to reconstruct the mandible. Panoramic radiograph of the reconstruction. (Courtesy of Larsen PE, Peterson LJ: *J Oral Maxillofac Surg* 51:62-69, 1993.)

tailed mapping of the lesion. This technique can demonstrate collateral flow and assess the rate of flow through the lesion. Subtraction techniques improve visualization (Fig 20-2). Aspiration of osseous defects is standard. There is no characteristic plain radiographic appearance. In preparing the patient for surgery, it should be remembered that high-flow lesions may lead to turbulent blood flow and produce adrionic consumption coagulopathy. Autologous blood donation should be used if possible. Hypotensive anesthesia helps reduce bleeding.

Treatment.—Embolization should be used to decrease blood flow within the malformation while avoiding disruption of flow through proximal feeders. Selective cannulation of the feeders with deposition of material within the vasculature of the lesion avoids the problem of increased flow through colateral vessels. A temporary, semipermanent, or permanent embolization material may be selected. At the time of embolization, the diminished flow is confirmed. Surgical removal of the lesion is scheduled 24-48 hours later before the development of new collateral vessels to the lesion (Fig 20-3). Complications of embolization include arterial spasm, vessel rupture, adverse effects of contrast medium, and others.

Surgery aims to remove the lesion completely while maintaining control of bleeding, then reconstructing the defect to an adequate level of function. Exposure of the ipsilateral external carotid artery before removing the lesion allows easy access should uncontrollable bleeding occur. The multiple vessels encountered in the involved bone often appear as a tangled mass and should be individually ligated. The lesion and the bone adjacent to it are resected in one piece. Immediate bone graft reconstruction carries a higher risk of infection, but its potential benefits recommend it, especially for young patients. Often the resected mandible is hollowed out, teeth are removed, and the mandible is packed with cancellous bone from the ilium before replacement to the area from which it was resected (Fig 20-4). Patients should have follow-up arteriography at 1 year. After the graft is healed and a recurrent vascular lesion is ruled out, endosseous implants may be placed.

Summary.—High-flow vascular malformations of the mandible carry high morbidity and mortality because of uncontrolled bleeding. Predictable results and minimal morbidity may be achieved by a sequential treatment approach, including careful planning, selective microembolization, and surgery.

▶ High-flow vascular malformations, arterial or arteriovenous, are potentially lifethreatening because of severe uncontrollable bleeding leading to exsanguination at the time of surgical removal of the lesion. Despite sophisticated monitoring procedures and the availability of blood replacement, surgical morbidity and mortality still occurs. In this article, the authors recommend embolizing the microvasculature within the lesion, leaving the feeder vessels clear before surgery. Surgical removal of the lesion should follow 24–48 hours later. This protocol significantly decreases the vasculature associated with the lesion and prevents the development of new feeder vessels to the lesion before surgical excision. The rationale is that the lower intravascular pressure usually found within the vessels of a typical lesion encourages an increase in collateral flow from other sources—feeders—when a feeder vessel is obstructed. Because mandibular vascular lesions can be supplied by branches from the internal carotid, the opposite external carotid and the vertebral basilar vessels, it is virtually impossible to obstruct all feeder vessels to a lesion. By obstructing the microvasculature by embolization, the lesion can be resected by ligating the feeder vessels that are usually visible at the surgical site without fear of collateral flow and uncontrollable bleeding. This approach seems very rational and should become the standard approach for the management of these life-threatening lesions.—S.M. Roser, D.M.D., M.D.

Diagnostic Imaging

Odontogenic Cysts: Improved Imaging With a Dental CT Software Program

Abrahams JJ, Oliverio PJ (Yale Univ, New Haven, Conn)
AJNR 14:367–374, 1993   105-94-20–4

Introduction.—In the evaluation of odontogenic cysts, obtaining a correct diagnosis and clearly delineating the extent of the cyst can have a significant impact on the treatment plan and surgical approach. In an attempt to improve radiographic assessment of odontogenic cysts, a dental (CT) software program was used called *DentaScan,* originally developed for evaluation of patients considering osseointegrated dental implants. The program uses axial scans to reformat systematically multiple cross-referenced panoramic and cross-sectional images. This allows clear delineation of the mandibular canal and cortical margins. The investigators compared the DentaScan program with conventional radiography in the imaging of 9 patients with proven odontogenic cysts of the mandible.

Methods.—The evaluation included 4 radicular cysts, 2 odontogenic keratocysts, 2 dentigerous cysts, and 1 calcifying odontogenic cyst. The DentaScan program and conventional radiography were compared for delineation of anatomy and detection of neurovascular bundle displacement, cortical bone involvement, and root involvement.

Findings.—The DentaScan program showed the mental foramen and inferior alveolar canal more clearly than the conventional films. It was also better able to determine the displaced neurovascular bundle, which was extremely difficult to see on plain films. The CT program was also better at demonstrating the position of the canal in relation to the lesion. It more frequently and clearly delineated cortical involvement and was instrumental in 1 case of odontogenic keratocyst in detecting buccolingual expansion. Although both modalities were good at evaluating root involvement, the DentaScan proved superior when teeth were superimposed on plain films. Contrast resolution was also better on the DentaScan images.

Conclusion.—This small study demonstrates the value of using the DentaScan CT software program in the evaluation of odontogenic cysts. The most valuable aspect appears to be cross-sectional imaging, which is unique to this program and allows differentiation of buccal from lingual cortical involvement and determination of the position of the neurovascular bundle. Dental CT software should be the imaging study of choice for the evaluation of odontogenic cysts and other bony lesions of the mandible.

▶ The authors, who are radiologists, recommend obtaining a CT scan, DentaScan, of large mandibular cysts before surgical management. Restorative dentists and surgeons using implants are familiar with value of the DentaScan, which permits viewing the mandible and maxilla in cross-sectional slices. The use of the DentaScan can be valuable in the management of pathologic conditions of the mandible because it provides useful information regarding the extent of the lesion, the involvement of the dentition, and the location of the mandibular neurovascular bundle. It should be considered only after standard panoramic, periapical, occlusal and posterior-anterior mandibular views are obtained and evaluated. It is an additional radiation exposure and expense to the patient.—S.M. Roser, D.M.D., M.D.

Sonography of Nonneoplastic Disorders of the Salivary Glands
Traxler M, Schurawitzki H, Ulm C, Solar P, Blahout R, Piehslinger E, Schadlbauer E (Univ of Vienna)
Int J Oral Maxillofac Surg 21:360–363, 1992   105-94-20–5

Classification of the Various Disorders and Their
Ocurrence in Our Group of Patients

Disorder	Patients
Sialolithiasis	192
Acute sialadenitis without calculi	72
Abscess formation without calculi	9
Chronic recurrent sialadenitis	45
Immunosialadenitis	36
Salivary gland cysts	13
	367

(Courtesy of Traxler M. Schurawitzki H, Ulm C, et al: *Int J Oral Maxillofac Surg* 21:360-363, 1992.)

Background.—Salivary gland disorders are detected primarily by palpation, plain films, sialography, CT, or MRI. Several authors have reported the efficacy of ultrasound in assessing salivary gland disease. The value of sonography in the diagnosis of nonneoplastic changes in the major salivary glands was studied.

Methods and Findings.—Six hundred thirty-seven patients with salivary gland disorders were examined by real-time sonography. The possibility of neoplasia could not be excluded by ultrasound in 270 cases. In the remaining patients, acute inflammation was diagnosed in 72 cases, Sjögren's syndrome or chronic inflammation in 81 cases, abscess in 9, sialolithiasis in 192, and cysts in 13 (table).

Conclusion.—Although it is possible to distinguish local tissue changes very well on sonography, not all salivary gland neoplasms have ill-defined borders. In diagnosing sialolithiasis, the value of sonography is greater than that of conventional radiography, as sonography can detect nonradiopaque salivary stones and define their location. Sonography also helps to confirm or exclude abscesses in cases of acute inflammation. In chronic recurrent inflammations and immunosialadenitis, however, sonography does not significantly contribute to the diagnosis.

▶ Sonography is a very useful noninvasive diagnostic imaging technique that has no harmful effects. Sound waves are generated and sent through the area being scanned. Tissues bounce (echo) the sound waves back to the surface to be recorded and transformed into an image. Different tissues echo sound waves differently. Sonography has been available for a long time and has been most commonly used to scan the developing fetus. Other familiar uses include diagnosing mitral valve prolapse and locating abdominal masses. In the early 1980s, reports began to appear in our literature about the use of sonography in the head and neck. This article is one of the larger studies undertaken in this area, and the results indicate that sonography is useful for diagnosing and locating parotid gland calculi, particularly radiolucent calculi. Other common pathologic entities, such as Sjögren's syndrome, also can be diagnosed. Sonography should all but eliminate sialography, a less benign study.—S.M. Roser, D.M.D., M.D.

Lichen Planus

Fluocinonide in an Adhesive Base for Treatment of Oral Lichen Planus: A Double-Blind, Placebo-Controlled Clinical Study

Voûte ABE, Schulten EAJM, Langendijk PNJ, Kostense PJ, van der Waal I (Free Univ, Amsterdam)
Oral Surg Oral Med Oral Pathol 75:181–185, 1993   105-94-20-6

Background.—Lichen planus, a common chronic inflammatory disease of squamous cell origin, affects the skin and mucosa. Treatment is only symptomatic, because the cause of this disease is unknown. The ef-

TABLE 1.—Results With Regard to Signs

Clinical types	Response (signs)			Number of patients		Total
	+++	++	+	0	−	
Erosive lichen planus (N = 12)						
Fluocinonide	1	2	1	0	1	5
Placebo	0	2	2	1	2	7
Reticular lichen planus (N = 13)						
Fluocinonide	2	3	1	0	0	6
Placebo	0	0	0	4	3	7
Combination of erosive and reticular changes (N = 15)						
Fluocinonide	1	4	1	2	1	9
Placebo	0	2	0	3	1	6
All types (N = 40)						
Fluocinonide	4	9	3	2	2	20 †
Placebo	0	4	2	8	6	20 †

Note: +++ = complete response; ++, good response; +, partial response; 0, no effect; and −, increase of signs.
†Statistically significant ($X^2 = 10.4$; $P = .0013$).
(Courtesy of Voûte ABE, Schulten EAJM, Langendijk PNJ, et al: Oral Surg Oral Med Oral Pathol 75:181–185, 1993.)

ficacy of a class 3 corticosteroid, fluocinonide in an adhesive base, in the treatment of symptomatic oral lichen planus was investigated.

Methods.—Forty consecutive patients with oral lichen planus were enrolled in the randomized, double-blind, placebo-controlled trial. The diagnosis of oral lichen planus was based on histopathologic and immunofluorescence findings. Topical .025% fluocinonide was used. Follow-up ranged from 3 to 17 months.

TABLE 2.—Results With Regard to Symptoms

Number of patients

Response (symptoms)

Clinical types	+++	++	+	0	–	Total
All types (N = 40)						
Fluocinonide	13	2	3	2	0	20 †
Placebo	6	1	5	6	2	20 †

Note: +++ = complete response; ++, good response; +, partial response; 0, no effect; and –, = increase of symptoms.
† Statistically significant (X_t^2 = 6.97; P = .008).
(Courtesy of Voûte ABE, Schulten EAJM, Langendijk PNJ, et al: *Oral Surg Oral Med Oral Pathol* 75:181–185, 1993.)

Findings.—Twenty percent of the patients receiving the active agent had complete remission, and 60% had a good or partial response. The corresponding figures in the placebo group were 0% and 30%. The signs and symptoms of 70% of the patients given placebo showed no response. No adverse effects occurred during follow-up (Tables 1 and 2).

Conclusion.—The topical application of fluocinonide in an adhesive base is an effective way to reduce the signs and symptoms of patients with oral lichen planus. The absence of adverse effects indicate that the treatment is also safe.

▶ This well-designed study supports the use of a potent corticosteroid, fluocinonide, in a topical preparation for treatment of oral lichen planus. Lichen planus is considered a disease of the cellular immune system in which lymphocytes become cytotoxic for basal cells of the epithelium. A similar immune etiology has been reported in erythema multiforme. Lichen planus is a chronic disease; treatment is symptomatic only and usually involves topical or systemic corticosteroids. Current steroid preparations are effective in reducing or eliminating the symptoms of lichen planus. Thus, the value of the fluocinonide preparation remains to determined by a study that compared it to currently used preparations rather than to a placebo as used in this study.—S.M. Roser, D.M.D., M.D.

Salivary Glands

Salivary Gland Calculi: Diagnostic Imaging and Surgical Management
Bodner L (Tel Aviv Univ, Israel)
Compend Contin Educ Dent 14:572–584, 1993   105-94-20–7

Background.—Sialothiasis, a common salivary gland disorder, is associated with salivary calculi. These calculi occur mainly in the submandibular gland and sometimes in the parotid gland. Peak incidence is be-

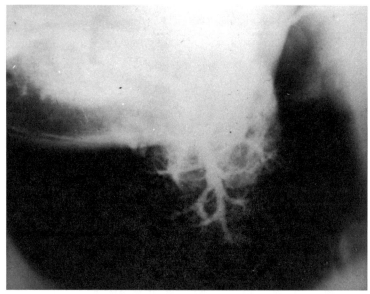

Fig 20–5.—Normal sialography, despite the sialolith in the posterior one third of the Wharton's duct. (Courtesy of Bodner L: *Compend Contin Educ Dent* 14:572–584, 1993.)

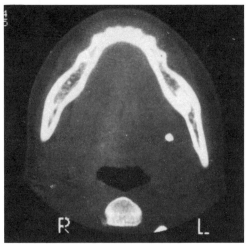

Fig 20–6.—Axial CT scan shows that the small radiopaque mass is a sialolith. (Courtesy of Bodner L: *Compend Contin Educ Dent* 14:572–584, 1993.)

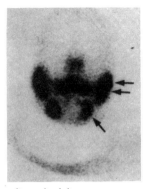

Fig 20–7.—Scintigraphy of the salivary gland demonstrates concentration of ^{99m}Tc in parotid (*upper arrows*) and submandibular (*lower arrow*) glands. (Courtesy of Bodner L: *Compend Contin Educ Dent* 14:572–584, 1993.)

tween the fourth and sixth decades, and there is a male predilection. The mechanism involved in salivary calculi formation is not well understood. Possibly, a mucous plug forms and becomes lodged against the duct's luminal wall. Imaging and surgical management of sialolithiasis were discussed.

Diagnostic Imaging.—The most common views for detecting calculi in the submandibular duct or gland on plain radiographs are the lower occlusal view of the floor of the mouth for sialoliths in the anterior two thirds of the Wharton's duct, a rotational panoramic radiograph for calculi in the duct or gland, and a 15-degree lateral oblique of the mandible for calculi in the posterior third of the duct or in the gland itself. Sialography is a well-established radiographic method for assessing diseases affecting the duct system of the parotid and submandibular glands (Fig 20–5). However, it is limited in its ability to detect masses of less than 2 cm. Computed tomography can detect any size mass. Although the indications for ultrasonography have been expanding, CT is still the method of choice for visualizing lesions affecting deeper structures (Figs 20–6 and 20–7).

Management.—Sialothithotomy—the removal of the calculus through the intraoral approach with the patient under local anesthesia—is the treatment of choice. When the calculus is further back in the duct, the duct must be incised. Usually, there is no need to suture the incised duct. Sialolithotomy can be done with a carbon dioxide laser. Intraglandular sialoliths or those in the hilus necessitate submandibular sialoadenectomy or partial parotidectomy. When a sialolith has obstructed a gland for a long time, causing irreversible damage to the secretory function, the gland should be surgically removed.

▶ The etiology, pathogenesis, and surgical approaches to treatment of salivary gland calculi are well established. Historically, the most commonly used imaging techniques for the detection of calculi have been plain films and sia-lography. The benefits of CT scans (detection of lesions of any size), scintig-raphy (evaluation of salivary gland dynamics), and ultrasonography (noninva-siveness and nonutilization of ionizing radiation) in the detection of salivary gland pathology are highlighted in this article.—S.M. Roser, D.M.D., M.D., and A. Schreiber, D.M.D.

Subject Index

A

Abutment
  UCLA, review of, 93: 95
Acetone
  penetration of composite resin, 93: 69
Acid
  containing drinks and dental health,
    93: 320
  etch composite resin technique for small
    occlusal defects, 94: 395
  etching of dentin, 93: 187
    to improve bond strength, 93: 61
  resistance and fluoride uptake from
    glass ionomer cement by dentin,
    93: 210
Acidic
  conditions, fluoride release from
    light-cured glass ionomers in,
    94: 440
Acidogenicity
  of plaque, and time and duration of
    sorbitol gum chewing, 94: 146
Acrylic resin (*see* Resin, acrylic)
Adenoidectomy
  incisor position after, normalization of,
    94: 78
Adhesion
  to dentin, and smear layer with wetness,
    93: 174
Adhesive, 93: 174
  All-Bond/no etch, dentin wetness and,
    93: 186
  base, fluocinonide in, for oral lichen
    planus, 94: 573
  bond strength, dentin wetness,
    permeability and thickness in,
    93: 185
  cements, and cementation, 94: 354
  ceramic inlay, marginal adaptation and
    fit of, 94: 463
  cervical abrasion lesions and, 93: 174
  Clearfil Photobond, dentin wetness and,
    93: 186
  comparison of four adhesives, 93: 182
  composite resin cement, luting of
    prefabricated posts with, 94: 422
  dentin, 94: 419
    bonding in resin composite
      restoration, 93: 184
  effect on sealant bond strength, 93: 183
  electron microscopy of, scanning,
    93: 179
  enamel dentin, 93: 184
  Fittydent, 93: 182
  liners in amalgam, compressive strength
    and creep, 93: 152

luting agents
  in marginal seating of cast
    restorations, 94: 349
  tensile strengths of, compressive and
    diametral, 94: 435
  materials to enamel and dentin, 93: 53
  resin, application to broken amalgam,
    93: 78
  Scotchbond, 93: 2, 176, 183
    dentin wetness and, 93: 186
    shear strength of, 93: 181
  shear strength of, 93: 179
  strength of BIS-GMA cement to
    tin-plated alloy, 94: 459
  Super Poligrip, 93: 182
  Super Wernet's, 93: 182
  Superbond, shear strength of, 93: 181
  system
    bonded to nickel-chromium-beryllium
      alloy, shear strength of, 93: 165
    evaluation, clinical, results, 93: 175
    for high-copper amalgam repair,
      94: 423
    Panavia, 93: 166
    Silicoater system, 93: 166
  Tenure, dentin wetness and, 93: 186
  tragacanth, 93: 182
Adolescence
  craniomandibular disorders, subjective
    symptom changes during, 94: 102
  malocclusion in, skeletal class II, surgical
    vs. orthodontic correction, 94: 107
  temporomandibular disorders in, and
    class II elastics and extractions,
    94: 105
Aerosols
  bacteria in, preprocedural antiseptic
    rinsing reducing, 94: 236
Age
  craniomandibular disorder increase
    with, 93: 302
Aged
  geriatric dentistry
    continuing education in, 93: 49
    methicillin-resistant *Staphylococcus
      aureus* and, 93: 11
  mandibular bone loss of, 93: 106
  smell disorders in, 94: 269
  taste disorders in, 94: 269
  teeth of, value of, and quality of life,
    94: 37
Aging
  in hydroxyapatite implant healing,
    94: 511
AIDS, 93: 388, 94: 236
  gingival status in, 93: 391
  head and neck tumors in, 94: 566
  periodontal status in, 93: 390

Metal
  castings, resins bonded to, 93: 165
  ceramic crown, marginal adaptation
      with, 93: 168
  core
    cementing ceramic restoration over,
        93: 71
    porcelain fusion over, 93: 72
  porcelain-fused-to-metal
    crown, marginal adaptation, 93: 162
    restorations, 94: 453
  post (see Post, metal)
Metastases
  of jaws, 94: 274
Methicillin
  resistant *Staphylococcus aureus* in
      geriatric dentistry, 93: 11
Microbes
  oral, laser killing, 94: 187
  species counts, relationship to clinical
      status at sample site, 93: 359
Microcracks
  on composite resin surface, 94: 408
Microfil
  posterior composite resin, 93: 142
Microflora
  of periodontal sites showing destructive
      progression, 93: 360
Microleakage
  of amalgam restoration, 93: 75
    using Amalgambond and Copalite,
        94: 428
  around composite inlay, direct, 93: 220
  of composite resin and glass ionomer
      cement restorations
    in cervical cavity preparations,
        94: 286
    laboratory study, bonding systems in,
        94: 289
  of composite resin restorations
    class II, matrix systems and
        polymerization techniques in,
        94: 402
    margins placed in dentin, 94: 290
  coronal, three materials as barriers to,
      after endodontic treatment,
      94: 170
  of crown
    full, and pulp, 94: 352
    with glass ionomer cement, 93: 199
  in high-copper amalgam repair with
      adhesive system, 94: 423
  in pneumatic vs. hand condensation of
      amalgam, 93: 74
Microorganisms
  in used ultrasound cleaning solutions,
      94: 32
Microscopy

electron (*see* Electron microscopy)
  light and electron, of implant
      osseointegration, 93: 449
Microstructure
  of dentin, 93: 189
Millon Adolescent Personality Inventory
  in orthodontic compliance, 93: 276
  three basic categories for test
      instrument, 93: 277
Mineralization
  of teeth, 93: 257
    regional variation in tempo, 93: 257
Miniplate
  fixation, for inferior maxillary
      repositioning, long-term stability
      after, 94: 492
  in maxillofacial surgery, 94: 543
Mirage Bond
  shear bond strength of, 94: 430
Model
  caries risk prediction, 93: 314
  Columbia University, for basic science
      instruction, 93: 42
  dentin bovine, of fluoride-releasing
      cements, 93: 210
  medical, of caries, 94: 132
  predictive, in orthodontics, 93: 275
  three-dimensional, for craniofacial
      surgery, endoplan, 93: 441
Molar
  first, ankylosed mandibular permanent,
      treatment, 93: 269
  mandibular
    anesthesia for, endodontic, 94: 160
    step-back preparation in, ultrasound
        efficacy after, 94: 165
  maxillary, electronic apex locator for,
      accuracy of, 94: 172
  permanent, secondary retention of,
      94: 80
  primary, ankylosis of, 94: 81
  third
    impaction, 93: 111
    impaction, asymptomatic, removal,
        93: 423
    impaction, removal, alveolar and
        lingual nerve damage during,
        93: 112
    impaction, removal risks and benefits,
        93: 421
    removal, complications, 93: 111
    removal, dexamethasone for sequelae
        reduction, 94: 471
    removal, for general practitioner,
        93: 110
    removal, oxygen saturation during
        local anesthetic and IV sedation,
        93: 437

Author Index

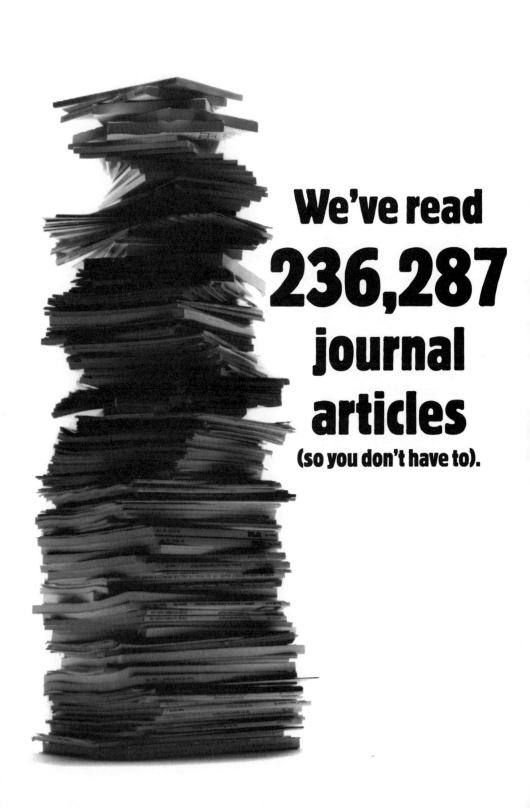

We've read
236,287
journal
articles
(so you don't have to).

The Year Books—
The best from 236,287 journal articles.

At Mosby, we subscribe to more than 950 medical and allied health journals from every corner of the globe. We read them all, tirelessly scanning for anything that relates to your field.

We send everything we find related to a given specialty to the distinguished editors of the **Year Book** in that area, and they pick out *the best*, the articles they feel *every practitioner in that specialty should be aware of.*

For the **1994 Year Books** we surveyed a total of 236,287 articles and found hundreds of articles related to your field. Our expert editors reviewed these and chose the developments you don't want to miss.

The best articles—condensed, organized, and with personal commentary.

Not only do you get the past year's most important articles in your field, you get them in a format that makes them easy to use.

Every article that the editors pick is condensed into a concise, outlined abstract, a summary of the article's most important points highlighted with bold paragraph headings. So you can quickly scan for exactly what you need.

In addition to identifying the year's best articles, the editors write concise commentaries following each article, telling whether or not the study in question is a reliable one, whether a new technique is effective, or whether a particular trend you've head about merits your immediate attention.

No other abstracting service offers this expert advice to help you decide how the year's advances will affect the way you practice.

With a special added benefit for Year Book subscribers.

In 1994, your **Year Book** subscription includes a new added benefit. Access to **MOSBY Document Express**, a rapid-response information retrieval service that puts copies of original source documents in your hands, in a little as a few hours.

With **MOSBY Document Express**, you have convenient, *around-the-clock-access to literally every article* upon which **Year Book** summaries are based. What's more, you can also order journal articles cited in references—or for that matter, virtually any medical or scientific article that can be located. Plus, at your direction, we will deliver the article(s) by FAX, overnight delivery service, or regular mail.

This new added benefit is just one of the enhanced services that makes your **Year Book** subscription an even better value—it's your key to the full breadth of health sciences information. For more details, see **MOSBY Document Express** instructions at the beginning of this book.